KEEPING PATIENTS SAFE

Transforming the Work Environment of Nurses

Committee on the Work Environment for Nurses and Patient Safety

Board on Health Care Services

Ann Page, *Editor*

INSTITUTE OF MEDICINE
OF THE NATIONAL ACADEMIES

THE NATIONAL ACADEMIES PRESS
Washington, D.C.
www.nap.edu

THE NATIONAL ACADEMIES PRESS   500 Fifth Street, N.W.   Washington, DC 20001

NOTICE: The project that is the subject of this report was approved by the Governing Board of the National Research Council, whose members are drawn from the councils of the National Academy of Sciences, the National Academy of Engineering, and the Institute of Medicine. The members of the committee responsible for the report were chosen for their special competences and with regard for appropriate balance.

Support for this project was provided by the Agency for Healthcare Research and Quality of the U.S. Department of Health and Human Services. The views presented in this report are those of the Institute of Medicine Committee on the Work Environment for Nurses and Patient Safety and are not necessarily those of the funding agency.

Library of Congress Cataloging-in-Publication Data

Keeping patients safe : transforming the work environment of nurses / Committee on the Work Environment for Nurses and Patient Safety, Board on Health Care Services ; Ann Page, editor.
    p. ; cm.
  ISBN 0-309-09067-9 (hardcover)
  1. Nursing—Safety measures. 2. Work environment—Safety measures. 3. Industrial safety. 4. Nursing errors—Prevention. 5. Medical care—Quality control. 6. Nurse and patient.
  [DNLM: 1. Safety Management—organization & administration. 2. Nurse's Role. 3. Nursing Care—organization & administration. 4. Workplace—organization & administration. WX 185 K26c 2004] I. Page, Ann. II. Institute of Medicine (U.S.). Board on Health Care Services. Committee on the Work Environment for Nurses and Patient Safety.
  RT87.S24K447 2004
  362.17'3—dc22

                                    2003022651

Additional copies of this report are available from the National Academies Press, 500 Fifth Street, N.W., Lockbox 285, Washington, DC 20055; (800) 624-6242 or (202) 334-3313 (in the Washington metropolitan area); Internet, http://www.nap.edu.

For more information about the Institute of Medicine, visit the IOM home page at: www.iom.edu.

*"Knowing is not enough; we must apply.
Willing is not enough; we must do."*
—Goethe

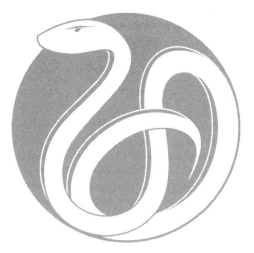

INSTITUTE OF MEDICINE
OF THE NATIONAL ACADEMIES

Shaping the Future for Health

THE NATIONAL ACADEMIES
Advisers to the Nation on Science, Engineering, and Medicine

The **National Academy of Sciences** is a private, nonprofit, self-perpetuating society of distinguished scholars engaged in scientific and engineering research, dedicated to the furtherance of science and technology and to their use for the general welfare. Upon the authority of the charter granted to it by the Congress in 1863, the Academy has a mandate that requires it to advise the federal government on scientific and technical matters. Dr. Bruce M. Alberts is president of the National Academy of Sciences.

The **National Academy of Engineering** was established in 1964, under the charter of the National Academy of Sciences, as a parallel organization of outstanding engineers. It is autonomous in its administration and in the selection of its members, sharing with the National Academy of Sciences the responsibility for advising the federal government. The National Academy of Engineering also sponsors engineering programs aimed at meeting national needs, encourages education and research, and recognizes the superior achievements of engineers. Dr. Wm. A. Wulf is president of the National Academy of Engineering.

The **Institute of Medicine** was established in 1970 by the National Academy of Sciences to secure the services of eminent members of appropriate professions in the examination of policy matters pertaining to the health of the public. The Institute acts under the responsibility given to the National Academy of Sciences by its congressional charter to be an adviser to the federal government and, upon its own initiative, to identify issues of medical care, research, and education. Dr. Harvey V. Fineberg is president of the Institute of Medicine.

The **National Research Council** was organized by the National Academy of Sciences in 1916 to associate the broad community of science and technology with the Academy's purposes of furthering knowledge and advising the federal government. Functioning in accordance with general policies determined by the Academy, the Council has become the principal operating agency of both the National Academy of Sciences and the National Academy of Engineering in providing services to the government, the public, and the scientific and engineering communities. The Council is administered jointly by both Academies and the Institute of Medicine. Dr. Bruce M. Alberts and Dr. Wm. A. Wulf are chair and vice chair, respectively, of the National Research Council.

www.national-academies.org

Reviewers

This report has been reviewed in draft form by individuals chosen for their diverse perspectives and technical expertise, in accordance with procedures approved by the National Research Council's Report Review Committee. The purpose of this independent review is to provide candid and critical comments that will assist the institution in making its published report as sound as possible and to ensure that the report meets institutional standards for objectivity, evidence, and responsiveness to the study charge. The review comments and draft manuscript remain confidential to protect the integrity of the deliberative process. We wish to thank the following individuals for their review of this report:

DONNA DIERS, Yale University School of Nursing, New Haven, Connecticut

COLLEEN GOODE, University of Colorado Hospital, Denver, Colorado

KERRY KILPATRICK, University of North Carolina at Chapel Hill, North Carolina

NANCY LANGSTON, Virginia Commonwealth University, Richmond, Virginia

ELAINE LARSON, Columbia University, New York, New York

MITCHELL RABKIN, Harvard Medical School, Boston, Massachusetts

JAMES REASON, Disley, Cheshire, United Kingdom

VINOD SAHNEY, Henry Ford Health System, Detroit, Michigan

FRANCOIS SAINFORT, Georgia Institute of Technology, Atlanta, Georgia

ROBYN STONE, Institute for the Future of Aging Services, Washington, D.C.

MARY WAKEFIELD, University of North Dakota School of Medicine and Health Sciences, Grand Forks, North Dakota

Although the reviewers listed above have provided many constructive comments and suggestions, they were not asked to endorse the conclusions or recommendations nor did they see the final draft of the report before its release. The review of this report was overseen by **ENRIQUETA BOND,** Burroughs Wellcome Fund, Research Triangle Park, North Carolina, and **GAIL L. WARDEN,** Henry Ford Health System, Detroit, Michigan. Appointed by the National Research Council and Institute of Medicine, they were responsible for making certain that an independent examination of this report was carried out in accordance with institutional procedures and that all review comments were carefully considered. Responsibility for the final content of this report rests entirely with the authoring committee and the institution.

Foreword

This report adds to our understanding of how to keep patients safe from the combined effects of the complexities of our technologically driven, compartmentalized, health care system and the fallibility of human health care providers, managers, and leadership within that system. Two prior Institute of Medicine reports—*To Err Is Human: Building a Safer Health System* and *Crossing the Quality Chasm: A New Health System for the 21st Century*—provide strong evidence on how the health care delivery system should be modified to compensate for these two error-conducive attributes. They speak to how the experiences of patients should be changed, how teams of health care workers should interact, how health care organizations can better design work and institute proactive error-reduction strategies, and how policy officials and health care purchasers can reshape health policy to create a safer health care system. The present report builds on these prior studies by examining patient safety from a new perspective—the characteristics of the work environment in which patient care is provided. It does so from the vantage point of the largest component of the health care workforce and a critical element of our health care system—nurses.

When we are hospitalized, in a nursing home, or managing a chronic condition in our own homes—at some of our most vulnerable moments—nurses are the health care providers we are most likely to encounter, spend the greatest amount of time with, and be dependent upon for our recovery. Nursing actions such as ongoing monitoring of patient health status have been shown to be directly related to better patient outcomes. In their other roles, nurses intercept health care errors before they can adversely affect patients. When there are not enough nurses in a hospital to monitor patients and provide therapeutic care, hospitals are forced to close beds, restrict admissions, and divert patients in need of emergency services, and patients are placed at risk. Good health care requires a nursing workforce appropriate in size and expertise, and unconstrained in its ability to provide patient care safely.

This report presents guidance on how to design nurses' work environments to enable them to provide safer patient care. It does so by explaining in detail how health care organizations should implement key recommendations of *To Err Is Human* and *Crossing the Quality Chasm*, examining aspects of work environments not addressed in those prior reports, and unifying the evidence from the two prior reports and this report into a strong framework for building work environments that promote the practice of safe nursing care. All health care organizations can follow this framework and the report's recommendations to construct work environments more conducive to patient safety. Because of the centrality of nursing care in achieving good patient outcomes, patient safety demands that the recommendations in this report be adopted by all health care organizations, labor organizations, nursing schools, governmental agencies, and nurses themselves.

Harvey V. Fineberg, M.D., Ph.D.
President, Institute of Medicine
November 4, 2003

Preface

Throughout this report, evidence is presented describing the critical role of nurses in the U.S. health care system. Nurses monitor patients' status, coordinate their care, educate them and their families, and provide essential therapeutic care. This report also documents the many changes that have taken place in health care delivery over the last two decades that have affected the way in which nurses provide this care and keep patients safe from the inevitable health care errors so well documented in an earlier Institute of Medicine (IOM) report *To Err Is Human: Building a Safer Health System.*

The Committee on the Work Environment for Nurses and Patient Safety identified plentiful threats to patient safety arising from every level and component of health care delivery, including the work processes, workload, work hours, and workspaces of nursing staff. Fortunately, the committee also identified findings from health services, nursing, organizational, and industrial research, as well as other empirical information on error production and prevention in a variety of industries, that provide clear guidance about how to reduce such threats.

While the committee was not charged to, and did not, address the current nursing shortage in the United States, it was mindful of this situation in developing its recommendations. While nursing shortages in this country tend to be recurrent, federal government analyses show a growing discrepancy between the supply of and demand for registered nurses. This shortage is predicted to worsen in the near future, fueled by a projected 18 percent growth in the U.S. population between 2000 and 2020 and a 65 percent growth in the population over age 65, which requires a disproportionately larger share of health care services.

In the face of the current and projected nursing shortage, the committee believes it is even more imperative that nurses' work and work environments be designed to facilitate the safe delivery of nursing care. If the supply of nurses is to be stretched thin, nurses must be supported by work processes, workspaces, work hours, staffing, and organizational cultures that better defend against the commission of errors and readily detect and mitigate errors when they occur. It may be tempting to think that these recommendations can wait for increases in the supply of nurses, but evidence on how better to retain nurses indicates that the converse is true. Nurses are more likely to stay in health care organizations that implement many of the management, workforce, and work design practices recommended in this report.

It is our hope that this report's recommended framework, actions, and material presented in two appendixes on safe work hours and interdisciplinary collaboration and team functioning will be useful tools to all health care organizations, labor organizations, policy officials, educators, and nurses who seek to create safer health care delivery. While this study focuses on nurses, predominantly in hospitals and nursing homes, many of the committee's recommendations are applicable to the work environments of all health care workers. Implementing these recommendations can greatly advance the safety of all individuals receiving health care.

Donald M. Steinwachs, Ph.D.   Ada Sue Hinshaw, Ph.D., R.N.
Chair   *Vice Chair*
November 4, 2003   **November 4, 2003**

Acknowledgments

The Committee on the Work Environment for Nurses and Patient Safety thanks the many individuals who generously contributed their time, knowledge, and expertise to this study. We are especially indebted to the nurses who shared with us patient safety stories that are either excerpted or originally presented in this report. Their forthrightness helps us all see clearly the real-life implications of the issues addressed in this report. Bonnie Jennings, RN, Ph.D., American Academy of Nursing/American Nurses Foundation Scholar-in-Residence at the Institute of Medicine, also contributed her strong knowledge of nursing, a literature review, and her writing skills to Chapter 3 of this report. Lieutenant Colonel Rachel Armstrong RN, U.S. Army Nurse Corps, additionally provided much assistance in literature review and analyses for several chapters of the report.

The committee commissioned nine papers to provide background information for its deliberations and to synthesize the evidence on particular issues. We thank Julie Sochalski, Ph.D., of the University of Pennsylvania School of Nursing for her paper, "The Nursing Workforce: Profile, Trends, Projections"; Barbara Mark, Ph.D., of the University of North Carolina at Chapel Hill School of Nursing for her paper, "The Work of Registered Nurses, Licensed Practical Nurses, and Nurses Aides in Acute Care Hospitals"; Barbara Bowers, Ph.D., of the University of Wisconsin-Madison School of Nursing Studies for her paper, "The Work of Nurses and Nurse Aides in Long Term Care Facilities"; Karen Martin of Martin Associates for her paper, "The Work of Nurses and Nursing Assistants in Home Care, Public Health, and Other Community Settings"; Ann Rogers, Ph.D., of the University of Pennsylvania School of Nursing for her paper, "Work Hour

Regulation in Safety-Sensitive Industries"; Gail Ingersoll, Ed.D., and Madeline Schmitt, Ph.D., both of the University of Rochester Medical Center, for their paper, "Interdisciplinary Collaboration, Team Functioning, and Patient Safety"; Ann Hendrich of Ascension Health and Nelson Lee of Rapid Modeling, Inc. for their paper, "Evidence-based Design of Nursing Workspace in Hospitals"; Pascale Carayon, Ph.D., Carla Alvarado, Ph.D., and Ann Hundt, Ph.D., all of the University of Wisconsin-Madison Department of Industrial Engineering, for their paper, "Reducing Workload and Increasing Patient Safety Through Work and Workspace Design"; and Murat Bayiz of the Anderson School of Management at the University of California, Los Angeles, for his paper, "Work and Workload Measurements in Nurse Staffing Models."

Many individuals and organizations also presented testimony to the committee on aspects of nurses' work environments that likely affect patient safety and potential improvements. We thank Barbara Blakeney, President of the American Nurses Association; Linda Burnes Boltin, Dr.P.H., of the American Academy of Nursing; Kathleen Long, Ph.D., President of the American Association of Colleges of Nursing; Phil Authier, President of the American Organization of Nurse Executives; Eileen Zungolo, Ed.D., President of the National League for Nursing; Jeanne Surdo, Secretary-Treasurer of United American Nurses; Martha Baker, President of the Service Employees International Union, Local 1991; Katherine Cox, Policy Analyst with the American Federation of State, County, and Municipal Employees; Gerry Shea, Assistant to the President for Government Affairs at the AFL-CIO; Jim Bentley, Senior Vice President for Strategic Policy Planning for the American Hospital Association; Steven Chies, Vice Chair of the American Health Care Association; Robin Stone, Ph.D., Executive Director of the Institute for the Future of Aging Services, an affiliate of the American Association of Homes and Services for the Aging; Tim Flaherty, M.D., of the American Medical Association and National Patient Safety Foundation; Steven Edelstein, J.D., of the Paraprofessional Institute; Donna Lenhoff, Esq., Executive Director of the National Citizens Coalition for Nursing Home Reform; Dennis O'Leary, President, and Margaret van Amringe, Vice President for External Relations, both of the Joint Commission on Accreditation of Healthcare Organizations; Cathy Rick, Chief Nursing Officer of the U.S. Department of Veterans Affairs; Sean Clarke, RN, Ph.D., of the University of Pennsylvania Center for Health Outcomes and Policy Research; Caryl Lee, RN, Program Manager for the National Center for Patient Safety of the U.S. Department of Veterans Affairs; Joyce Berger, Senior Advisor at the Health Technology Center; Daved van Stralen, M.D., Medical Director of Totally Kids® Specialty Healthcare, the American Association of Critical Care Nurses; Philip Greiner, past Chair, and Sonda Oppewal, Chair, of the Public Health Nursing Section of the American

Public Health Association; Laurence Wellikson, Executive Director, and Janet Nagamine of the National Association of Inpatient Physicians; and John Hoff, Deputy Assistant Secretary for Disability, Aging, and Long Term Care Policy, and Jennie Harvel and Marvin Feuerberg, both Senior Policy Analysts, all with the U.S. Department of Health and Human Services. We also thank Paul Ginsburg, Ph.D., President of the Center for Studying Health System Change, and Cheryl Peterson of the American Nurses Association.

At the Institute of Medicine, we would especially like to thank Bill McLeod, Adrienne Davis, Roberta Gooding, and all the staff of the George E. Brown Jr. Library for their patience and expert assistance in voluminous reference retrieval and formatting. Gooloo Wunderlich and Karen Adams of the Board on Health Care Services offered their wisdom and guidance throughout multiple stages of this study. Tony Burton was ever ready with his expert logistical support and problem-solving abilities, and Sue Barron ensured that this study complied with all Institute of Medicine study procedures. Bronwyn Schrecker at the Institute of Medicine and Jennifer Pinkerman at the National Research Council facilitated the external review process with great efficiency and attention to detail. We are very grateful to them all.

Rona Briere of Briere Associates, Inc. provided expert editorial assistance and Alisa Decatur excellent proofreading and manuscript preparation assistance.

Finally, we thank the Agency for Healthcare Research and Quality, whose funding made this study possible. We especially thank Helen Burstin, M.D., Director of the Center for Primary Care Research, and Sally Phillips, RN, Ph.D., Nurse Scholar within that center, for their very valuable insights and assistance.

Contents

Tables, Figures, and Boxes

TABLES

Executive Summary

PATIENT SAFETY CONTINUES TO BE THREATENED

In its report *To Err Is Human: Building a Safer Health System*, the Institute of Medicine (IOM) estimated that as many as 98,000 hospitalized Americans die each year—not as a result of their illness or disease, but as a result of errors in their care (IOM, 2000). This alarming number, which reflects only deaths occurring in hospital settings, exceeds the numbers of fatalities due to motor vehicle accidents, breast cancer, or AIDS. Moreover, this figure does not reflect the many patients who survive, but sustain serious injuries.

This high volume of errors was recently affirmed by some with first-hand knowledge of errors—practicing physicians, patients, and their families. Fully 35 percent of practicing physicians and 42 percent of members of the American public responding to a 2002 national survey reported having experienced an error either in their own care or in that of a family member. Moreover, 18 percent of the physicians and 24 percent of the members of the public responding cited an error that had serious health consequences, including death, long-term disability, and severe pain (Blendon et al., 2002).

This profusion of health care errors has received attention from federal and state policy makers, health care organizations (HCOs), individual health care practitioners, and experts on safety from a variety of disciplines. Key stimuli for this increased attention have included actions undertaken by the federal government to fund more research on why such errors occur and how to prevent them, to collect data on patient safety, to support new information technology for health care delivery, and to disseminate patient safety information to consumers and providers (Clancy and Scully, 2003).

1

In this context, and in recognition of evidence on the key role of nurses in patient safety, the U.S. Department of Health and Human Services' (DHHS) Agency for Healthcare Research and Quality (AHRQ) asked the IOM to conduct a study to identify:

- Key aspects of the work environment for nurses that likely have an impact on patient safety.
- Potential improvements in health care working conditions that would likely increase patient safety.

AHRQ further directed that the study be conducted "in the context of current policy debates on regulation of nursing work hours and nursing workload . . . [and] cover such topics as: extended work hours and fatigue, including mandatory overtime; workload issues, including state regulation of nurse-to-bed ratios; workplace environmental issues, including poorly designed care processes; . . . workplace systems, including reliance on memory and lack of support systems for decision-making; and workplace communication, including social, physical, and other barriers to effective communication among care team members." The IOM convened the Committee on the Work Environment for Nurses and Patient Safety to conduct this study.

THE CRITICAL ROLE OF NURSES IN PATIENT SAFETY

The 2.8 million licensed nurses and 2.3 million nursing assistants providing patient care in this country represent approximately 54 percent of all health care workers and provide patient care in virtually all locations in which health care is delivered—hospitals; nursing homes; ambulatory care settings, such as clinics or physicians' offices; private homes; schools; and employee workplaces. When people are hospitalized, in a nursing home, having a baby, or learning to manage a chronic condition in their own home—at some of their most vulnerable moments—nurses are the health care providers they are most likely to encounter; spend the greatest amount of time with; and, along with other health care providers, depend on for their recovery.

Research is now beginning to document what physicians, patients, other health care providers, and nurses themselves have long known: how well we are cared for by nurses affects our health, and sometimes can be a matter of life or death. As physicians in the American College of Critical Care Medicine have noted: "Critical care nurses do the majority of patient assessment, evaluation, and care in the ICU [intensive care unit]" (Brilli et al., 2001:2011). Nursing actions, such as ongoing monitoring of patients' health status, are directly related to better patient outcomes (Kahn et al., 1990;

Mitchell and Shortell, 1997; Rubenstein et al., 1992). Nursing vigilance also defends patients against errors. A study of medication errors in two hospitals over a 6-month period found that nurses were responsible for intercepting 86 percent of all medication errors made by physicians, pharmacists, and others involved in providing medications for patients before the error reached the patient (Leape et al., 1995).

In reviewing evidence on acute hospital nurse staffing published from 1990 to 2001, the AHRQ report *Making Health Care Safer: A Critical Analysis of Patient Safety Practices* (Seago, 2001:430) concluded that "leaner nurse staffing is associated with increased length of stay, nosocomial infection (urinary tract infection, postoperative infection, and pneumonia), and pressure ulcers. . . . These studies . . . taken together, provide substantial evidence that richer nurse staffing is associated with better patient outcomes." Subsequent studies have added to this evidence base and substantiate the observation that greater numbers of patient deaths are associated with fewer nurses to provide care (Aiken et al., 2002), and less nursing time provided to patients is associated with higher rates of infection, gastrointestinal bleeding, pneumonia, cardiac arrest, and death from these and other causes (Needleman et al., 2002). In caring for us all, nurses are indispensable to our safety.

NURSES' WORK ENVIRONMENTS:
A THREAT TO PATIENT SAFETY

In conducting this study, the committee reviewed evidence on the work and work environments of nurses; related health services, nursing, behavioral, and organizational research; findings from human factors analysis and engineering; and studies of safety in other industries. This evidence revealed that the typical work environment of nurses is characterized by many serious threats to patient safety. These threats are found in all four of the basic components of all organizations—organizational management practices, workforce deployment practices, work design, and organizational culture.

Frequent Failure to Follow Management Practices Necessary for Safety

Certain management practices are essential to the creation of safety within organizations and to the success of the organizational changes often needed to build stronger patient safety defenses. These practices include (1) balancing the tension between production efficiency and reliability (safety), (2) creating and sustaining trust throughout the organization, (3) actively managing the process of change, (4) involving workers in decision making pertaining to work design and work flow, and (5) using knowledge management practices to establish the organization as a "learning organization." Evidence shows that these practices are not employed in many nursing work environments.

In particular, many hospital restructuring and redesign initiatives[1] that have been widely adopted over the last two decades have changed the ways in which licensed nurses and nurse assistants are organized to provide patient care. Many of these changes have been focused largely on increasing efficiency and have been undertaken in ways that have damaged trust between nursing staff and management. Changes often have been poorly managed so that intended results have not been achieved, infrequently have involved nurses in decision making pertaining to the redesign of their work, and have not employed practices that encourage the uptake and dissemination of knowledge throughout the organization. The committee found, for example, that:

* **Loss of trust in hospital administration is widespread among nursing staff** (Decker et al., 2001; Ingersoll et al., 2001; Kramer and Schmalenberg, 1993). This loss of trust stems in part from a perception that initiatives in patient care and nursing work redesign have emphasized efficiency over patient safety. Poor communication practices have also led to mistrust (Walston and Kimberly, 1997). This loss of trust has serious implications for the ability of hospitals and other HCOs to make the fundamental changes essential to providing safer patient care.

* **Clinical nursing leadership has been reduced at multiple levels, and the voice of nurses in patient care has diminished.** Hospital reengineering initiatives often have resulted in the loss of a separate department of nursing (Gelinas and Manthey, 1997). At the same time, nursing staff have perceived a decline in chief nursing executives with power and authority equal to that of other top hospital officials, as well as in directors of nursing who are highly visible and accessible to staff (Aiken et al., 2000). These changes—along with losses of chief nursing officers without replacement; decreases in the numbers of nurse managers; and increased responsibilities of remaining nurse managers for more than one patient care unit, as well as for supervising personnel other than nursing staff (e.g., housekeepers, transportation staff, dietary aides) (Aiken et al., 2001; Sovie and Jawad, 2001)— have had the cumulative effect of reducing direct management support available to patient care staff. This situation hampers nurses' ability to fix problems in their work environments that threaten patient safety (Tucker and Edmondson, 2002).

---

[1]The terms "restructuring," "reengineering," and "redesigning" are used interchangeably in the literature.

Unsafe Workforce Deployment

Despite the strong and accumulating evidence that higher nurse staffing levels in hospitals and nursing homes result in safer patient care, there is wide variation in nurse staffing levels across hospitals and nursing homes. Data from 135 hospitals contacted in 2002 show that although a nurse working in a medical–surgical unit on the day shift typically is assigned six patients to care for, that number is sometimes much higher for individual nurses. Fully 23 percent of hospitals reported that nurses in their medical–surgical units on the day shift were each responsible for caring for 7 to 12 patients (Cavouras and Suby, 2003). Nursing homes also vary in the number of patients assigned to nursing staff.

Currently available methods for achieving safer staffing levels in hospitals, such as authorizing nursing staff to halt admissions to their unit when staffing is inadequate for safe patient care, are not employed uniformly by hospitals or nursing homes. Federal regulations governing nursing home staffing are over a decade old and do not reflect new knowledge on safe staffing levels. Minimum standards for registered nurses require only the presence of one licensed nurse in a nursing home, regardless of its size. Moreover, the regulations do not specify minimum staffing levels for nurse assistants, who provide most of the nursing care in these facilities.

Additionally, not all HCOs have taken steps to compensate for the widely acknowledged fact that, like newly licensed physicians, newly licensed nurses need additional training and education once they enter the workforce, and that experienced nurses similarly need ongoing education and training to keep up with the continuing growth of new medical knowledge and technology. Surveys of nursing administrators from acute care hospitals and nursing homes and newly licensed nurses themselves report the same finding: many newly licensed nurses do not possess the overall educational preparation to provide safe, effective care. Registered nurses (RNs) are viewed as especially lacking skills in recognizing abnormal physical and diagnostic findings and responding to emergencies (Smith and Crawford, 2002a,b).

Despite these findings, hospitals are reported to have scaled back orientation programs for newly hired nurses, as well as ongoing in-service training and continuing education programs, as a result of financial pressures (Berens, 2000). A federally sponsored study of staffing in long-term care facilities similarly found that current initial certification education for nurse assistants is insufficient (CMS, 2002). The committee found evidence that all health care professionals (nurses and physicians alike) need better training, as well as organizational practices that promote and support interdisciplinary collaboration and teamwork. Decision support technology is also needed in all nursing work environments.

Unsafe Work and Workspace Design

Several aspects of the way in which nurses' work is designed pose threats to patient safety. The long work hours of some nurses represent one of the most serious threats. While most nurses typically work 8- or 12-hour shifts, some work much longer hours. In one study, 3.5 percent of scheduled shifts exceeded 12 hours, including "shifts" as long as 22.5 hours.[2] In another study, 27 percent of full-time hospital and nursing home nurses reported working more than 13 hours at a stretch one or more times a week.[3] The effects of fatigue on human performance are well known. Prolonged periods of wakefulness (e.g., 17 hours without sleep) can produce performance decrements equivalent to a blood alcohol concentration (BAC) of 0.05 percent, the BAC level defined as alcohol intoxication in many western industrialized countries (Dawson and Reid, 1997; Lamond and Dawson, 1998).[4]

Other nursing work processes, such as medication administration, are often carried out in ways that are conducive to the commission of errors and without the support of newer technologies that can prevent errors in medication administration. One study of preventable adverse drug events in hospitals found that 34 percent of medication errors took place in the course of administering the drug (a nursing role), as opposed to occurring as a part of ordering, transcribing, or dispensing the drug (Bates et al., 1995). A similar 6-month study of all adverse drug events in two tertiary care hospitals found that 38 percent occurred during the administration of the drug by nursing staff (Pepper, 1995).

Other inefficient care processes and workspace design features decrease patient safety by reducing the amount of time nurses have for monitoring patients and providing therapeutic care. For example, while not intrinsically dangerous to patients, documentation of patient information and care processes consumes an estimated 13–28 percent of a hospital nurse's time (Pabst et al., 1996; Smeltzer et al., 1996; Upenieks, 1998; Urden and Roode, 1997). For home care nurses, the time required is estimated to be much greater as a result of regulatory requirements for patient information and assessment (Trossman, 2001). Other inefficiencies arise from interruptions

---

[2]Unpublished data from Ann Rogers, Ph.D., University of Pennsylvania (manuscript in preparation).

[3]Unpublished data from Alison Trinkoff, Ph.D., University of Maryland at Baltimore, National Institute for Occupational Safety and Health grant R01OH3702 (personal communication. April 9, 2003).

[4]In the United States, BAC-level definitions of intoxication are set by the states. Limits of 0.08 and 0.10 are typical for adult drivers; the majority of states set lower levels for drivers under 21 years of age (e.g., 0.00–0.07) (Wagenaar et al., 2001).

and distractions associated with nursing tasks; workspaces not designed to facilitate nursing organization and activities; limited access to information systems; and other common work practices, including using nurses to perform such non-nursing duties as picking up blood products and delivering laboratory specimens.

Punitive Cultures That Hinder the Reporting and Prevention of Errors

To Err Is Human also calls attention to the need to create organizational cultures of safety that promote the reporting, analysis, and prevention of errors within all HCOs. The committee finds that while some progress has been made in fostering such cultures, full implementation has not yet been achieved. Incidents have been reported in which nurses who were involved in the commission of an error but found blameless by a number of independent authoritative bodies were unjustly disciplined by state regulatory agencies. HCOs need the assistance of state and federal oversight organizations if they are to create fully effective programs for detecting and preventing patient care errors in their organizations.

NEED FOR BUNDLES OF MUTUALLY REINFORCING PATIENT SAFETY DEFENSES IN NURSES' WORK ENVIRONMENTS

No single action can, by itself, keep patients safe from health care errors. Because multiple components and processes of HCOs create situations that nurture errors in the work environments of nurses, multiple, mutually reinforcing changes in those environments are needed to substantially reduce errors and increase patient safety. To this end, defenses must be created in all organizational components: (1) leadership and management, (2) the workforce, (3) work processes, and (4) organizational culture. Bundles of changes are needed within each of these components to strengthen patient safety.

Transformational Leadership and Evidence-Based Management

Creating work environments for nurses that are most conducive to patient safety will require fundamental changes throughout many HCOs in terms of how work is designed, how personnel are deployed, and how the very culture of the organization understands and acts on the science of safety. These changes require leadership capable of transforming not just physical environments, but also the beliefs and practices of both nurses and other health care workers providing patient care and those in the HCO who establish the policies and practices that shape those environments—the individuals who constitute the management of the organization.

Leadership will need to assure the effective use of practices that (1) balance the tension between production efficiency and reliability (safety), (2) create and sustain trust throughout the organization, (3) actively manage the process of change, (4) involve workers in decision making pertaining to work design and work flow, and (5) use knowledge management practices to establish the organization as a "learning organization." To this end, the committee makes the following recommendations:

Recommendation 4-1.[5] HCOs should acquire nurse leaders for all levels of management (e.g., at the organization-wide and patient care unit levels) who will:

- Participate in executive decisions within the HCO.
- Represent nursing staff to organization management and facilitate their mutual trust.
- Achieve effective communication between nursing and other clinical leadership.
- Facilitate input of direct-care nursing staff into operational decision making and the design of work processes and work flow.
- Be provided with organizational resources to support the acquisition, management, and dissemination to nursing staff of the knowledge needed to support their clinical decision making and actions.

Recommendation 4-2. Leaders of HCOs should take action to identify and minimize the potential adverse effects of their decisions on patient safety by:

- Educating board members and senior, midlevel, and line managers about the link between management practices and safety.
- Emphasizing safety to the same extent as productivity and financial goals in internal management planning and reports and in public reports to stakeholders.

Recommendation 4-3. HCOs should employ management structures and processes throughout the organization that:

- Provide ongoing vigilance in balancing efficiency and safety.
- Demonstrate trust in workers and promote trust by workers.

---

[5]For ease of reference, the committee's recommendations are numbered according to the chapter of the main text in which they appear.

- Actively manage the process of change.
- Engage workers in nonhierarchical decision making and in the design of work processes and work flow.
- Establish the organization as a "learning organization."

Because HCOs vary in the extent to which they currently employ the above practices and in their available resources, the committee also makes the following recommendation:

> **Recommendation 4-4. Professional associations, philanthropic organizations, and other organizational leaders within the health care industry should sponsor collaboratives that incorporate multiple academic and other research-based organizations to support HCOs in the identification and adoption of evidence-based management practices.**

Maximizing Workforce Capability

Monitoring patient health status, performing therapeutic treatments, and integrating patient care to avoid health care gaps are nursing functions that directly affect patient safety. Accomplishing these activities requires an adequate number of nursing staff with the clinical knowledge and skills needed to carry out these interventions and the ability to effectively communicate findings and coordinate care with the interventions of other members of the patient's health care team. Nurse staffing levels, the knowledge and skill level of nursing staff, and the extent to which workers collaborate in sharing their knowledge and skills all affect patient outcomes and safety.

Regulatory, internal HCO, and marketplace (consumer-driven) approaches are traditionally advocated as methods to achieve appropriate staffing levels. The committee determined that each of these approaches has limitations as well as strengths; their coordinated and combined use holds the most promise for achieving safe staffing levels. The committee also took particular note of the need for more accurate and reliable staffing data for hospitals and nursing homes to help make these efforts more effective and to facilitate additional needed research on staffing. Finally, the committee identified a need for more research on hospital staffing for specific types of patient care units, such as medical–surgical and labor and delivery units. The committee therefore makes the following recommendations:

> **Recommendation 5-1. The U.S. Department of Health and Human Services (DHHS) should update existing regulations established in 1990 that specify minimum standards for registered and licensed**

nurse staffing in nursing homes. Updated minimum standards should:

- Require the presence of at least one RN within the facility at all times.
- Specify staffing levels that increase as the number of patients increase, and that are based on the findings and recommendations of the DHHS report to Congress, *Appropriateness of Minimum Nurse Staffing Ratios in Nursing Homes—Phase II Final Report.*
- Address staffing levels for nurse assistants, who provide the majority of patient care.

Recommendation 5-2. Hospitals and nursing homes should employ nurse staffing practices that identify needed nurse staffing for each patient care unit per shift. These practices should:

- Incorporate estimates of patient volume that count admissions, discharges, and "less than full-day" patients in addition to a census of patients at a point in time.
- Involve direct-care nursing staff in determining and evaluating the approaches used to determine appropriate unit staffing levels for each shift.
- Provide for staffing "elasticity" or "slack" within each shift's scheduling to accommodate unpredicted variations in patient volume and acuity and resulting workload. Methods used to provide slack should give preference to scheduling excess staff and creating cross-trained float pools within the HCO. Use of nurses from external agencies should be avoided.
- Empower nursing unit staff to regulate unit work flow and set criteria for unit closures to new admissions and transfers as nursing workload and staffing necessitate.
- Involve direct-care nursing staff in identifying the causes of nursing staff turnover and in developing methods to improve nursing staff retention.

Recommendation 5-3. Hospitals and nursing homes should perform ongoing evaluation of the effectiveness of their nurse staffing practices with respect to patient safety, and increase internal oversight of their staffing methods, levels, and effects on patient safety whenever staffing falls below the following levels for a 24-hour day:

- In hospital ICUs—one licensed nurse for every 2 patients (12 hours of licensed nursing staff per patient day).
- In nursing homes, for long-stay residents—one RN for every 32 patients (0.75 hours per resident day), one licensed nurse for every 18 patients (1.3 hours per resident day), and one nurse assistant for every 8.5 patients (2.8 hours per resident day).

Recommendation 5-4. DHHS should implement a nationwide, publicly accessible system for collecting and managing valid and reliable staffing and turnover data from hospitals and nursing homes. Information on individual hospital and nursing home staffing at the level of individual nursing units and the facility in the aggregate should be disclosed routinely to the public.

- Federal and state nursing home report cards should include standardized, case-mix–adjusted information on the average hours per patient day of RN, licensed, and nurse assistant care provided to residents and a comparison with federal and state standards.
- During the next 3 years, public and private sponsors of the new hospital report card to be located on the federal government website should undertake an initiative—in collaboration with experts in acute hospital care, nurse staffing, and consumer information—to develop, test, and implement measures of hospital nurse staffing levels for the public.

Moreover, the knowledge base on effective clinical care and new health care technologies is increasing rapidly, making it impossible for nurses (and other clinicians) to incorporate this information into their clinical decision making and practice without organizational support. Organizational studies and research on exemplary work environments indicate the importance of investment in ongoing employee learning by employers. The committee therefore makes the following recommendation:

Recommendation 5-5. HCOs should dedicate budgetary resources equal to a defined percentage of nursing payroll to support nursing staff in their ongoing acquisition and maintenance of knowledge and skills. These resources should be sufficient for and used to implement policies and practices that:

- Assign experienced nursing staff to precept nurses newly practicing in a clinical area to address knowledge and skill gaps.

- Annually ensure that each licensed nurse and nurse assistant has an individualized plan and resources for educational development within health care.
- Provide education and training of staff as new technology or changes in the workplace are introduced.
- Provide decision support technology identified with the active involvement of direct-care nursing staff to enable point-of-care learning.
- Disseminate to individual staff organizational learning as captured in clinical tools, algorithms, and pathways.

Finally, in response to evidence on inconsistent interprofessional collaboration among nursing staff and other health care providers, the committee makes the following recommendation:

Recommendation 5-6. HCOs should take action to support interdisciplinary collaboration by adopting such interdisciplinary practice mechanisms as interdisciplinary rounds, and by providing ongoing formal education and training in interdisciplinary collaboration for all health care providers on a regularly scheduled, continuous basis (e.g., monthly, quarterly, or semiannually).

Design of Work and Workspace to Prevent and Mitigate Errors

Nurses' work processes and workspaces need to be designed to make them more efficient, less conducive to the commission of errors, and more amenable to detecting and remedying errors when they occur. The work hours of a minority of nurses, in particular, are identified as a serious threat to the safety of patients. The effects of fatigue include slowed reaction time, lapses of attention to detail, errors of omission, compromised problem solving, reduced motivation, and decreased energy for successful completion of required tasks. Other safety-sensitive industries have acknowledged and taken action to defend against these effects by limiting the number of shifts or hours worked in a week.

Changing work patterns will require attention from HCOs, regulatory bodies, state boards of nursing, schools of nursing, and nurses themselves. Accordingly, the committee makes the following recommendation:

Recommendation 6-1. To reduce error-producing fatigue, state regulatory bodies should prohibit nursing staff from providing patient care in any combination of scheduled shifts, mandatory overtime, or voluntary overtime in excess of 12 hours in any given 24-hour period and in excess of 60 hours per 7-day period. To this end:

- HCOs and labor organizations representing nursing staff should establish policies and practices designed to prevent nurses who provide direct patient care from working longer than 12 hours in a 24-hour period and in excess of 60 hours per 7-day period.
- Schools of nursing, state boards of nursing, and HCOs should educate nurses about the threats to patient safety caused by fatigue.

Enabling nursing staff to collaborate with other health care personnel in identifying high-risk and inefficient work processes and workspaces and (re)designing them for patient safety and efficiency is also essential. Moreover, documentation practices are in great need of redesign. However, this cannot be accomplished solely by nursing staff and internal HCO efforts. Because many documentation practices are driven by external parties, such as regulators and oversight organizations, these entities will need to assist in the redesign of documentation practices. To address these needs, the committee makes the following recommendations:

Recommendation 6-2. HCOs should provide nursing leadership with resources that enable them to design the nursing work environment and care processes to reduce errors. These efforts must directly involve direct-care nurses throughout all phases of the work design and should concentrate on errors associated with:

- Surveillance of patient health status.
- Patient transfers and other patient hand-offs.
- Complex patient care processes.
- Non–value-added activities performed by nurses, such as locating and obtaining supplies, looking for personnel, completing redundant and unnecessary documentation, and compensating for poor communication systems.

Recommendation 6-3. HCOs should address handwashing and medication administration among their first work design initiatives.

Recommendation 6-4. Regulators; leaders in health care; and experts in nursing, law, informatics, and related disciplines should jointly convene to identify strategies for safely reducing the burden associated with patient and work-related documentation.

Creating and Sustaining a Culture of Safety

Employing a nursing workforce strong in numbers and capabilities and designing their work to prevent errors will not be sufficient to fully safeguard patients. The largest and most capable workforce is still fallible, and the best-designed work processes are still designed by fallible individuals. Patient safety also requires an organizational commitment to vigilance to prevent potential errors, and to the detection, analysis, and redress of errors when they occur.

A variety of safety-conscious industries have made such a commitment and achieved substantially lower rates of errors by doing so. These organizations place as high a priority on safety as they do on production; all employees are fully engaged in the process of detecting high-risk situations before an error occurs. Management is so responsive to employees' detection of risk that it dedicates time, personnel, budget, and training resources to bring about changes needed to make work processes safer. Employees also are empowered to act in dangerous situations to reduce the likelihood of adverse events. These attitudes and employee engagement are so pervasive and observable in the behaviors of these organizations and their employees that an actual *culture of safety* exists within the organization. These organizational cultures are effective because they (1) recognize that the majority of errors are created by systemic organizational defects in work processes, not by blameworthy individuals; (2) support staff; and (3) foster continuous learning by the organization as a whole and its employees.

HCOs should redouble their efforts to create such cultures of safety within their work environments. Such efforts require a long-term commitment because they necessitate changes in the attitudes and behaviors of both organizations and people. Time is needed to enact an initial change, evaluate, refine, and enact further change. Strong organizational leadership is also essential. The safety of patients needs to be a stated and visible priority, with every organizational member understanding that each is fallible, even with the best of intentions, as are the processes used. Moreover, establishing a fair and just culture in responding to errors reduces workers' fear and disincentives to report errors and near misses. As a result, all nursing staff are more inclined to be vigilant for errors and near misses, with a view toward learning from each event and strengthening the culture of safety accordingly. Action also is needed from state boards of nursing and Congress to enable strong and effective cultures of safety to exist. To these ends, the committee makes the following recommendations:

Recommendation 7-1. HCO boards of directors, managerial leadership, and labor partners should create and sustain cultures of safety by implementing the recommendations presented previously and by:

- Specifying short- and long-term safety objectives.
- Continuously reviewing success in meeting these objectives and providing feedback at all levels.
- Conducting an annual, confidential survey of nursing and other health care workers to assess the extent to which a culture of safety exists.
- Instituting a deidentified, fair, and just reporting system for errors and near misses.
- Engaging in ongoing employee training in error detection, analysis, and reduction.
- Implementing procedures for analyzing errors and providing feedback to direct-care workers.
- Instituting rewards and incentives for error reduction.

Recommendation 7-2. The National Council of State Boards of Nursing, in consultation with patient safety experts and health care leaders, should undertake an initiative to design uniform processes across states for better distinguishing human errors from willful negligence and intentional misconduct, along with guidelines for their application by state boards of nursing and other state regulatory bodies having authority over nursing.

Recommendation 7-3. Congress should pass legislation to extend peer review protections to data related to patient safety and quality improvement that are collected and analyzed by HCOs for internal use or shared with others solely for purposes of improving safety and quality.

Summary

Implementing all of the above recommendations will create the necessary bundles of mutually reinforcing patient safeguards in the work environments of nurses listed in Box ES-1.

IMPLEMENTING THE COMMITTEE'S RECOMMENDATIONS

The Recommendations Build on Two Prior IOM Reports

The committee's recommendations build on those contained in two prior IOM reports: *To Err Is Human: Building a Safer Health System* (IOM, 2000) and *Crossing the Quality Chasm: A New Health System for the 21st*

BOX ES-1   Necessary Patient Safeguards in the Work Environment of Nurses

Governing Boards That Focus on Safety

- Are knowledgeable about the link between management practices and patient safety.
- Emphasize patient safety to the same extent as financial and productivity goals.

Leadership and Evidence-Based Management Structures and Processes

- Provide ongoing vigilance in balancing efficiency and patient safety.
- Demonstrate and promote trust in and by nursing staff.
- Actively manage the process of change.
- Engage nursing staff in nonhierarchical decision making and work design.
- Establish the organization as a "learning organization."

Effective Nursing Leadership

- Participates in executive decision making.
- Represents nursing staff to management.
- Achieves effective communication between nurses and other clinical leadership.
- Facilitates input from direct-care nursing staff into decision making.
- Commands organizational resources for nursing knowledge acquisition and clinical decision making.

Adequate Staffing

- Is established by sound methodologies as determined by nursing staff.
- Provides mechanisms to accommodate unplanned variations in patient care workload.

Century (IOM, 2001). The authors of the *Quality Chasm* report identify four different levels for intervening in the delivery of health care: (1) the experience of patients; (2) the functioning of small units of care delivery ("microsystems"), such as surgical teams or nursing units; (3) the functioning of organizations that house the microsystems; and (4) the policy, payment, regulation, accreditation, and other external factors that shape the environment in which HCOs deliver care. *To Err Is Human* speaks mainly

- Enables nursing staff to regulate nursing unit work flow.
- Is consistent with best available evidence on safe staffing thresholds.

Organizational Support for Ongoing Learning and Decision Support

- Uses preceptors for novice nurses.
- Provides ongoing educational support and resources to nursing staff.
- Provides training in new technology.
- Provides decision support at the point of care.

Mechanisms That Promote Interdisciplinary Collaboration

- Use interdisciplinary practice mechanisms, such as interdisciplinary patient care rounds.
- Provide formal education and training in interdisciplinary collaboration for all health care providers.

Work Design That Promotes Safety

- Defends against fatigue and unsafe and inefficient work design.
- Tackles medication administration, handwashing, documentation, and other high-priority practices.

Organizational Culture That Continuously Strengthens Patient Safety

- Regularly reviews organizational success in achieving formally specified safety objectives.
- Fosters a fair and just error-reporting, analysis, and feedback system.
- Trains and rewards workers for safety.

to the fourth level (i.e., policy, payment, regulation, accreditation, and other external factors) in its articulation of a national agenda for patient safety. *Crossing the Quality Chasm* addresses primarily how the experiences of patients and the work of microsystems of care should be changed (Berwick, 2002). The present report, which focuses on the third level (i.e., HCOs and their work environments), complements the work of the two prior IOM reports in three ways:

- It provides greater detail about how HCOs can and should implement key recommendations from *To Err Is Human* and *Crossing the Quality Chasm* in such areas as creating cultures of safety and addressing work design.
- It addresses aspects of the work environment that are critical to patient safety but are not addressed in either of the two prior reports, such as the adequacy of staffing levels and worker fatigue.
- It unifies the work of the prior two IOM reports and this report into a framework that all HCOs can use to construct work environments more conducive to patient safety.

Piecemeal Approaches Will Not Be Successful

With respect to this report's recommendations, the committee wishes to underscore that none of these recommendations is "less important." Redesigned work practices will still be unsafe if the number of nurses available to perform the work as designed is insufficient. Nor will an apparently sufficient number of nurses perform as needed if they are suffering from the effects of fatigue, inexperienced in a given work process, or unfamiliar with the work processes because they have been secured from a temporary agency. Moreover, even when the most capable workforce provides care using the best-designed work processes, errors will still occur because neither the nurse nor the work process is perfect. Defenses against human errors can be developed and put in place only if nursing staff are not afraid of reporting those errors and are involved in designing even stronger defenses. Finally, instituting all of these defense strategies can be accomplished only by individuals who have a vision of and command resources for the organization as a whole—an organization's leadership and management. Their actions are the essential precursor to creating safer health care environments by addressing all sources of threats to patient safety (see Figure ES-1).

Additional Research Necessitates Ongoing Change

Finally, the committee notes that changing health care delivery practices to increase patient safety must be an ongoing process. Research findings and dissemination of practices that other HCOs have found successful in improving patient safety will help HCOs as learning organizations add to their repertoire of patient safety practices. This report calls attention to several areas in which, at present, information is limited about how to design nurses' work and work environments to make them safer for patients. Research is needed to provide better information on nursing-related errors, means of achieving safer work processes and workspace design, a standard-

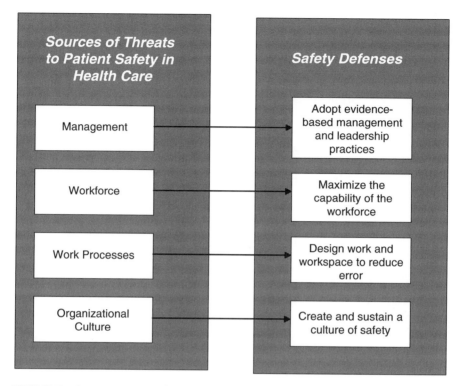

FIGURE ES-1   Sources of threats to patient safety in the work environment and corresponding safety defenses.

ized approach to measuring patient acuity, safe staffing levels for different types of patient care units, effective methods to help night shift workers compensate for fatigue, what limits should be imposed on successive days of working sustained work hours, and collaborative models of care. Accordingly, the committee makes the following recommendation:

> **Recommendation 8-1. Federal agencies and private foundations should support research in the following areas to provide HCOs with the additional information they need to continue to strengthen nurse work environments for patient safety:**
>
> - **Studies and development of methods to better describe, both qualitatively and quantitatively, the work nurses perform in different care settings.**
> - **Descriptive studies of nursing-related errors.**

- Design, application, and evaluation (including financial costs and savings) of safer and more efficient work processes and work-space, including the application of information technology.
- Development and testing of a standardized approach to measuring patient acuity.
- Determination of safe staffing levels within different types of nursing units.
- Development and testing of methods to help night shift workers compensate for fatigue.
- Research on the effects of successive work days and sustained work hours on patient safety.
- Development and evaluation of models of collaborative care, including care by teams.

REFERENCES

Aiken L, Clarke S, Sloane D. 2000. Hospital restructuring: Does it adversely affect care and outcomes? *Journal of Nursing Administration* 30(10):457–465.

Aiken L, Clarke S, Sloane D, Sochalski J, Busse R, Clarke H, Giovannetti P, Hunt J, Rafferty A, Shamian J. 2001. Nurses' reports on hospital care in five countries. *Health Affairs* 20(3):43–53.

Aiken L, Clarke S, Sloane D, Sochalski J, Silber J. 2002. Hospital nurse staffing and patient mortality, nurse burnout, and job dissatisfaction. *Journal of the American Medical Association* 288:1987–1993.

Bates D, Cullen D, Laird N, Petersen L, Small S, Servi D, Laffel G, Sweitzer B, Shea B, Hallisey R, Vander Vleit M, Nemeskal R, Leape L. 1995. Incidence of adverse drug events and potential adverse drug events: Implications for prevention. *Journal of the American Medical Association* 274:29–34.

Berens M. 2000, September 11. Training often takes a back seat; budget pressures, lack of state laws aggravate trend. *Chicago Tribune*. News. p. 7.

Berwick D. 2002. A user's manual for the IOM's "Quality Chasm" report. *Health Affairs* 21(3):80–90.

Blendon R, DesRoches C, Brodie M, Benson J, Rosen A, Schneider E, Altman D, Zapert K, Herrmann M, Steffenson A. 2002. Views of practicing physicians and the public on medical errors. *The New England Journal of Medicine* 347(24):1933–1940.

Brilli R, Spevetz A, Branson R, Campbell G, Cohen H, Dasta J, Harvey M, Kelley M, Kelley K, Rudis M, St. Andre A, Stone J, Teres D, Weled B, Peruzzi W, the members of the American College of Critical Care Medicine Task Force on Models of Critical Care Delivery, the members of the American College of Critical Care Medicine Guidelines for the Definition of an Intensivist, and the Practice of Critical Care Medicine. 2001. Critical care delivery in the intensive care unit: Defining clinical roles and the best practice model. *Critical Care Medicine* 29(10):2007–2019.

Cavouras C, Suby C. 2003. Perspectives on Staffing and Scheduling. *2003 Survey of Hours Report: Direct and Total Hours per Patient Day (HPPD) by Patient Care Units*. Phoenix, AZ: Labor Management Institute.

Clancy C, Scully T. 2003. A call to excellence. *Health Affairs* 22(2):113–115.

CMS (Centers for Medicare and Medicaid Services). 2002. *Report to Congress: Appropriateness of Minimum Nurse Staffing Ratios in Nursing Homes—Phase II Final Report:* U.S. Department of Health and Human Services. [Online]. Available: www.cms.gov/medicaid/reports/rp1201home.asp "last modified on Wednesday, June 12, 2002" [accessed on June, 25, 2002].

Dawson D, Reid K. 1997. Fatigue, alcohol and performance impairment. *Nature* 388:235.

Decker D, Wheeler G, Johnson J, Parsons R. 2001. Effect of organizational change on the individual employee. *The Health Care Manager* 19(4):1–12.

Gelinas L, Manthey M. 1997. The impact of organizational redesign on nurse executive leadership. *Journal of Nursing Administration* 27(10):35–42.

Ingersoll G, Fisher M, Ross B, Soja M, Kidd N. 2001. Employee response to major organizational redesign. *Applied Nursing Research* 14(1):18–28.

IOM (Institute of Medicine). 2000. *To Err Is Human: Building a Safer Health System.* Washington, DC: National Academy Press.

IOM. 2001. *Crossing the Quality Chasm: A New Health System for the 21st Century.* Washington, DC: National Academy Press.

Kahn K, Rogers W, Rubenstein L, Sherwood M, Reinisch E, Keeler E, Draper D, Kosecoff J, Brook R. 1990. Measuring quality of care with explicit process criteria before and after implementation of the DRG-based prospective payment system. *Journal of the American Medical Association* 264(15):1969–1973.

Kramer M, Schmalenberg C. 1993. Learning from success: Autonomy and empowerment. *Nursing Management* 24(5):58–64.

Lamond N, Dawson D. 1998. *Quantifying the Performance Impairment Associated With Sustained Wakefulness.* South Australia: The Centre for Sleep Research, The Queen Elizabeth Hospital. [Online]. Available: http://cf.alpha.org/internet/projects/ftdt/backgr/Daw_Lam.html [accessed July 7, 2003].

Leape L, Bates D, Cullen D, Cooper J, Demonaco H, Gallivan T, Hallisey R, Ives J, Laird N, Laffel G, Nemeskal R, Petersen L, Porter K, Servi D, Shea B, Small S, Sweitzer B, Thompson B, Vander Vleit M. 1995. Systems analysis of adverse drug events. *Journal of the American Medical Association* 274(1):35–43.

Mitchell P, Shortell S. 1997. Adverse outcomes and variations in organization of care delivery. *Medical Care* 35:NS 19–32.

Needleman J, Buerhaus P, Mattke S, Stewart M, Zelevinsky K. 2002. Nurse-staffing levels and the quality of care in hospitals. *The New England Journal of Medicine* 346(22):1715–1722.

Pabst M, Scherubel J, Minnick A. 1996. The impact of computerized documentation on nurses' use of time. *Computers in Nursing* 14(1):25–30.

Pepper G. 1995. Errors in drug administration by nurses. *American Journal of Health-System Pharmacy* 52:390–395.

Rubenstein L, Chang B, Keeler E, Kahn K. 1992. Measuring the quality of nursing surveillance activities for five diseases before and after implementation of the drug-based prospective payment system. In: *Patient Outcomes Research: Examining the Effectiveness of Nursing Practice.* Proceedings of the State of the Science Conference. Bethesda, MD: NIH, National Center for Nursing Research. Washington, DC: U.S. Government Printing Office.

Seago J. 2001. Nurse staffing, models of care delivery, and interventions. In: Shojania K, Duncan B, McDonald K, Wachter R, eds. *Making Health Care Safer: A Critical Analysis of Patient Safety Practices.* Evidence Report/Technology Assessment No. 43. Rockville, MD: AHRQ.

Smeltzer C, Hines P, Beebe H, Keller B. 1996. Streamlining documentation: An opportunity to reduce costs and increase nurse clinicians' time with patients. *Journal of Nursing Care Quality* 10(4):66–77.

Smith J, Crawford L. 2002a. *Report of Findings from the 2001 Employers Survey.* NCSBN Research Brief. 3. Chicago, IL: National Council of State Boards of Nursing, Inc.

Smith J, Crawford L. 2002b. *Report of Findings from the Practice and Professional Issues Survey—Spring 2001.* NCSBN Research Brief. 2. Chicago, IL: National Council of State Boards of Nursing, Inc.

Sovie M, Jawad A. 2001. Hospital restructuring and its impact on outcomes. *Journal of Nursing Administration* 31(12):588–600.

Trossman S. 2001. The documentation dilemma: Nurses poised to address paperwork burden. *The American Nurse,* 33(5): 1, 9, 18.

Tucker A, Edmondson A. 2002. Managing routine exceptions: A model of nurse problem solving behavior. *Advances in Health Care Management* 3:87–113.

Upenieks V. 1998. Work sampling: Assessing nursing efficiency. *Nursing Management* 29(4): 27–29.

Urden L, Roode J. 1997. Work sampling: A decision-making tool for determining resources and work redesign. *Journal of Nursing Administration* 27(9):34–41.

Wagenaar A, O'Malley P, LaFond C. 2001. Lowered legal blood alcohol limits for young drivers: Effects on drinking, driving, and driving-after-drinking behaviors in 30 states. *American Journal of Public Health* 91(5):801–804.

Walston S, Kimberly J. 1997. Reengineering hospitals: Evidence from the field. *Hospital and Health Services Administration* 42(2):143–163.

1

Nursing: Inseparably Linked to Patient Safety

Over the last two decades, substantial changes have been made in the organization and delivery of health care. These fast-paced changes have resulted from multiple, concurrent events, including (1) major modifications in the ways in which government and private health insurance programs reimburse health care providers (including hospitals, nursing homes, home health care agencies, and individual practitioners); (2) cost-containment efforts of health care organizations (HCOs) in response to these changes in reimbursement; (3) growth in and increased demand for new health care technologies; and (4) changes in the health care workforce. HCOs have responded in a variety of ways that, in turn, have affected the work and work environment of nurses. Some of these changes have resulted, for example, in greater numbers of more acutely ill and technology-dependent patients being assigned to individual nurses; changes in how licensed and unlicensed nursing staff are deployed; and a growing number of competing demands on nurses' time, such as increased paperwork and documentation requirements. Many individuals and organizations have expressed concern that these and other changes have adversely affected nurses' ability to provide safe patient care (Aiken et al., 2001a; Service Employees International Union, 2001; Shindul-Rothschild et al., 1996).

In response to such concerns, the U.S. Department of Health and Human Services' Agency for Healthcare Research and Quality (AHRQ) asked the Institute of Medicine (IOM) to conduct a study to identify key aspects of the work environment for nurses that likely have an impact on patient safety, and to identify potential improvements in health care working conditions that would likely increase patient safety. AHRQ further directed that the study be conducted "in the context of current policy debates on regulation of nursing work hours and nursing workload . . . [and] cover such topics as: extended work hours and fatigue, including mandatory overtime; workload issues, including state regulation of nurse-to-bed ratios; workplace environmental issues, including poorly designed care processes; . . . workplace systems, including reliance on memory and lack of support systems for decision-making; and workplace communication, including social, physical, and other barriers to effective communication among care team members." The Committee on the Work Environment for Nurses and Patient Safety was formed to carry out this study. This report presents the study results.

In responding to its charge, the committee reviewed and built upon recommendations for increasing patient safety contained in two earlier IOM reports—*To Err Is Human: Building a Safer Health System* (IOM, 2000) and *Crossing the Quality Chasm: A New Health System for the 21st Century* (IOM, 2001). In this introductory chapter, we first summarize and update the evidence presented in *To Err Is Human* about the magnitude and etiology of health care errors affecting patient safety. We then present evidence of the key role played by nurses in patient care and safety, and briefly describe some of the characteristics of the current health care delivery system that shape the work and work environment of nurses, particularly in in-patient facilities. Evidence is then presented showing that nurses are not immune to the problems that plague health care delivery in the United States—problems that foster the occurrence of errors in which all health care providers, not just nurses, are involved. The chapter ends with a call for a substantial transformation in the work environment of nurses to better safeguard patients.

THOUSANDS OF HEALTH CARE ERRORS

I was a "new" nurse. I'd been practicing only a few months when I was assigned an elderly patient who was scheduled for abdominal surgery that morning and needed a urinary catheter inserted. I knew about, but hadn't performed, this procedure before, and neither had the other nurses on the floor—we all were new graduates and fairly inexperienced. I asked my head nurse if she would supervise me while I placed the catheter, but she was late for a meeting and assured me that it wasn't difficult and I would be fine.

I went to get the supplies I needed, but there were no prepackaged catheterization trays on the floor. I ran the stairs to the floors above and below me, but they were out, too. As I passed the nursing station, the clerk called out to me that the OR [operating room] wanted to know where the patient was. I began to round up the materials needed on an item-by-item basis.

I got a sterile prep tray (the last one), sterile catheter and gloves, antiseptics for cleansing, and drainage bag. I opened the sterile prep tray, prepared the patient, put on the sterile gloves, and realized I hadn't opened the bottles of antiseptic before putting on the sterile gloves and that the routine sterile prep tray didn't contain what I had expected. There were no more gloves in the patient's room. I went to get more, cautioning the patient to not move, and leaving my sterile field unattended.

As I passed the nurses' station, the clerk again called out: "The OR called again and they are really angry and want to know what's keeping your patient. You are backing up the entire OR schedule!" I got the gloves and with trembling hands, uncertainty about the sterility of my "sterile field," and not the best of technique, inserted the catheter.

A day or two later, I was charting on my patients and seated next to the patient's resident, who exclaimed, "Mrs. X has the worst UTI [urinary tract infection] I've ever seen!"

I didn't say anything. I was ashamed and afraid, and besides, the resident was already writing an order for antibiotics. There was nothing more to be done. What would be gained if I told anyone?

What happened to Mrs. X in the above (true) incident was a mistake—an *error*. Her urinary tract infection was an *adverse event* likely resulting from (at least in the opinion of the nurse performing the procedure) that error. While this error involved an inexperienced nurse, errors are committed by individuals with all levels of experience.

To Err Is Human helped the United States (and other countries) come to a better understanding of the likely hundreds of thousands of health care errors and adverse events that occur in the United States every year in which nurses, physicians, pharmacists, dentists, nurse aides, and assistants—in fact, all health care providers—are involved. First, *To Err Is Human* presented the vocabulary necessary to begin to better understand the problem:

- *Errors* are failures of planned actions to be completed as intended, or the use of wrong plans to achieve what is intended.
- *Adverse events* are injuries caused by medical intervention, as opposed to the health condition of a patient. A large proportion of adverse events are the result of errors. When the adverse event is the result of an error, it is considered a *preventable adverse event*.

Sometimes an error, such as giving a patient the wrong medication, may lead to no detectable adverse event. Other errors can temporarily or permanently harm the health of the patient or cause the person's death. In the incident described above, the catheterization of the patient was not completed as intended. The process was replete with errors, including the nurse's technique in catheterization, the nurse manager's assumption that the new nurse could perform the procedure safely, and the supply department's failure to stock prepackaged catheterization trays on the floor. The patient received an injury—a urinary tract infection—an adverse event that was likely preventable. The infection likely caused discomfort and possibly even pain. It required the administration of antibiotics, which carries the risk of side effects, adverse reactions, and medication errors. Moreover, the administration of antibiotics may have prolonged the patient's stay in the hospital. Urinary tract infections can also lead to more serious kidney infections and, if undetected or occurring in a patient with a weakened immune system, can lead to sepsis (an infection in the blood), which can cause death.

To Err Is Human also calls attention to the magnitude of adverse events that occur every day to patients in the hospital. The report estimates that adverse events (involving all health care providers) occur in 2.9 to 3.7 percent of acute care hospitalizations, and that approximately half of these events are likely due to errors (i.e., preventable adverse events). The report further estimates that each year, between 44,000 and 98,000 hospitalized Americans die as a result of medical errors—more than die from motor vehicle accidents, breast cancer, or AIDS. Indeed, To Err Is Human presents evidence that these numbers are likely underestimates of the numbers of people injured by errors in health care. These numbers also do not include persons injured as a result of medical errors in nursing homes, home health care, and other health care settings. Earlier studies of medical errors have indicated similarly high rates of adverse events (Steel et al., 1981).

The IOM's estimates of high rates of errors have been reaffirmed more recently by two different sources—practicing physicians and the public at large. In a 2002 national survey of practicing physicians and the American public, 35 percent of surveyed U.S. physicians and 42 percent of the public reported experiencing an error either in their own care or in that of a family member. Moreover, 18 percent of the physicians and 24 percent of the public reported an error that had caused serious health consequences, including death (reported by 7 percent of physicians and 10 percent of the public), long-term disability (6 percent and 11 percent, respectively), and severe pain (11 percent and 16 percent). These were not the biased perceptions of distraught family members. About one-third of the respondents who reported experience with an error stated that the health professionals involved had told them about the error or apologized to them (Blendon et al., 2002).

The United States is not alone in its high rate of health care errors; research in other countries also has found high error rates. It is estimated that 10 percent of hospital patients in Great Britain and 16.6 percent of such patients in Australia experience an adverse event (WHO, 2002). No one receiving health care—young or old; severely or slightly ill; patients in hospitals, in nursing homes, or in their doctors' offices; wealthy, middle class, poor, or near poor; those receiving health insurance through Medicare, Medicaid, or private health insurance—is immune to health care errors and adverse events.

Most important, *To Err Is Human* has helped concerned individuals and organizations better understand the reasons behind this profusion of health care errors and how it can best be addressed.

WHY HEALTH CARE ERRORS OCCUR

Two very different views are often held about why errors in health care, like errors in other industries, occur (Reason, 2000).

The first view holds *individuals* as primarily responsible for any error or unsafe action. Unsafe acts are viewed as arising principally from an individual's faulty mental processes or weaknesses of character, such as forgetfulness, inattention, poor motivation, carelessness, negligence, and recklessness. Bad outcomes are viewed largely as the result of bad behavior by people, behavior that should be corrected through workplace policies and procedures, safety campaigns, disciplinary measures, the threat of litigation, retraining, and "naming, blaming, and shaming." In this view, when workplace errors occur, the person most directly involved in the work at the time the error is thought to have taken place (often known as "the last person to touch the patient") might well be blamed. In the above example, the nurse inserting the urinary catheter would be blamed for causing the urinary tract infection. After all, she inserted the catheter—a highly likely candidate for the introduction of bacteria causing the infection.

Such assignment of blame is the approach historically used in health care, as has been the case in other industries, and is deeply rooted in Western civilization (Reason, 2000). The 2002 survey of practicing physicians and the public cited earlier revealed that the public believes individuals, and not organizations, should be held responsible for errors with serious consequences through lawsuits, fines, and suspension of their professional licenses. Similarly, the majority of physicians surveyed believe that individual health professionals, as opposed to health care institutions, are more likely responsible for preventable medical errors (Blendon et al., 2002). This human tendency to blame bad outcomes on an individual's personal inadequacies rather than on situational factors beyond the individual's control (identified in social psychology as "fundamental attribution error") is a serious obstacle to preventing or mitigating the inevitable errors that occur in complex organizations such as those delivering health care (Reason, 1990). It fails to acknowledge that, indeed, "to err is human."

The contrasting *systems* view of errors and error prevention is based on research findings from a variety of fields, including studies of accidents and breaches of safety in a variety of industries, studies of "high-reliability organizations," and research into effective organizational and managerial practices. In all of this work, the interdependent interaction of multiple human and nonhuman (equipment, technologies, policies, and procedures) elements of any effort to achieve a stated purpose is regarded as a "production process" or "system." These interrelated human and nonhuman system elements are required to operate in synchrony if a given goal is to be achieved. As the elements of the production process or system are changed, the likelihood of error also changes. This research has revealed that errors typically result from problems within the system in which people work—*not* from poor individual worker performance—and typically originate in multiple areas within and external to an organization. Error results when these multiple problems converge and impair an organization's performance (Perrow, 1984; Reason, 2000). Not surprisingly, errors increasingly are attributed to the hyper-complex organizations that emerged in the last half of the twentieth century in response to technological and social changes (Perrow, 1984).

A fundamental principle of the systems approach to error reduction is the recognition that all humans make mistakes and that "errors are to be expected, even in the best organizations" (Reason, 2000:768). *To Err Is Human* endorses the systems approach to understanding and reducing errors and notes that failures in large systems, such as hospitals or their various patient care units, nursing homes, or ambulatory practice sites, are most often due to unanticipated events or factors occurring within multiple parts of the system. In most cases, the accumulation of these factors, as opposed to the actions of a single individual, is what leads to an error or accident. In the above example, these multiple factors include the inexperience of the nurse; the lack of available supervision; the unavailability of the tools needed to perform the task; and the nurse's possible perception of her lack of authority to call attention to and change the unsafe situation by, for example, sending the patient to the OR without a catheter and directing OR staff to catheterize the patient. Addressing any one of these factors might have prevented the urinary tract infection. Blaming the individual nurse would not change these factors and would not result in increased safety for the next patient in need of catheterization on the nursing unit. As Reason notes, when an error occurs, the question should not be "Who is at fault?" but rather "Why did our defenses fail?" (Reason, 2000).

At the same time, even though errors are understood to be the result of multiple factors within a system, the human component of systems in all industries has been identified as one of the largest contributors to the occurrence of accidents. Reason explains that since people design, manufacture, operate, maintain, and manage complex technological systems, it is hardly surprising that human decisions and actions are implicated in all organizational accidents. Human beings contribute to the commission of errors in two ways: through the commission of active failures and the creation of latent conditions[1] (Reason, 1997).

Active failures occur at the level of the front-line worker (e.g., airplane pilots; control room operators; health care workers, such as nurses, physicians, and pharmacists; and other operators of technology interfacing with people). Such failures are sometimes called the "sharp end" of an error. The types of errors committed by front-line workers involve such phenomena as lapses in memory, misreading or misinterpretation of written data, incorrect performance of a routine activity as a result of a distraction or interruption, or simply human variations in fine motor skills. The consequences of these actions are experienced almost immediately. In the above example, the nurse is the front-line worker at the sharp end of the work process. Her insertion of the catheter using poor processes and tools represents an active failure.

In contrast, latent conditions are factors in the production process or system that are not under the direct control of front-line workers. These factors include poor design of work or equipment, inadequate training, gaps in supervision, insufficient supply of equipment to perform work, undetected manufacturing defects or faulty maintenance, inadequate personnel deployment, and poorly structured operations. They arise from strategic and other top-level decisions made by entities at the "blunt end" of an organization or production system, such as government regulators, manufacturers, system designers, and high-level managers and decision makers.

The error described above resulted from multiple latent conditions. First, the new nurse had not had practical experience in either her nursing school or her workplace in the performance of this specific task. A mechanism for identifying the presence or absence of core nursing skill competencies would have detected this lack of experience, so that the nurse could have received instruction to fill this gap in her skill set. Further, the mechanism used to deploy staff created a situation in which all the nurses on duty in the unit at the time of the event were similarly new and inexperienced. Thus the nurse committing the error had no source of clinical expertise to whom she could turn for advice. Necessary supplies also were not available; the nurse was forced to improvise using equipment not specifically designed for the procedure, thereby creating opportunities for faulty technique. It is important to note, moreover, that the nurse did not give evidence of feeling

---

[1]*To Err Is Human* employs the terminology "active and latent errors" used in Reason's 1990 publication, *Human Error*. Reason's subsequent (1997) publication, *Managing the Risks of Organizational Accidents*, refines that terminology and now refers to active "failures" and latent "conditions." We adopt this more recent terminology here.

empowered to call a halt to an unsafe practice that was putting the patient at risk. Finally, the nurse's statement that she felt ashamed and afraid indicates that the workplace environment did not possess a culture of safety that would encourage the reporting, analysis, and remediation of error-producing situations. Because the nurse did not come forward, none of these latent conditions were recognized as threats to patient safety, and the potential remained that future patients admitted to this unit would face a similar risk to their safety. Indeed, latent conditions such as these are present in all organizations and have been identified as posing the greatest risk to safety in complex or high-technology systems because of their capacity to result in multiple types of active failures. Their impact spreads throughout an organization, creating error-producing factors within individual workplaces (Reason, 1990).

Unfortunately, when errors are discovered, attention tends to focus on the more visible "sharp end" of the activity (the person associated with the error) because latent conditions are less visible, often hidden in routine practices or in the structure or management of an organization. As a result, responses to errors tend to focus on retraining, "discipline" (reprimanding, firing, or suing), or other responses aimed at specific individuals. Although a punitive response may be appropriate in cases of willful wrongdoing, evidence has shown that it is not an effective way to prevent subsequent errors. Focusing only on the sharp end allows latent conditions to remain undetected in the system, and their accumulation makes the system more prone to additional accidents and errors in the future.

Efforts to discover and fix latent system conditions are more likely to result in safer systems than attempts to minimize active errors at the point at which they occur (Institute of Medicine, 2000). Reason (2000:769) uses the analogy of mosquito control to illustrate this argument: "Active failures are like mosquitoes. They can be swatted one by one, but they will still keep coming." The best remedies involve creating more effective defenses to target and prevent the conditions that allow them to breed and flourish in the first place.

However, viewing errors as resulting solely from either individual or systemic errors has its dangers. Attributing errors predominantly to the deficiencies of individuals fails to recognize the findings of safety studies estimating that the majority of unsafe acts—90 percent or more—arise from system failures in which individuals are not to blame (Reason, 1997). Focusing exclusively on individuals misses an essential part of the error story, and blocks the path to effective remediation.

On the other hand, an extreme systems perspective that recognizes no individual contributions to patient safety presents problems such as "learned helplessness" and failure to address instances of individual deficits in competencies or willful wrongdoing. With regard to the phenomenon of "learned helplessness," although most health professionals are highly motivated to provide safe patient care, there is a possibility that if the systems perspective becomes the sole explanation for unsafe practices, health care practitioners may be tempted to lessen their personal vigilance and striving for personal excellence and think, "It's the system—there's nothing I can do about it." But safe and effective health care depends upon each professional continuing the struggle under less-than-ideal local circumstances (Reason, 1997). Further, health care practitioners vary in their expertise, competency, and exercise of necessary care. To attribute all adverse events to system failings ignores the fact that some erroneous actions, albeit a relatively small proportion of the total, are the product of reckless or incompetent individual behaviors. An exclusive focus on the systems approach will not remedy these few, but significant, threats to patient safety. It also ignores the unsung and undocumented heroes.

Thus a number of patient safety experts believe we need to strive for fair and just systems of safety that acknowledge both the individual and system contributions to successful as well as adverse events while emphasizing the systems approach to error reduction (Reason, 1997). This perspective is reflected in *To Err Is Human*, which concludes that efforts to prevent errors and improve patient safety will be most successful if they emphasize a systems over an individual approach, focused on modifying the conditions within the system that contribute to errors. Protecting patients from errors and adverse events therefore requires an examination of health care delivery systems to identify defects and create stronger system-level defenses. As nurses are the largest component of the health care workforce, and are also strongly involved in the commission, detection, and prevention of errors and adverse events, they and their work environment are critical elements of stronger patient safety defenses.

THE CENTRAL ROLE OF NURSES IN PATIENT SAFETY

Nurses: The Largest Component of the Health Care Workforce

Nursing personnel represent the largest component of the health care workforce. Licensed nurses[2] and unlicensed nursing assistants (NAs) repre-

---

[2]In this report, "licensed nurse" refers to individuals licensed by a state to perform nursing duties—both registered nurses (RNs) and licensed practical or vocational nurses (LPNs or LVNs). "Nursing assistant" (NA) refers to unlicensed health care personnel who supplement the work of licensed nurses by performing routine patient care activities under the supervision of an RN or LPN/LVN. A variety of titles are used for these unlicensed nursing personnel, including nurse assistants, nurse aides, home health aides, personal care aides, ancillary nursing personnel, unlicensed nursing personnel, unlicensed assistive personnel (UAPs), nurse extenders, and nursing support personnel.

sent approximately 54 percent of all U.S. health care workers (e.g., physicians, nurses, dentists, allied health professionals, technicians and technologists, and other health care assistants) (Bureau of Labor Statistics, undated). Registered nurses (RNs) alone constitute approximately 23 percent of the entire health care workforce. These 2.2 million RNs, along with 683,800 licensed practical nurses (LPNs) or licensed vocational nurses (LVNs) and 2.3 million nursing aides, orderlies, attendants, and personal and home care aides, provide health care to individuals in virtually all locations in which health care is delivered—hospitals; long-term care facilities; ambulatory care settings, such as clinics or physicians' offices; and other settings, including the private homes of individuals, schools, and employee workplaces. In most of these settings, the nurse or NA is the health care provider who has the greatest amount of direct contact with patients. In U.S. hospitals, approximately one of every four hospital employees is a licensed nurse (AHA, 2002). In nursing homes, the majority of patient care is provided by NAs, under the supervision of a licensed nurse. Efforts to detect and remedy error-producing defects in health care systems will be severely constrained without the assistance of the eyes, ears, cognitive powers, and interventions of over half the health care workforce.

Surveillance and "Rescue" of Patients

A primary activity performed by nursing staff in all hospitals, long-term care facilities, and ambulatory settings is ongoing patient surveillance (sometimes referred to as patient "assessment," "evaluation," or "monitoring")—an important mechanism for the detection of errors and the prevention of adverse events. If a patient's status begins to decline, the decline will be detectable though the nurse's observation of changes in the patient's physical or cognitive status. Performance of this patient monitoring requires great attention, knowledge, and responsiveness on the part of the nurse.

Patient assessment is the basis for all licensed nursing care (ANA, 1998). Indeed, ongoing patient assessment and evaluation are the two guideposts of licensed nursing care between which hands-on nursing treatments, patient education, and care planning are delivered. In acute care hospitals, this bedside monitoring or surveillance of the condition of patients prior to, during, and following medical procedures such as surgery, initiation of new medications, or a course of medical therapy typically includes, for example, monitoring patients' vital signs (temperature, heart rate and rhythm, breathing rate and character, blood pressure), airway, risk/presence of infection, fluid intake and output, electrolytes, and pain (Bulechek et al., 1994). In intensive care units, the monitoring is more frequent, invasive, and technologically complex, as illustrated in Box 1-1.

BOX 1-1   Patient Monitoring in an Intensive Care Unit: An Example

Another nurse and I were assigned two patients: a 2-day-old infant born 3½ months prematurely and a full-term, 3-day-old infant named Dan. A congenital bacterial infection had invaded Dan's blood and lungs after his birth, and his condition had deteriorated so badly during the night that he had to be placed on a heart-lung bypass machine known as extra-corporeal membrane oxygenation, or ECMO. In his brief life, Baby Dan already had suffered multiple ruptures of his lung tissue, the result of the high pressures needed by the mechanical ventilator to push air into his diseased lungs. Two tubes, inserted between his ribs on both sides, re-moved the air leaking into his chest cavity. A third tube, exiting below his sternum, removed fluid collecting in the sac around his heart to prevent compression of the heart. The ECMO machine, used only as a last resort in dire cases, functionally replaced Dan's failing heart and lungs. The machine drained his blood from a small tube inserted into a vein in his neck, passed it through plastic tubing to an artificial lung for gas ex-change, and returned it under pressure to his body through a second tube in his aorta.

Blood flowing outside the body involves a great risk of clotting, which is controlled by continuous infusion of a blood-thinning medication, hep-arin, into the ECMO circuit. However, too much thinning of the blood can lead to uncontrolled bleeding, and the fluid oozing from Dan's incision sites showed that his blood's ability to clot was already severely impaired. I had to test his blood's clotting ability every 10 minutes to adjust the heparin infusion. In addition, he was on two other medication infusions to address his failing blood pressure and required frequent transfusions of various blood products to supply clotting factors and improve his blood pressure. He further was receiving several antibiotics to combat the in-fection and required constant sedation to keep him from fighting us. Car-ing for an ECMO patient typically required two nurses—one trained as a specialist to monitor the ECMO circuit continuously, the other to provide constant assessment of the patient's vital signs and other health status indicators and manage the other aspects of patient care.

Over the course of our 12-hour shift, we started to rein in his many problems, and Baby Dan slowly improved. Although he would remain on ECMO several more days to recuperate, he eventually overcame his in-fection and was discharged.

SOURCE: Bingham (2002).

A review of 81 research papers published predominantly since 1990 examining the relationship between organizational structures/processes and patient mortality/adverse events revealed that nursing surveillance was one of three organizational process variables consistently related to lower mortality (Mitchell and Shortell, 1997). Studies of quality of care before and after implementation of the Medicare prospective payment system for hospitals found better-quality nursing surveillance to be predictive of lower severity-adjusted Medicare mortality (Kahn et al., 1990; Rubenstein et al., 1992).

Although the type and frequency of patient assessment and monitoring activities carried out by licensed nurses vary by the setting of care, the clinical condition, and other characteristics of the patient, such activities are performed by nurses for each patient in every setting in which health care is delivered—ambulatory primary care sites, hospitals, schools, workplace health sites, home health agencies, and nursing homes. In nursing homes, each resident receives a comprehensive assessment performed or coordinated by an RN upon admission and at regularly scheduled intervals thereafter. This assessment employs a federally prescribed minimum data set (MDS)[3] to document each resident's diagnoses and health conditions, dental and nutritional status, skin condition, medications, discharge potential and other special treatments or conditions needed, customary routines, cognitive patterns, communication, vision, mood and behavior patterns, psychosocial well-being, physical functions, continence, and other physical and psychosocial characteristics. When this assessment detects areas of concern, a more detailed resident assessment protocol is initiated (Morris et al., 1995).

For chronically ill homebound patients, home health nurses assess the health status and responses to treatments of individuals too ill to leave their home using a wide array of assessment instruments and tools. Examples of these include stethoscopes, sphygmomanometers (blood pressure measurement devices), Doppler fetal monitors, depression screening tools, Denver Developmental Screening tests, pain scales, the Braden scale for pressure ulcer prevention, wound measurement instruments, diet recall checklists, glucose tests, urine tests, fall risk assessment tools, an Alcohol Consumption Questionnaire, functional independence measurements, safety checklists, the SF-12 and other health surveys, tools for measuring activities of daily living (ADLs) and instrumental ADLs, a Mini-Mental Status Examination, a Family Assessment for School Nurses, and vision and hearing assessment tools (Martin, 2002). In addition, since 1999 the Medicare pro-

---

[3]Code of Federal Regulations, Chapter 42, Part 483, Subpart B, "Requirements for Long Term Care Facilities."

gram has required that an RN perform a comprehensive, detailed assessment of each Medicare beneficiary receiving Medicare-covered home health care at the initiation of home health care services and at regular intervals thereafter.[4] The nurse performing this assessment must assess the patient's health status and health care and support needs, as well as items included in the Medicare Outcome and Assessment Information Set (OASIS) that address the patient's history, and "sensory status, integumentary status, respiratory status, elimination status, neuro/emotional/behavioral status, activities of daily living, [and] medications," among other information.[5]

While performing these assessments (and also when delivering therapeutic treatment and patient education), nurses are functioning at the "sharp end" of the health care system because of their immediate link to the patient. This ongoing vigilance function often thrusts nurses into a role that has been described as the "front line" of patient defense (JCAHO, 2001). Studies of organizations with a strong track record of high reliability and safety have shown that such vigilance by front-line workers is essential for detecting threats to safety before they actually become errors and adverse events (Roberts, 1990; Roberts and Bea, 2001). Because licensed nurses and NAs work at the "sharp end" of health care delivery, they are key instruments for carrying out such vigilance in health care.

The goal of this nursing surveillance or vigilance function is the early detection of a downturn in a patient's health status or the advent of an adverse event, and the initiation of activities to "rescue" the patient and restore health. When this does not happen, "failure to rescue" is said to occur. The concept of failure to rescue has been tested and validated as an indicator of the quality of acute hospital care for surgical patients (Silber et al., 1992). When higher levels of nurse staffing are present, the incidence of failure to rescue is reduced (Aiken et al., 2002; Needleman et al., 2002). Further evidence of the effectiveness of nurse surveillance is found in studies of medication errors. A systems analysis of 334 medication errors associated with 264 preventable adverse events occurring in two hospitals over a 6-month period revealed that nurses were the health care personnel most likely to intercept errors in the ordering of a medication by a physician, the transcription of the drug order by a clerk, or the dispensing of the drug by a pharmacist before such errors resulted in an adverse event. Nearly half of all physician errors examined in this study had been intercepted before they resulted in an adverse event; 87 percent of those interceptions were by nurses. About one-third of transcription and dispensing errors had been

---

[4]When speech, physical, or occupational therapy is the only home health service ordered by the physician, the comprehensive assessment may be performed by a licensed therapist of that service instead of by an RN.

[5]Code of Federal Regulations, Chapter 42, Part 484.55, revised as of October 1, 2002.

intercepted prior to administration, again largely by nurses. Overall, nurses were responsible for intercepting 86 percent of all medication errors made by those in all disciplines (Leape et al., 1995).

Coordination and Integration of Care and Services from Multiple Providers

In addition to providing surveillance of patients, therapeutic nursing interventions, and treatments to carry out medical orders, licensed nurses serve as the integrator or coordinator of patient care. These integrating activities include implementing physician treatment orders and explaining them to the patient; planning for patients' discharge from hospitals or other health care facilities to enable continued care in the home, school, or nursing home; providing health care treatment in the home or other setting of care; and educating the patient and family about the patient's disease, course of therapy, medications, self-care activities, and other areas of concern to the patient. In addition, while such practices are not desirable, nurses are also pressed into performing a variety of non-nursing patient care activities because of their ever-present availability in inpatient facilities. For example, when delivery of medications, medical equipment or supplies, blood products, or laboratory specimens is required for the patient, and transport staff are not available for the purpose, this activity often is carried out by the nurse. This practice, relying on the "inevitable availability" of nurses, occurs frequently (Prescott et al., 1991; Upenieks, 1998). Large proportions of nurses report spending time delivering and retrieving food trays; performing housekeeping duties; transporting patients; and ordering, coordinating, or performing ancillary services (Aiken et al., 2001a).

The amount of time nurses spend integrating or coordinating care is suggested by the amount of time they spend on "indirect" as opposed to "direct" patient care. Direct patient care encompasses activities carried out in the presence of the patient and family, such as performing a physical examination and other assessments of the patient, administering medications, and performing treatments and procedures. Indirect care involves those activities that are performed away from but on behalf of the patient, such as documenting care, communicating with other health care providers, seeking consultations, and preparing medications (Division of Nursing, 1978). Although numerous work sampling studies of nursing care have been conducted—with varying degrees of divergence from these definitions—and the location of some indirect care activities may be shifting to the bedside (as is the case with automated patient records), the vast majority of studies agree that nurses spend a greater percentage of their time in indirect versus direct care (Hendrickson et al., 1990; Linden and English, 1994; Upenieks, 1998). As a result of all these indirect activities, nurses have substantial contact with all health care personnel providing care to the patient—across multiple units, divisions, services, institutions, and providers constituting the health care delivery system—and are able to detect and take action to fill gaps in patient care in order to protect the patient.

Distinguished physician and author Lewis Thomas, former Dean of the Yale and New York University medical schools and chief executive officer of the Sloan-Kettering Institute in New York City at the time of his death in 1993, well describes this integrating and coordinating function of nurses in *The Youngest Science: Notes of a Medicine Watcher*:

> One thing the nurses do is to hold the place together. It is an astonishment, which every patient feels from time to time, observing the affairs of a large, complex hospital from the vantage point of his bed, that the whole institution doesn't fly to pieces. A hospital operates by the constant interplay of powerful forces pulling away at each other in different directions, each force essential for getting necessary things done, but always at odds with each other. . . . My discovery, as a patient . . . is that the institution is held together, glued together, enabled to function as an organism, by the nurses and nobody else. (Thomas, 1983:66–67)

PATIENT SAFETY RISK FACTORS IN NURSES' WORK AND WORK ENVIRONMENTS

Because nurses carry out the responsibilities described above, they potentially are well positioned to observe and influence how the health care system functions across all aspects of patient care, and thereby to detect and address threats to patient safety. However, nurses' work and work environments have changed over the last two decades, and these changes have been cited as having implications for patient safety.

More Acutely Ill Patients

Nurses, health care industry associations, and numerous other entities have observed that hospital and nursing home patients are more severely ill than in the recent past. Although the truth of this observation is widely accepted, its extent and its implications for nursing are difficult to determine. First, there is no standard method used across hospitals to measure the severity of illness of all hospital patients. Although many hospitals use patient acuity systems to estimate the amount of nursing care their patients will require, those systems are not standardized, and there is no external reporting to produce national trend data. Second, where other severity-of-illness measurements are collected (i.e., for Medicare patients), the severity of a patient's medical illness does not necessarily correlate with the level of nursing care that a patient requires. For example, a patient with pneumonia might not have a high score on a medical severity-of-illness algorithm but still could require a large amount of nursing care.

Nonetheless, Medicare data and a limited amount of state-specific hospital data support the observation that, beginning in the mid-1980s following implementation of the Medicare prospective payment system (PPS) for hospitals and continuing into the late 1990s, patients admitted to hospitals were increasingly more acutely ill. Data on all Medicare hospital admissions for 1985–1997 show an annual increase in the complexity of cases treated in acute care hospitals as measured by the Medicare case mix index (CMI),[6] while a review of patient data for all payors and all acute care general hospitals in Pennsylvania during 1994–1997 revealed that the severity of illness of patients admitted to those hospitals increased in the aggregate by 4.5 percent over the 4-year period (Unruh, 2002b). The annual increases were highest in the early years just after implementation of the PPS and slowed fairly steadily until 1998, when a decline in severity as measured by the CMI was observed. This decline continued into 1999, the last year for which these data are available. It was determined that the CMI decrease of 0.5 percent in 1998 likely reflected changes in coding practices; however, this was not the case for the 0.4 percent CMI decline in 1999 (Medicare Payment Advisory Commission, 2001).

This increase in the severity of illness of hospital patients has had a ripple effect throughout all health care settings. Evidence indicates that patients receiving care in long-term care facilities, in their homes, and in other community-based settings are more ill and debilitated and/or require more technologically complex medical care than in the past. In nursing homes, the proportion of patients who are more frail (i.e., need assistance with three or more ADLs, such as bathing, dressing, eating, and toileting) and therefore need more skilled and/or specialized care increased from 72 percent in 1987 to 83 percent in 1996. As a consequence, over the last few years, nursing homes have developed specialized units to care for patients who need more extensive care, such as those with dementia, rehabilitation needs, ventilator dependency, or brain injury. Approximately 12.6 percent of all nursing homes in 1996 had units devoted to the specialized care of

---

[6]A hospital's CMI represents the average diagnosis-related group (DRG) relative weight for that hospital. It is calculated by summing the DRG weights for all Medicare discharges during a fiscal year, and dividing by the number of discharges (CMS, 2003). The Medicare CMI is calculated annually based on charges submitted to the Medicare program for all hospital patients. While the CMI is therefore a direct measure of costliness, it is often used as a surrogate indicator of severity of illness because more acutely ill patients typically are higher-cost patients. However, this is not always the case, especially because technology is often costly, but may not always be used by the most acutely ill. The CMI is therefore an imperfect indicator of severity of illness and patients' need for nursing care.

individuals with Alzheimer's disease (the most common type of specialized unit); more than half had been in operation for 5 years or less (Rhoades and Krauss, 2001).

While there is no precise way to measure trends in the numbers of nursing home patients having more complex *medical* needs—necessitating intervention from a licensed nurse as opposed to ADL support from an NA—changes can be inferred from the proportion of residents whose care is covered by Medicare, because Medicare coverage of nursing home care is limited to payment for rehabilitation care and skilled nursing services. Between 1987 and 1996, the percentage of nursing home patients whose care was paid for by Medicare increased from 3 to 9 percent, and the proportion of nursing homes certified to receive Medicare reimbursement increased from 28 to 73 percent, indicating that the number of nursing homes planning to take in residents with more acute illness or more complex needs increased substantially (Rhoades and Krauss, 2001). This increase in resident dependency and medical complexity has important implications for the work of nurses and NAs. Staff time required to meet basic patient care needs (such as feeding, toileting, and ambulation) increases with the level of dependency of residents (CMS, 2002). Since Medicare residents often have complex health conditions or are recovering from serious health events, a more sophisticated knowledge base is required to care for these residents, and a higher level of vigilance and monitoring is required.

Shorter Hospital Stays

In addition to the likelihood that patients in hospitals are sicker, evidence is clear that when patients are admitted to the hospital, their hospital stays are for shorter periods of time than in the past. This combination of increased patient severity of illness and shorter inpatient stays has given rise to the expression that nurses are asked to care for patients "sicker and quicker." From 1980 to 2000, the average length of a patient's stay in the hospital (for nonfederal short-term general hospitals and other special hospitals) declined from 7.6 to 5.8 days (AHA, 2002). Although it is likely that these shorter stays in part reflect improvements in care, their implication in the context of nursing is that as patients' lengths of stay decrease, the less demanding initial patient workup and post-treatment recovery periods are foregone. The remaining patient days in the hospital involve caring for patients in need of a greater intensity of care. Further, these reduced lengths of stay allow less time for nurses to become acquainted with their patients' baseline health and to readily detect changes in health status, educate patients and families about health conditions, and fully prepare patients and families for discharge. Shorter lengths of inpatient stays also transfer the risk for adverse events from the hospital setting to the home, where such events may be less readily detected and result in more serious consequences for the patient.

Redesigned Work

Labor costs are the largest component of hospital expenses, and nursing staff represent the largest category of hospital labor (AHA, 2002). As hospitals tried to respond to the cost pressures generated by new reimbursement methods in the 1980s, many of their approaches targeted more efficient use of nursing staff. These initiatives (referred to as restructuring, reengineering, or redesign initiatives)[7] continued through the 1990s into the present and have been widely adopted (Gelinas and Manthey, 1997). Redesign initiatives typically have changed the ways in which licensed nurses and NAs are organized to provide patient care, through, for example, personnel reductions; cross-training of personnel to perform additional duties; changes in the mix of nursing staff (RN, LPN/LVN, or unlicensed staff); reassignment of support services (e.g., laboratory, radiology) to nursing units; redistribution of patients across nursing units; redesign of patient care processes; and other changes in organization structure, decision-making processes, and the responsibilities of management and patient care staff (Aiken et al., 2000; Norrish and Rundall, 2001; Ritter-Teitel, 2002; Walston et al., 2000; Walston and Kimberly, 1997). Use of multiskilled workers who are not RNs to perform such activities as making beds, giving patients baths, positioning patients too ill to position themselves, performing electrocardiograms, and drawing blood was identified as a core feature of redesign initiatives by 61 percent of 360 hospital nurse executives surveyed in 1995 (Gelinas and Manthey, 1997).

The outcomes of these redesign initiatives are not clear (Walston et al., 2000). Formal measurements of the results of these multifaceted restructuring, reengineering, and redesign initiatives have been few, and findings have been contradictory with respect to the consequences for nurses' work and work environment, including nursing staff satisfaction, control over work environment, concern over changes in responsibilities, and work group relationships. However, role conflict and ambiguity are consistent issues in redesigned work settings (Ingersoll et al., 2001; Walston et al., 2000), and such changes have been well documented as contributing to error-producing situations because they involve departures from well-established routines and create new situations for which workers have no preplanned solutions (Reason, 1990).

---

[7]The terms "restructuring," "reengineering," and "redesigning" are used interchangeably in the literature.

Changes in Deployment of Nursing Personnel to Care for Patients

Declining numbers of nursing staff available to care for inpatients in health care facilities have been widely reported by the press, labor publications, and professional journals (Aiken et al., 2001b; Hurley, 2000; Shindul-Rothschild et al., 1996). Quantitative analyses to explore this perception have been hampered by the limitations of available data on nurse staffing[8] and patient acuity. As a result, national studies have not yet produced a fully clear picture of changes in nurse staffing levels. An analysis of national hospital staffing data from 1981 through 1993 (while total hospital employment was growing steadily) revealed that total nursing personnel (RNs, LPNs, and NAs) per 1,000 adjusted patient days, also adjusted for case mix, declined nationally by 7.3 percent. This decrease in the number of nursing caregivers per patient was accomplished primarily through the loss of non-RN personnel (Aiken et al., 1996). A follow-up study of RN staffing between 1990 and 1996 found that the number of hospital RNs increased nationally by 15 percent, and that the percentage of RNs among all hospital employees increased from approximately 22 percent to 25 percent. During this period, however, LPN full-time equivalents (FTEs) decreased by 14 percent (data were not available on NAs) (Kovner et al., 2000).

Several explanations have been advanced for the mismatch between reports of declining RN staffing and the quantitative data generated by analyses such as those cited above. The first is that while levels of RN staffing may have held constant or even increased, they have not been adequate to compensate for the loss of LPN/LVN and NA staff whose duties likely have fallen to RNs. The further increase in patient acuity and shortened hospital stays compounds the workload of RNs. Another explanation is that inadequate staffing data cannot fully document the extent to which RNs are or are not available to provide direct care to patients. Data on RN hospital staffing often include RNs engaged in administrative duties who have no patient care responsibilities, as well as RNs providing care in outpatient hospital settings, and therefore cannot provide a clear picture of changes in the numbers of RNs providing direct care to inpatients. Finally, these studies have not always distinguished between full-time and part-time nurses; two part-time nurses may be counted as two nurses despite equaling only one full-time nurse.

Another important factor is the extent to which national statistics mask the variation that exists across individual hospitals. A recent and detailed analysis of nurse staffing levels at the aggregate level across facilities and at

---

[8]For example, commonly used data sources do not always distinguish between nursing staff in outpatient and inpatient care units or between nurses in administrative positions providing no direct patient care and nurses providing bedside patient care, or collect data on NAs.

the level of individual hospitals illustrates this point. This study of nurse staffing in all general, acute care Pennsylvania hospitals from 1991 to 1997 found that, although the statewide ratio of all nursing staff (RNs, LPNs, and NAs) to patient days of care increased from 3.86 to 4.04 between 1991 and 1997, examination of staffing at each hospital individually revealed that 32 percent of hospitals reduced the ratio of all nurses (RNs, LPNs, and NAs) to patients by more than 10 percent; and, with adjustments for the increased acuity of patients, more than 50 percent of hospitals decreased their ratio of nursing staff to patient days by more than 10 percent (Unruh, 2002a). Such declines are worrisome because health services research continues to produce strong evidence that nurse staffing in the aggregate is an important factor in the prevention of adverse events in both acute hospitals (Kovner et al., 2002; Needleman et al., 2002; Seago, 2001) and nursing homes (CMS, 2002).

Frequent Patient Turnover

High patient turnover rates contribute to increased workload for hospital nurses. Patient turnover refers to the phenomenon in which a given hospital bed may be occupied by more than one patient in a 24-hour period. For example, a patient may be discharged at 10:00 in the morning and a new patient admitted to the same bed during the same nursing shift. The number of patients in need of care is typically counted at a point in time during a 24-hour period (e.g., midnight). However, this patient census does not indicate the true number of patients in need of care because it does not reflect the actual number of patients cared for or the admissions and discharges taking place on a given day. Assessment and stabilization of patients upon admission and patient education and planning upon discharge are time- and personnel-intensive.

The patient turnover rate has increased as the numbers of available hospital beds and lengths of stay have declined. In one study of 20 medical–surgical units in five hospitals, the number of admissions, discharges, and transfers averaged between 25 and 70 percent of the midnight census (Lawrenz, 1992). Patient turnover rates as high as 40–50 percent also have been reported during an 8- to 12-hour period (Norrish and Rundall, 2001).

High Staff Turnover

High rates of turnover characterize the nursing staff of both hospitals and nursing homes. Such high turnover can have adverse consequences for patient safety. Evidence from non–health care industries shows that new or substitute staff are less familiar with work processes, and that the potential for errors thereby increases (Rousseau and Libuser, 1997). In nursing homes, high turnover rates have been hypothesized to result in low staff morale, staff shortages, and poor quality of care (CMS, 2002).

A 2001 survey of directors of nursing of all U.S. nonfederal acute care hospitals found (for the 14.7 percent of hospitals responding) that, on average, 21.3 percent of all full-time registered hospital nurses had resigned or been terminated during the preceding year. While most hospitals reported turnover rates of 10–30 percent, some cited much higher rates. For example, 2 percent of responding hospitals reported turnover rates of 50 percent or higher (The HSM Group, 2002). Turnover rates among nursing staff in nursing homes are even greater. A national survey conducted by the American Health Care Association (AHCA) in 2001 found annual turnover rates of 78 percent for NAs, 56 percent for staff RNs, 54 percent for LPNs/ LVNs, and 43–47 percent for directors of nursing and RNs with administrative duties (AHCA, 2002).

Long Work Hours

Nursing staff working in in-patient facilities traditionally have worked in 8-hour shifts, but increasingly work longer hours. Reasons include a desire for increased compensation ("elective overtime"), requirements by facilities to work overtime ("mandatory overtime") to compensate for insufficient staffing, and a desire for more flexible work hours (e.g., 10- or 12-hour shifts) to accommodate the needs of either facilities or nurses or both. Scheduled shifts may be 8, 10, or 12 hours, and may not follow the traditional pattern of day, evening, or night shifts. Moreover, nurses working on specialized units, such as the OR, dialysis units, and some intensive care units, may be required to be on call in addition to their regularly scheduled shifts (Rogers, 2002).

A 2002 study funded as part of AHRQ's initiative to examine the effects of working conditions on patient safety documented the work patterns of a national sample of hospital staff nurses who are members of the American Nurses Association. The study measured each nurse's work hours, length of shifts, and amount of overtime hours worked and the effects of these factors on nurses' commission of errors. It was found that although the majority (84.3 percent) of scheduled shifts were 8 or 12 hours in duration, 3.5 percent were for periods greater than 12 hours, some lasting as long as 22.5 hours.[9]

---

[9]Ann Rogers, Ph.D., University of Pennsylvania, unpublished data (manuscript in preparation).

Research on the work hours of nursing staff in nursing homes also has revealed extended work hours. In site visits to 17 nursing facilities in Ohio, Colorado, and Texas in 2001, researchers found that double shifts (i.e., two consecutive 8-hour shifts totaling 16 hours) and extra shifts were performed in many of these facilities on a regular basis. Double shifts in particular were pervasive. In 13 of the 17 facilities, at least one nursing staff member, but frequently more, had worked between one and three double shifts in the previous 7 days. In five facilities, at least one staff member had worked between four and seven double shifts in the last 7 days. In one of the facilities, more than a third of the interviewed nursing staff had worked between eight and eleven double shifts in the last 14 days (CMS, 2002).

The number of hours worked has been identified as a contributing factor to the commission of errors by nurses (Narumi et al., 1999). The AHRQ-funded study mentioned above found that shift durations of greater than 12 hours were significantly associated with increased errors among nurses.

Rapid Increases in New Knowledge and Technology

The IOM (2001) report *Crossing the Quality Chasm* cites the growing complexity of science and technology, resulting from the tremendous advances made in clinical knowledge, drugs, medical devices, and technologies for use in patient care, as one of the four main attributes of the U.S. health system affecting health care quality. Since the results of the first randomized controlled clinical trial were published more than 50 years ago, health care practitioners have been increasingly inundated with information about what does and does not work to achieve good clinical outcomes. Over the last 30 years, such trials have increased in number from 100 to nearly 10,000 annually. The first 5 years of this 30-year period accounts for only 1 percent of all the articles in the medical literature, while the last 5 years accounts for almost half. Although part of this growth in the literature can be attributed to factors other than new findings and knowledge, there is no doubt that as the knowledge base has expanded, so, too, has the number of drugs, medical devices, and other technological supports (IOM, 2001).

Such increases in technology are beneficial and likely to continue. In a study of hospital organizational and structural features associated with patient mortality, only the presence of high technology or its proxies has been consistently associated with lower mortality (Mitchell and Shortell, 1997). However, these developments also have implications for patient safety and health care providers, including nursing staff. First, as stated in the *Quality Chasm* report, "Today, no one clinician can retain all the information necessary for sound, evidence-based practice. No unaided human being can read, recall, and act effectively on the volume of clinically relevant scientific literature" (IOM, 2001:25). If nurses are not aided with information and decision support at the point of care delivery, the likelihood of errors increases. Second, this growth of technology, much of it involving high-risk systems, creates changes in the work nurses are asked to perform. In particular, as systems (e.g., medication administration) become more automated, the technology makes work less transparent and creates opportunities for new types of errors (Reason, 1990).

Increased Interruptions and Demands on Nurses' Time

Interruptions

Changes such as those described above have resulted in increases in the types and amount of work required of nurses. In addition to the heavier patient care loads borne by nursing staff, evidence cited above indicates that large proportions of nurses spend time performing activities that can disrupt their primary patient care responsibilities, such as delivering and retrieving food trays; performing housekeeping duties; transporting patients; and ordering, coordinating, or performing ancillary services, such as delivery of medical equipment or supplies, blood products, or laboratory specimens (Aiken et al., 2001a; Prescott et al., 1991; Upenieks, 1998). It is clear that interruptions and interference occur frequently in nursing care from these and other nursing unit activities (Bowers et al., 2001; O'Shea, 1999; Wakefield et al., 1998; Walters, 1992). To the extent that such interruptions and distractions take place, patient safety is threatened. When health professionals have been asked to report their perceptions of why medical errors occur, interruptions and distractions have frequently been cited (Ely et al., 1995; Gladstone, 1995).

Documentation and Paperwork

Documenting nursing work and other activities to meet facility, insurance, private accreditation, state, and federal requirements, as well as to furnish information needed by other providers, is uniformly cited across all care delivery settings as imposing a heavy demand on nurses' time. The types of required documentation vary. Some may be characterized as administrative, that is, not treatment-specific; examples are providing insurance certifications, obtaining permission for the release of information, and informing patients of their rights. Other documentation pertains to nursing care; examples here are recording medications and treatment given, performing nursing assessments, and preparing discharge plans. Nurses in particular settings must also complete setting-specific documentation. For example, as discussed earlier, home health care nurses must complete a federally required OASIS assessment instrument for each Medicare beneficiary receiving Medicare home health care services, while nursing home nurses must complete a similar federally prescribed MDS for nursing home residents. These data sets are not always maximally compatible with internal documentation systems used by HCOs (e.g., the OMAHA system for home health care) and can create redundancies. Finally, nurses sometimes practice lengthy narrative charting as a defense against increasing litigation.

To the extent that paperwork and other documentation requirements lessen the time nurses have for direct contact with patients, they contribute to the reduced availability of nurses that has been shown to affect patient safety. Estimates from work sampling studies and surveys of nurses within individual hospitals of the amount of time spent in patient care documentation range from 13 to 28 percent (Korst et al., 2003; Pabst et al., 1996; Smeltzer et al., 1996; Upenieks, 1998; Urden and Roode, 1997). Home care nurses are estimated to spend a much greater proportion of their time in documenting care. According to some estimates, home health nurses spend approximately twice as much time in documenting patient care as do hospital nurses, in part because of more prescriptive federal regulatory requirements (Trossman, 2001). Completion of required paperwork is also cited as one reason nurses work overtime; because it cannot be accomplished in an 8-hour shift, it becomes a form of unpaid mandatory overtime (Trossman, 2001).

THREATS TO PATIENT SAFETY POSED BY WORK ENVIRONMENT FACTORS

All of the changes affecting the work environment of nurses described above can constitute latent factors conducive to health care errors. This fact is dramatically expressed in the text, but not the title, of a widely cited *Chicago Tribune* article, "Nursing Mistakes Kill, Injure Thousands Annually" (Berens, 2000). This article reports the results of an analysis of records from the U.S. Food and Drug Administration and other Department of Health and Humans Services agencies, federal and state files of annual hospital surveys and complaint investigations, court and private health care files, and nurse disciplinary records for every state. The analysis detected 1,720 deaths and 9,584 injuries among hospital patients resulting from the actions or inactions of RNs over a 5-year period, and 119 deaths and 564 patient injuries due to errors on the part of unlicensed NAs. Because of incomplete reporting, the article notes that these numbers should be interpreted as underestimates. Despite its title, the article does not point to willful wrongdoing or carelessness on the part of the RNs and NAs associated with these errors. Instead, it calls attention to their working conditions as the underlying causes (latent conditions) of the errors, prominently citing inadequate nurse training and insufficient monitoring of patients because of too few nurses being assigned to patient care.

These findings are underscored by an analysis of data on serious health care errors that are reported to the Joint Commission on the Accreditation of Healthcare Organizations (JCAHO) database on sentinel events. JCAHO defines a sentinel event as an "unexpected occurrence involving death or serious physical or psychological injury, or the risk thereof" (JCAHO, 2003:53). The JCAHO database is relatively small and subject to under-reporting. Nevertheless, for 19 percent of the total errors reported to the database from 1995 to 2002, nurse staffing levels are cited as one of the four major causal factors for reported serious errors/adverse events, such as patient falls, medication and transfusion errors, delays in treatment, and operative and postoperative complications. Inadequate staff orientation and training and competency assessment, as well as breakdowns in communication, were also revealed as frequent contributors to errors; communication-related factors were the most frequently identified root cause of all types of sentinel events (Croteau, 2003).

Preventing errors associated with such conditions requires that strong defenses be built into the work environment of nurses. As noted by Reason (2000:769), "We cannot change the human condition, but we can change the conditions under which humans work."

TRANSFORMING NURSES' WORK ENVIRONMENTS: ESSENTIAL TO PATIENT SAFETY

The evidence cited above and in succeeding chapters makes clear that (1) patient safety continues to be threatened; (2) latent conditions in work environments are the primary sources of those threats; and (3) nurses are the largest contingent of health care workers and perform critical patient safety functions while operating at the "sharp end" of health care. Given these facts, it is clear that the latent conditions present in the work environment of nurses must be addressed if patient safety is to be improved. This conclusion validates AHRQ's charge to the IOM to identify key aspects of the work environment for nurses likely to have an impact on patient safety, and potential improvements in health care working conditions that would likely increase patient safety.

In carrying out this charge, the committee reviewed published research and other evidence from a variety of disciplines: health services and nursing research; behavioral and organizational research on work and workforce effectiveness; human factors analysis and engineering; studies of organizational disasters and their evolution; and studies of high-risk industries (e.g., nuclear power production, chemical processing, transportation) with low accident rates (often called "high-reliability organizations"). The committee also commissioned papers and received expert testimony. (Appendix A contains a description of the committee's membership and the process used to conduct this study.)

This process revealed that identifying and remediating latent factors in the work environment of nurses and increasing patient safety are not likely to be achieved by any single action. Instead, it will be necessary to implement *bundles* of mutually reinforcing practices—changes that support each other in altering the context of worker behavior within a work environment. Such bundles of changes are needed within each of the four fundamental components of all organizations: (1) management and leadership, (2) workforce deployment, (3) work processes, and (4) organizational culture. The changes needed in each of these components are essential to building stronger patient safety defenses in HCOs. Evidence also indicates that they are basic to efficient organization practices in the twenty-first century and to recruitment and retention of nurses in a time of nursing shortages, and indeed are fundamental to the effective deployment of all health care workers, not just nurses. However, evidence further indicates that many of these fundamental changes have not yet occurred in the work environments of nurses; thus there is a need not merely for small changes in those environments, but for a broad transformation.

Many individual aspects of the necessary transformation in these four bundles of practices are identified in *To Err Is Human* (IOM, 2000) and *Crossing the Quality Chasm* (IOM, 2001). This report is intended to serve as a companion to those earlier reports. It delves more deeply into some of their recommendations, and addresses some issues not discussed in those reports, such as worker fatigue and staffing levels. It also emphasizes the role health care organizations can play in increasing patient safety—a role addressed less fully in *To Err Is Human* and *Crossing the Quality Chasm* (Berwick, 2002; IOM, 2001).

In Chapter 2, we focus on the underlying framework linking the needed bundles of changes in management and leadership, workforce deployment, work processes, and organizational culture. We also describe further how this report relates to *To Err Is Human* and *Crossing the Quality Chasm*. Chapter 3 describes the characteristics of the nursing workforce and its work that are important factors in reshaping nursing work environments. Chapters 4 through 7 address the above four organizational components and the evidence base supporting the committee's recommendations for change: Chapter 4 examines the need for evidence-based management and leadership; Chapter 5 calls for strengthening workforce capability; Chapter 6 speaks to the need to design nurses' work and workspace to prevent errors; and Chapter 7 describes the need to create and sustain cultures of safety within organizations. Finally, Chapter 8 reviews the study findings in light of the turbulence that is characteristic of the U.S. health care system. It presents a case for making these changes despite the many difficulties facing HCOs, policy makers, and other components of the health care system. It asserts the committee's position that it is not just necessary, but also possible, to transform the work environment of today's nurses. It further provides evidence that in addition to benefiting patients, such changes will benefit nurses, other health care workers, and the organizations in which they practice.

REFERENCES

AHA (American Hospital Association). 2002. *Hospital Statistics 2002.* Chicago, IL: Health Forum LLC, an affiliate of AHA.

AHCA (American Health Care Association). 2002. *Results of the 2001 AHCA Nursing Position Vacancy and Turnover Survey.* Washington, DC: AHCA.

Aiken L, Sochalski J, Anderson G. 1996. Downsizing the hospital nursing workforce. *Health Affairs* 15(4):88–92.

Aiken L, Clarke S, Sloane D. 2000. Hospital restructuring: Does it adversely affect care and outcomes? *Journal of Nursing Administration* 20(10):457–465.

Aiken L, Clarke S, Sloane D, Sochalski J, Busse R, Clarke H, Giovannetti P, Hunt J, Rafferty A, Shamian J. 2001a. Nurses' reports on hospital care in five countries. *Health Affairs* 20(3):43–53.

Aiken L, Clarke S, Sloane D, Sochalski J. 2001b. An international perspective on hospital nurses' work environments: The case for reform. *Policy, Politics, & Nursing Practice* 2(4):255–263.

Aiken L, Clarke S, Sloane D, Sochalski J, Silber J. 2002. Hospital nurse staffing and patient mortality, nurse burnout, and job dissatisfaction. *Journal of the American Medical Association* 288:1987–1993.

ANA (American Nurses Association). 1998. *Standards of Clinical Nursing Practice.* Washington, DC: ANA.

Berens M. 2000 (September 10). Nursing Mistakes Kill, Injure Thousands. *Chicago Tribune.* News Section. P. 20.

Berwick D. 2002. A user's manual for the IOM's "Quality Chasm" report. *Health Affairs* 21(3):80–90.

Bingham R. 2002. Leaving nursing. *Health Affairs* 21(1):211–217.

Blendon R, DesRoches C, Brodie M, Benson J, Rosen A, Schneider E, Altman D, Zapert K, Herrmann M, Steffenson A. 2002. Views of practicing physicians and the public on medical errors. *The New England Journal of Medicine* 347(24):1933–1940.

Bowers B, Lauring C, Jacobson N. 2001. How nurses manage time and work in long term care facilities. *Journal of Advanced Nursing* 33:484–491.

Bulechek G, McCloskey J, Titler M, Denehey J. 1994. Report on the NIC project: Nursing interventions used in practice. *American Journal of Nursing* 94(10):59–62, 64, 66.

Bureau of Labor Statistics, Department of Labor. Undated. *2001 National Occupational Employment Statistics.* [Online]. Available: http://stats.bls.gov/oesdate [accessed December 13, 2002].

CMS (Centers for Medicare and Medicaid Services). 2002. *Report to Congress: Appropriateness of Minimum Nurse Staffing Ratios in Nursing Homes—Phase II Final Report:* U.S. Department of Health and Human Services. [Online]. Available: www.cms.gov/medicaid/reports/rp1201home.asp [accessed June 25, 2002].

CMS. 2003. *Acute Inpatient Prospective Payment System:* U.S. Department of Health and Human Services. [Online]. Available: "Last modified on Tuesday, September 9, 2003." Available: www.cms.gov/providers/hipps/ippspufs.asp [accessed October 4, 2003].

Croteau R. 2003 (March 26). *Lessons Learned From Review of Sentinel Events 1995–2002: Issues Relevant to Nursing.* Joint Commission on the Accreditation of Healthcare Organization Nursing Advisory Council Meeting.

Division of Nursing. 1978. *Methods for Studying Nurse Staffing in a Patient Unit.* DHEW Publication No. HRA 78-3. Washington, DC: U.S. Government Printing Office.

Ely J, Levinson W, Elder N, Mainous A, Vinson D. 1995. Perceived causes of family physicians' errors. *Journal of Family Practice* 40(4):337–344.

Gelinas L, Manthey M. 1997. The impact of organizational redesign on nurse executive leadership. *Journal of Nursing Administration* 27(10):35–42.

Gladstone J. 1995. Drug administration errors: A study into the factors underlying the occurrence and reporting of drug errors in a district general hospital. *Journal of Advanced Nursing* 22(4):628–637.

Hendrickson G, Doddato T, Kovner C. 1990. How do nurses use their time? *Journal of Nursing Administration* 20(3):31–37.

Hurley M. 2000. Workload, UAPs, and you. *RN* 63(12):47–49.

Ingersoll G, Fisher M, Ross B, Soja M, Kidd N. 2001. Employee response to major organizational redesign. *Applied Nursing Research* 14(1):18–28.

IOM (Institute of Medicine). 2000. *To Err Is Human: Building a Safer Health System.* Washington, DC: National Academy Press.

IOM. 2001. *Crossing the Quality Chasm: A New Health System for the 21st Century.* Washington, DC: National Academy Press.

JCAHO (Joint Commission on Accreditation of Healthcare Organizations). 2001. *Front Line of Defense: The Role of Nurses in Preventing Sentinel Events.* Oakbrook Terrace, IL: Joint Commission Resources.

JCAHO. 2003. *2003 Hospital Accreditation Standards.* Oakbrook Terrace, IL: Joint Commission Resources.

Kahn K, Rogers W, Rubenstein L, Sherwood M, Reinisch E, Keeler E, Draper D, Kosecoff J, Brook R. 1990. Measuring quality of care with explicit process criteria before and after implementation of the DRG-based prospective payment system. *Journal of the American Medical Association* 264(15):1969–1973.

Korst L, Eusebio-Angeja A, Chamorro T, Aydin C, Gregory K. 2003. Nursing documentation time during implementation of an electronic medical record. *Journal of Nursing Administration* 33(1):24–30.

Kovner C, Jones C, Gergen P. 2000. Nurse staffing in acute care hospitals, 1990–1996. *Policy, Politics, & Nursing Practice* 1(3):194–204.

Kovner C, Jones C, Zhan C, Gergen P, Basu J. 2002. Nurse staffing and post surgical adverse events: An analysis of administrative data from a sample of U.S. hospitals, 1990–1996. *Health Services Research* 37(3):611–629.

Lawrenz E. 1992. Are patient classification systems still the best way to measure workload? *Perspectives on Staffing and Scheduling* XI(5):1–4.

Leape L, Bates D, Cullen D, Cooper J, Demonaco H, Gallivan T, Hallisey R, Ives J, Laird N, Laffel G, Nemeskal R, Petersen L, Porter K, Servi D, Shea B, Small S, Sweitzer B, Thompson B, Vander Vliet M. 1995. Systems analysis of adverse drug events. *Journal of the American Medical Association* 274(1):35–43.

Linden L, English K. 1994. Adjusting the cost-quality equation: Utilizing work sampling and time study data to redesign clinical practice. *Journal of Nursing Care Quality* 8(3):34–42.

Martin K. 2002 (September 24). *The Work of Nurses and Nursing Assistants in Home Care: Public Health, and Other Community Settings.* Paper commissioned by the Institute of

Medicine Committee on the Work Environment for Nurses and Patient Safety and presented to the Committee.

Medicare Payment Advisory Commission. 2001. *Report to the Congress: Medicare Payment Policy.* [Online]. Available: www.medpac.gov/publications/congressional_reports/Mar01 %Entire%20report.pdf [accessed February 24, 2003].

Mitchell P, Shortell S. 1997. Adverse outcomes and variations in organization of care delivery. *Medical Care* 35(Supplement 11):NS19–32.

Morris J, Murphy K, Nonemaker S. 1995. *Long Term Care Resident Assessment Instrument User's Manual, Version 2.0.* Baltimore, MD: Health Care Financing Administration, U.S. DHHS.

Narumi J, Miyazawa S, Miyata H, Suzuki A, Kohsaka S, Kosugi H. 1999. Analysis of human error in nursing care. *Accident Analysis & Prevention* 31(6):625–629.

Needleman J, Buerhaus P, Mattke S, Stewart M, Zelevinsky K. 2002. Nurse-staffing levels and the quality of care in hospitals. *The New England Journal of Medicine* 346(22):1715–1722.

Norrish B, Rundall T. 2001. Hospital restructuring and the work of registered nurses. *Milbank Quarterly* 79(1):55.

O'Shea E. 1999. Factors contributing to medication errors: A literature review. *Journal of Clinical Nursing* 8(5):496–505.

Pabst M, Scherubel J, Minnick A. 1996. The impact of computerized documentation on nurses' use of time. *Computers in Nursing* 14(1):25–30.

Perrow C. 1984. *Normal Accidents.* New York, NY: Basic Books.

Prescott P, Phillips C, Ryan J, Thompson K. 1991. Changing how nurses spend their time. *Image* 23(1):23–28.

Reason J. 1990. *Human Error.* Cambridge, UK: Cambridge University Press.

Reason J. 1997. *Managing the Risks of Organizational Accidents.* Burlington, VT: Ashgate Publishing Company.

Reason J. 2000. Human error: Models and management. *British Medical Journal* 320(7237): 768–770.

Rhoades J, Krauss N. 2001. *Chartbook #3: Nursing Home Trends, 1987 and 1996.* [Online]. Available: http://www.meps.ahrq.gov/papers/cb3_99-0032/cb3.htm [accessed October 4, 2003]. Rockville, MD: Agency for Healthcare Research and Quality.

Ritter-Teitel J. 2002. The impact of restructuring on professional nursing practice. *The Journal of Nursing Administration* 32(1):31–41.

Roberts K. 1990. Managing high reliability organizations. *California Management Review* Summer:101–113.

Roberts K, Bea R. 2001. When systems fail. *Organizational Dynamics* 29(3):179–191.

Rogers A. 2002. *Work Hour Regulation in Safety-Sensitive Industries.* Paper commissioned by the Institute of Medicine Committee on the Work Environment for Nurses and Patient Safety. Washington, DC: IOM.

Rousseau D, Libuser C. 1997. Contingent workers in high risk environments. *California Management Review* 39(2):103–123.

Rubenstein L, Chang B, Keeler E, Kahn K. 1992. Measuring the quality of nursing surveillance activities for five diseases before and after implementation of the drug-based prospective payment system. In: *Patient Outcomes Research: Examining the Effectiveness of Nursing Practice.* Proceedings of the State of the Science Conference. Bethesda, MD: NIH, National Center for Nursing Research. Washington, DC: U.S. Government Printing Office.

Seago J. 2001. Nurse staffing, models of care delivery, and interventions. In: Shojania K, Duncan B, McDonald K, Wachter R, eds. *Making Health Care Safer: A Critical Analysis of Patient Safety Practices.* Evidence Report/Technology Assessment No. 43. Rockville, MD: AHRQ.

Service Employees International Union. 2001. *The Shortage of Care: A Study by the SEIU Nurse Alliance.* Washington, DC: Service Employees International Union.

Shindul-Rothschild J, Berry D, Long-Middleton E. 1996. Where have all the nurses gone? Final results of our patient care survey. *American Journal of Nursing 96* 11:25–39.

Silber J, Williams S, Krakauer H, Schwartz S. 1992. Hospital and patient characteristics associated with death after surgery: A study of adverse occurrence and failure to rescue. *Medical Care* 30(7):615–627.

Smeltzer C, Hines P, Beebe H, Keller B. 1996. Streamlining documentation: An opportunity to reduce costs and increase nurse clinicians' time with patients. *Journal of Nursing Care Quality* 10(4):66–77.

Steel K, Gertman P, Crescenzi C, Anderson J. 1981. Iatrogenic illness on a general medical service at a university hospital. *The New England Journal of Medicine* 304(638-42):100–110.

The HSM Group. 2002. *Acute Care Hospital Survey of RN Vacancy and Turnover Rates.* Chicago, IL: American Organization of Nurse Executives.

Thomas L. 1983. *The Youngest Science: Notes of a Medicine-Watcher.* New York, NY: The Viking Press.

Trossman S. 2001. The documentation dilemma: Nurses poised to address paperwork burden. *The American Nurse* 33(5):1, 9, 18.

Unruh L. 2002a. Nursing staff reductions in Pennsylvania hospitals: Exploring the discrepancy between perceptions and data. *Medical Care Research and Review* 59(2):197–214.

Unruh L. 2002b. Trends in adverse events in hospitalized patients. *Journal for Healthcare Quality* 24(5):4–10.

Upenieks V. 1998. Work sampling: Assessing nursing efficiency. *Nursing Management* 29(4):27–29.

Urden L, Roode J. 1997. Work sampling: A decision-making tool for determining resources and work redesign. *Journal of Nursing Administration* 27(9):34–41.

Wakefield B, Wakefield D, Uden-Holman T, Blegen M. 1998. Nurses' perceptions of why medication administration errors occur. *MEDSURG Nursing* 7(1):39–44.

Walston S, Kimberly J. 1997. Reengineering hospitals: Evidence from the field. *Hospital and Health Services Administration* 42(2):143–163.

Walston S, Burns J, Kimberley J. 2000. Does reengineering really work? An examination of the context and outcomes of hospital reengineering initiatives. *Health Services Research* 34(6):1363–1388.

Walters J. 1992. Nurses' perceptions of reportable medication errors and factors that contribute to their occurrence. *Applied Nursing Research* 5(2):86–88.

WHO (World Health Organization). 2002. *Quality of Care: Patient Safety.* [Online]. Available: www.who.int/gb/EB_WHA/PDF/WHA55/ea5513.pdf [accessed February 6, 2003].

2

A Framework for Building
Patient Safety Defenses into
Nurses' Work Environments

BUILDING ON *TO ERR IS HUMAN* AND
CROSSING THE QUALITY CHASM

As noted in Chapter 1, this study builds upon the findings of two prior Institute of Medicine (IOM) reports that address mechanisms for improving patient safety—*To Err Is Human: Building a Safer Health System* (IOM, 2000) and *Crossing the Quality Chasm: A New Health System for the 21st Century* (IOM, 2001). *To Err Is Human* identifies a national agenda for change, specifying actions that entities—primarily those external to organizations directly delivering health care (Congress, regulators, accreditors, public and private purchasers, health professional licensing bodies, and professional societies)—should take to better safeguard patients. The report additionally devotes a chapter and two recommendations to actions that health care organizations (HCOs)—those organizations employing health care workers to deliver direct patient care—should take to improve patient safety. The first recommendation calls for HCOs to establish "patient safety programs with defined executive responsibility" that:

- provide strong, clear and visible attention to safety;
- implement non-punitive systems for reporting and analyzing errors within their organizations;
- incorporate well understood safety principles, such as standardizing and simplifying equipment, supplies, and processes; and
- establish interdisciplinary team training programs for providers that incorporate proven methods of team training such as simulation. (IOM, 2000:156)

The second recommendation calls on HCOs to "implement proven medication safety practices" (IOM, 2000:157).

Crossing the Quality Chasm further addresses patient safety as one of six highlighted aims for U.S. health care: that it be safe, effective, patient-centered, timely, efficient, and equitable. To achieve these six aims, the report specifies actions that HCOs and other entities should take to improve all aspects of health care quality—not just patient safety. The report's recommendations call on HCOs to (1) redesign care processes; (2) make effective use of information technologies; (3) manage clinical knowledge and skills; (4) develop effective teams; (5) coordinate care across patient conditions, services, and settings over time; and (6) incorporate performance and outcome measurements for improvement and accountability.

The authors of *Crossing the Quality Chasm* identify four different levels for intervening in the delivery of health care: (1) the experience of patients; (2) the functioning of small units of care delivery ("microsystems"), such as surgical teams or nursing units; (3) the functioning of organizations that house the microsystems; and (4) the environment of policy, payment, regulation, accreditation, and similar external factors that shape the environment in which health care delivery organizations deliver care. Whereas *To Err Is Human* speaks mainly to the fourth level, *Crossing the Quality Chasm* addresses primarily the first and second levels—how the experiences of patients and the work of microsystems of care, such as health care teams, nursing units, or individual health care workers delivering care to patients, should be changed (Berwick, 2002). Both of these reports direct less attention to the third level above—the organizations (HCOs) that house the microsystems.

This report emphasizes this level of the HCO. HCOs—by virtue of their employment of health care providers, establishment of work processes, and management of the resources used to deliver health care—are the primary developers of the structures and processes used by health care workers to deliver care. For purposes of this study, the committee defines these internal HCO structures and processes as the "work environment." We recognize that organizations and factors external to HCOs also shape work environments, but note that these external elements have been strongly addressed in the two prior IOM reports.

This report, with its focus on HCOs and the work environments they contain, therefore complements the work of the two prior IOM reports in three ways:

• It provides greater detail on how HCOs can and should implement key recommendations of *To Err Is Human* and *Crossing the Quality Chasm* in such areas as cultures of safety and work design.

- It addresses aspects of the work environment that are critical to patient safety but are not addressed in either of the two prior reports, such as the adequacy of staffing levels and worker fatigue.
- It unifies the prior two IOM reports and this report into a framework that all HCOs can use to construct work environments more conducive to patient safety. This framework integrates the multiple, mutually reinforcing strategies that are needed within various components of the work environment to keep patients safe from the ever-present latent conditions and human errors that pose risks to patient safety (as described in Chapter 1).

THE NEED FOR BUNDLES OF MULTIPLE, MUTUALLY REINFORCING PATIENT SAFETY DEFENSES

Research from a variety of disciplines clearly documents that errors and adverse events, especially those that are difficult to correct, often result from multiple, interdependent factors that converge to impair the performance of organizations (Goodman, 2001; Perrow, 1984; Ramanuajm, forthcoming). Errors and accidents often originate within multiple steps in work design and implementation—in fact, in all steps of a production process—and in several components simultaneously. Consequently, reducing error and increasing patient safety are not likely to be achieved by any single action; rather, a comprehensive approach, addressing all components of health care delivery within an organization, is required.

Evidence in support of this contention comes from health services and nursing research; behavioral and organizational research on work and workforce effectiveness; human factors analysis and engineering; studies of organizational disasters and their evolution; and studies of high-reliability organizations.[1] For example, intensive study of individual disasters has yielded valuable information about the circumstances leading up to each catastrophic error. The combined knowledge obtained from multiple case studies yields a body of principles that, when applied, can reasonably be expected to reduce the occurrence of errors, their adverse consequences, or both (Reason, 1990). This approach is employed in the Joint Commission on Accreditation of Healthcare Organizations' (JCAHO) analyses of the root causes of sentinel events.

Similarly, organizational research conducted by social scientists has provided a multilevel view of organizations by focusing on the complex levels of human organizing, including individuals, dyads, groups, networks, firms,

---

[1]As noted in Chapter 1, high-reliability organizations are defined as high-risk industries (e.g., nuclear power production) with low accident rates.

and interfirm arrangements (House et al., 1995). This research has identified sets of practices and contextual factors that support or impede effective organizing. For example, the characteristics of world-class manufacturing systems have been identified not in terms of any one practice, but as bundles of mutually reinforcing practices (e.g., quality improvement structures; participative decision making; worker training; and access to unit or organization quality, financial, and managerial information) (MacDuffie, 1995). Such research has found that focusing on only one piece of the problem can backfire. Implementing a single practice, such as teamwork or new incentives, without supporting practices, such as access to pertinent information or education, may yield few practical consequences. In health care settings, for example, changes in work procedures without attention to their impact on staffing demand and existing workflow may actually reduce patient safety.

Studies of high-reliability organizations also have identified multiple, related practices associated with the achievement of high levels of safety in production processes. These include ensuring ongoing vigilance of workers to detect unexpected sequences of events that pose the risk of errors; constantly training workers in knowing how to detect errors in the making and respond to errors once they occur; incorporating personnel and equipment redundancy in work design; managing work flow, especially in interdependent work components; and practicing nonhierarchical decision making so that decisions are made at that point in the organization where expertise is greatest—often the point where the action is to be implemented, which can often be at lower levels of the organization's hierarchy (Roberts, 1990; Roberts and Bea, 2001).

As discussed in Chapter 1 and reinforced by the above research, then, reducing errors and increasing patient safety require multiple, mutually reinforcing changes—bundles of changes that support each other in altering the context of worker behavior within a work environment—not isolated interventions or a single "silver bullet" (Itner and MacDuffie, 1995; Pil and MacDuffie, 1996). These bundles of changes need to be applied throughout an organization's production processes. Fortunately, an evidence-based model for applying error-defense strategies throughout organizational work processes has been developed. This framework, based on empirical research on organizational safety for health care and other industries, is described below.

AN EVIDENCE-BASED MODEL
FOR SAFETY DEFENSES IN WORK ENVIRONMENTS

An old fable describes a group of blind men touching an elephant. Each alternatively describes the elephant as "a massive wall," "a thin cylindrical whip-like animal," a "muscular, tubular creature," or a "hard, rock-like being with sharp knife-like protuberances." As the fable illustrates, all of these characterizations are correct, just incomplete when isolated from each other. Early in the course of this study, it became apparent that the work environment of nurses as related to patient safety is similarly multidimensional. The committee noted evidence that patient safety is threatened by inadequate staffing levels, long work hours, poor education and training, unsafe work practices, underutilization of information technology, and a variety of other work conditions. It also quickly became apparent that these are not competing, but complementary views of the threats to patient safety.

The complementarity of these threats to safety is validated by the work of James Reason, whose analyses and writings provided much of the evidence base used by the IOM committee that produced *To Err Is Human*. In his widely cited book, *Human Error*, Reason (1990) reviews the basic components of and contributors to any organization's production processes and describes how errors arise in each. He notes that the concept of "production" is one on which there is wide agreement. All enterprises are involved in some form of production, whether the product is energy, chemical substances, the mass transport of people, or health care. Using the basic components of production, Reason develops a multifaceted model of organizational errors that has been used to analyze and develop error-defense strategies for health care settings (Meurier, 2000), as well as other lines of business (Helmreich, 2000).

Figure 2-1 identifies the basic elements of any organization's production process. In this model:

- **Decision makers** are both the designers and high-level managers of the organization. They set the goals for the organization as a whole in response to inputs from the external environment. They also direct, at a strategic level, the means by which organizational goals should be met. A large part of their function is concerned with the allocation of finite resources—money, equipment, people, and time. Their aim is to deploy these resources to maximize both productivity and the welfare of the organization's resources.
- **Line management** consists of departmental specialists who implement the strategies of decision makers.
- **Preconditions** include the necessary resources and environmental conditions for production, such as reliable and appropriate equipment, a skilled and knowledgeable workforce, an appropriate set of attitudes and motivators, work schedules, environmental conditions that permit efficient and safe operations, and codes of practice that give clear guidance to workers regarding desirable and undesirable performance.

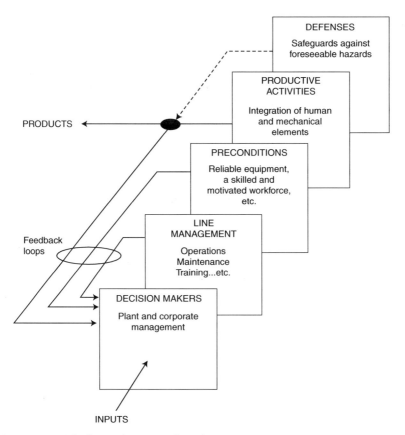

FIGURE 2-1   The basic elements of production.
SOURCE: Reprinted with the permission of Cambridge University Press from
Human Error by James Reason, copyright 1990.

  • **Productive activities** are the actual performance of humans and machines used to "deliver the right product at the right time."
  • **Defenses** include structural and procedural safeguards to prevent
foreseeable injury, damage, or costly outages.

Reason notes that each of the above elements of the production process is
shaped by the fallible decisions and actions of humans, thereby creating the
ever-present risk of error.[2]

---

[2]While Reason notes that a similar schema could be presented for purely mechanical or
technical failures, he, like the committee, focuses on human factors because accident analyses
reveal these to be the dominant factors in the production of errors.

In Figure 2-2, Reason maps the human decisions that are made within the various production elements, and identifies the role played by each in creating latent error-producing conditions or active errors at "the sharp end" (see Chapter 1) both of which ultimately lead to accidents when organizational defenses are inadequate.

Using Reason's model and the strong and convergent evidence obtained from studies of highly reliable organizations, research on work and work-

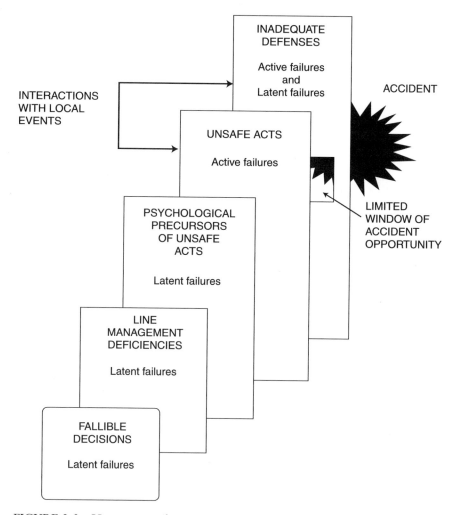

FIGURE 2-2 Human contributions to error within each production component. SOURCE: Reprinted with the permission of Cambridge University Press from *Human Error* by James Reason, copyright 1990.

force effectiveness, health services research, and human factors analysis and engineering, the committee has sought to identify those evidence-based, mutually reinforcing practices essential to successful error reduction and patient safety within each of the four fundamental components of all organizations introduced in Chapter 1: (1) management and leadership, (2) workforce deployment, (3) work processes, and (4) organizational culture. These safety defenses are summarized in Figure 2-3. These interventions map to Reason's schema and together constitute a framework for increasing patient safety through the modification of nurses' work environments. The committee notes that this framework applies to all HCOs, and has made recommendations that, unless explicitly stated otherwise in the recommendation itself, also are intended to apply to all HCOs. As Figure 2-3 illustrates, these recommendations are aimed at creating work environments with built-in patient safety defenses that include (1) adopting transformational leadership and evidence-based management practices, (2) maximiz-

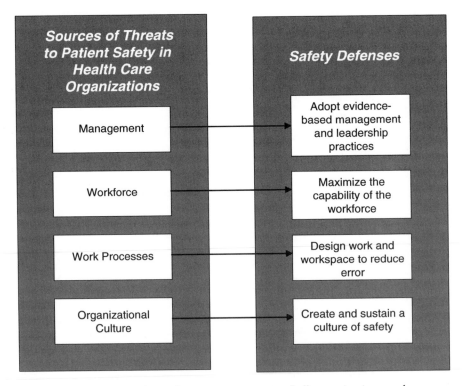

FIGURE 2-3 Basic work production components of all organizations and corresponding patient safety defenses.

ing the capability of the workforce, (3) designing work and workspace to defend against errors, and (4) creating and sustaining cultures of safety.

The evidence with respect to these practices and recommendations for their application by HCOs are discussed in Chapters 4 through 7, respectively. The implementation of these recommendations should recognize the unique features of health care that make it especially vulnerable to error production and escape from detection and remediation.

UNIQUE FEATURES OF HEALTH CARE THAT HAVE IMPLICATIONS FOR PATIENT SAFETY DEFENSES

In his more recent studies of patient safety, Reason has identified characteristics of the health care industry that distinguish it from other high-risk industries and make it more vulnerable to the production and effects of errors.[3] These include the greater diversity and associated risks of actions undertaken in health care, the greater vulnerability of health care consumers, differences in the delivery of health care services in contrast to other human services, the uncertainty of the health care knowledge base, and the less explicit and open investigation of errors.

Diversity of Tasks and Tools

Much of the complexity of health care systems stems from the enormous diversity of the tasks to be performed and the tools to be used in performing them. By contrast, aviation, nuclear power generation, and railway systems are relatively homogeneous in terms of both their functions and the equipment they use. Transport systems move people and goods from point A to point B, mainly in a tightly scheduled fashion, while power-generating systems produce megawatts in as stable a manner as possible. Each domain has a very limited number of equipment types. In modern commercial aviation, for example, two manufacturers—Boeing and Airbus—supply the vast majority of aircraft. Less standardization of activities and tools is found in health care activities. Health care encompasses a large, complex set of tailored services, as opposed to fewer, standardized products.

Greater Risk Associated with Health Care Activities

Human performance in complex systems can be assigned to one of three categories: routine operations, coping with abnormal or emergency condi-

---

[3]Personal communication, James Reason, August 11, 2003.

tions, and maintenance-related tasks (inspection, repair, calibration, and testing) (Reason and Hobbs, 2003). In the commercial aviation and nuclear power production industries, pilots and nuclear power plant operators spend the greater part of their time performing routine control and monitoring activities (mostly the latter). Health care professionals, in contrast, are more often dealing with abnormal, person-specific conditions and performing maintenance-equivalent work. Both of these operational modes are considerably more error-provocative and risk-laden than routine control. Two factors in particular are important in shaping error probabilities and their consequences: (1) the amount of "hands-on" work and (2) its safety criticality (i.e., the degree of hazard associated with less-than-adequate performance). Error opportunity is a function of the amount of immediate human involvement. Both emergency conditions and maintenance-related activities involve more direct physical contact than do routine operations. And in both cases, the safety criticality of errors is high.

Vulnerability of the Consumers of Production

In health care, individuals (i.e., patients) are an integral part of the "production process" in addition to being the recipients of health care services. Unlike passengers or the consumers of electrical power, however, patients are, by definition, vulnerable people. They are sick, injured, old, or very young. In nursing homes, for example, nearly half of all residents have some type of dementia. This vulnerability makes them much less able to participate in their own care and more liable to being seriously damaged by unsafe acts. Moreover, even when they are receiving safe and appropriate care, some patients' underlying physical condition can make that care ineffective. These poor outcomes are not the same as adverse events resulting from inappropriate and unsafe care.

Mode of Delivering Health Care

The processes and products of commercial transportation, nuclear power, and other industries often are delivered to end-users in a fairly impersonal "few-to-many" fashion; that is, few individuals are involved in transmitting the service to many individuals. In contrast, the delivery from the health care professional to the patient is mainly "one-to-one" or "few-to-one." This makes health care delivery a very personal, face-to-face transaction. The individual characteristics of the professional are likely to play a greater part in service delivery than in these other domains. Whether the health care professional chooses to go the extra mile is likely to have a far greater impact in health care than elsewhere.

Uncertainty of the Knowledge Base

Compared with many other highly technical hazardous endeavors, health care activities—despite many advances—are inexact procedures based upon incomplete knowledge, and are performed in a rapidly changing world on an increasingly aging population. Uncertainty is large, and error margins are small. Health care professionals and their patients both possess incomplete medical knowledge. As one surgeon recently noted:

> We look for medicine to be an orderly field of knowledge and procedure. But it is not. It is an imperfect science, an enterprise of constantly changing knowledge, uncertain information, fallible individuals, and at the same time lives on the line. There is science in what we do, yes, but also habit, intuition, and sometimes plain old guessing. The gap between what we know and what we aim for persists. And this gap complicates everything we do (Gawande, 2002:7).

Event Investigation

Accidents in non–health care domains, such as transportation, are newsworthy and publicly investigated, and the results are widely disseminated. In contrast, mishaps in health care, again with some exceptions (e.g., radiological events), tend to be investigated quietly at the local level, and, until recently, findings were neither shared nor made available for public scrutiny.

Summary

In summary, health care institutions are complex systems, and their complexity includes features that are less often present in the kinds of hazardous hi-tech systems that are often used as models for effective safety management. This does not mean that health care professionals cannot learn valuable safety lessons from these other domains; rather, HCOs, policy officials, nurses, and all parties working to increase patient safety need to be mindful of the distinctive features of health care delivery that make it even more susceptible to the production of errors.

REFERENCES

Berwick D. 2002. A user's manual for the IOM's "Quality Chasm" report. *Health Affairs* 21(3):80–90.

Gawande A. 2002. *Complications: A Surgeon's Notes on an Imperfect Science.* New York, NY: Metropolitan Books, Henry Holt and Company.

Goodman P. 2001. *Missing Organizational Linkages: Tools for Cross-Level Organizational Research.* Thousand Oaks, CA: Sage Publications.

Helmreich R. 2000. On error management: Lessons from aviation. *British Medical Journal* 320:781–785.

House R, Rousseau D, Thomas-Hunt M. 1995. The meso-paradigm: A framework for integration of micro and macro organizational behavior. In: *Research in Organizational Behavior* (Vol. 17). Greenwich, CT: JAI Press. Pp. 71–114.

IOM (Institute of Medicine). 2000. *To Err Is Human: Building a Safer Health System.* Washington, DC: National Academy Press.

IOM. 2001. *Crossing the Quality Chasm.* Washington, DC: National Academy Press.

Itner C, MacDuffie J. 1995. Explaining plant-level differences in manufacturing overhead: Structural and executional cost drivers in the world auto industry. *Production and Operations Management* 4:312–334.

MacDuffie J. 1995. Human resource bundles and manufacturing performance: Organizational logic and flexible production systems in the world auto industry. *Industrial and Labor Relations Review* 48:197–221.

Meurier C. 2000. Understanding the nature of errors in nursing: Using a model to analyse critical incident reports of errors which had resulted in an adverse or potentially adverse event. *Journal of Advanced Nursing* 32(1):202–207.

Perrow C. 1984. *Normal Accidents.* New York, NY: Basic Books.

Pil F, MacDuffie J. 1996. The adoption of high-involvement work practices. *Industrial Relations* 35:423–455.

Ramanuajm R. Forthcoming. The effects of discontinuous change on latent errors in organizations: The moderating role of risk. *Academy of Management Journal.*

Reason J. 1990. *Human Error.* Cambridge, UK: Cambridge University Press.

Reason J, Hobbs A. 2003. *Managing Maintenance Error: A Practical Guide.* Hampshire, UK: Ashgate.

Roberts K. 1990. Managing high reliability organizations. *California Management Review* Summer:101–113.

Roberts K, Bea R. 2001. When systems fail. *Organizational Dynamics* 29(3):179–191.

3

Nurses Caring for Patients:
Who They Are, Where They Work,
and What They Do[1]

An organization's workers and their work environment have a reciprocal relationship, each influencing the other in an ongoing, dynamic interplay that affects the level of safety within the organization (Cooper, 2000). To construct a nursing work environment that maximizes patient safety, the characteristics of the nursing workforce, the settings in which they provide care, and the nature of their work, as well as the implications of these elements for patient safety, need to be considered. This chapter does so, focusing predominantly on the role of nurses in hospitals and nursing homes, where the greatest amount of study has been conducted on patient safety.

WHO IS DOING THE WORK OF NURSING?

"When average citizens report that 'I saw the nurse,' or 'I talked to the nurse,' they could mean any of a vast array of workers" (Ward and Berkowitz, 2002:44). The word "nurse" is often used to refer to registered

---

[1]Portions of this chapter draw on four papers commissioned by the committee: "The Nursing Workforce: Profile, Trends and Projections" by Julie Sochalski, Ph.D., of the University of Pennsylvania School of Nursing; "The Work of Registered Nurses, Licensed Practical Nurses, and Nurses Aides in Acute Care Hospitals" by Barbara Mark, Ph.D., of the University of North Carolina at Chapel Hill School of Nursing; "The Work of Nurses and Nurse Aides in Long Term Care Facilities" by Barbara Bowers, Ph.D., of the University of Wisconsin-Madison School of Nursing; and "The Work of Nurses and Nurse Assistants in Home Care, Public Health, and Other Community Settings" by Karen Martin of Martin Associates.

nurses (RNs), licensed practical nurses/licensed vocational nurses (LPNs/LVNs), or nursing assistants (NAs). In this report, we refer collectively to all three of these groups of personnel as nursing staff.

There are over 5 million nursing staff in the United States. Of these, 2.2 million are actively employed as RNs[2] and 683,800 as LPNs/LVNs. RNs and LPNs/LVNs are licensed by the state in which they provide nursing care. Another 2.3 million unlicensed health care workers (Bureau of Labor Statistics, undated) supplement the work of licensed nurses by performing basic patient care activities under the supervision of an RN or LPN/LVN. These unlicensed health care personnel hold a variety of job titles, including nurse assistants, nurse aides, home health aides, personal care aides, ancillary nursing personnel, unlicensed nursing personnel, unlicensed assistive personnel, nurse extenders, and nursing support personnel. In this report, we refer collectively to these workers as NAs. Jobs for NAs are expected to be among the most rapidly expanding in the workforce as the overall U.S. population ages, and the need for postacute and chronic care increases. Indeed, the number of employed NAs increased by 40 percent between 1980 and 1990, more than twice the growth rate of the overall U.S. workforce. The greatest growth was in aides working in home care, whose numbers more than doubled from 1988 to 1998. From 1998 to 2008, a 36 percent increase in NA jobs is predicted, compared with a 14 percent increase in all workforce jobs (GAO, 2001b).

Variations in Education and in Experience and Expertise Among Members of the Nursing Workforce

Education

Each type of nursing personnel is educated differently. An overview of the education received by each is provided below.

Education for RNs Basic RN education can be attained through three routes: 3-year diploma programs, 2-year associates degree (AD) nursing programs, and 4-year baccalaureate degree programs. In addition to any of these three types of academic preparation, individuals must pass a state examination to be licensed as an RN.

The route chosen to receive entry-level, prelicensure RN education has changed considerably over the past two decades, with decreasing use of 3-year diploma programs and increased use of AD and baccalaureate programs. Between 1980 and 2000, the proportion of nurses receiving their

---

[2]Although there were approximately 2.7 million RNs in the United States in 2000, only approximately 2.2 million of them were working actively as nurses.

basic education from a diploma program decreased from 60 to 30 percent, while the proportion of those receiving basic education from AD or baccalaureate programs increased from 19 to 40 percent and 17 to 29 percent, respectively. However, these data do not fully characterize the educational level of the RN workforce, as many RNs pursue additional education after being licensed. In 2000, the distribution of RNs according to their highest degree was as follows: diploma preparation (23 percent), AD (34.3 percent), baccalaureate degree (32.7 percent), and master's or doctoral degree (10 percent). The educational level of RNs varies by place of employment. RNs in nursing homes generally have a lower level of education than those in other settings. In 2000, only 27 percent of RNs employed by nursing homes were prepared at the baccalaureate level, compared with 43 percent in hospitals. Nurses with advanced-practice credentials are also less well represented in nursing homes: 7.6 percent of hospital nurses were prepared at the masters or doctorate level, compared with 4.3 percent of nursing home nurses (Spratley et al., 2000).

Research on the effect of different educational paths to RN licensure on nurse performance and patient outcomes has been inconclusive. Such research has examined the characteristics, abilities, and work assignments of nurses with and without baccalaureate degrees, but has not been as thorough in examining the quality of the care they provide (including patient safety) (Blegen et al., 2001). However, an analysis of educational preparation and years of experience in the nursing workforce from the National Sample Survey of Registered Nurses (NSSRN) suggests that baccalaureate-prepared nurses have tended to stay in the workforce longer and accrue more years of work experience than those not thus prepared (Sochalski, 2002). Further, limited data from studies of magnet hospitals (i.e., hospitals characterized by their ability to attract and retain nurses) indicate that those hospitals have higher percentages of baccalaureate-prepared nurses (50 percent) as compared with the national hospital average of 34 percent (Aiken et al., 2000a).

Education for LPNs/LVNs   LPN/LVN training programs are shorter than those for RNs, taking 12 to 18 months, and emphasize technical nursing tasks such as monitoring vital signs, administering medications, and completing treatments (GAO, 2001b). In 2000, approximately 1,100 state-approved programs provided LPN/LVN education. Students attending these programs were enrolled predominantly in vocational/technical schools and community and junior colleges. A state licensing examination also must be completed successfully following the LPN/LVN training program (Bureau of Labor Statistics, 2003).

Education for NAs   Training for NAs depends on their place of employment. Those working in Medicare- or Medicaid-reimbursed nursing homes (the majority) and home health agencies must meet certain minimum training requirements and competency standards and acquire state certification to become certified nurse aides (CNAs). An individual may become a CNA either by completing a nurse aide training program and a competency evaluation (a written or oral test and skills demonstration) or by passing a competency evaluation alone. A minimum of 75 hours of training is required through a state-approved CNA program, although many state programs exceed the minimum. At least 16 of the 75 hours must be practical training under the direct supervision of an RN or LPN. For CNAs working in nursing homes, states are required to keep a registry of those who have passed their competency evaluations (GAO, 2001b). There are no similar federal requirements regarding training, certification, competency evaluation, or registries for NAs working in hospitals (GAO, 2001b).

Experience and Expertise

Experience and expertise refer to the knowledge and skill obtained apart from (often subsequent to) formal preparation in an academic institution. Experience is acquired when an actual practice situation "refines," "elaborates," or "disconfirms" knowledge that has been acquired previously through the study of theory or principles or participation in events. Expertise is the result of an individual's accumulation of knowledge and skill from such experiences (Benner, 1984:3–5). Thus, workers with similar formal education can possess varying degrees of expertise. A new graduate and a seasoned nurse of 20 years are both nurses, but their experience and expertise are very different.

The varying levels of expertise and skill acquired by learners have been identified through studies of different types of workers and learners within and outside of health care. These levels have been labeled as "novice," "advanced beginner," "competent," "proficient," and "expert" (Dreyfus and Dreyfus, 1986). As applied to nursing, they have been described as (1) novice—beginners who have no experience with the situations in which they must perform; (2) advanced beginners—individuals who have marginally acceptable performance based on a foundation of experience with real situations; (3) competent—individuals with 2 or 3 years in a similar situation; (4) proficient—wherein perception allows meanings to be understood in terms of the "big picture" rather than as isolated observations; and (5) expert—based on a wealth of experience enabling an intuitive grasp of situations and quick targeting of problem areas (Benner, 1984). According to this framework, expertise is subject matter–specific; thus, for example, RNs may be expert in one area of practice, such as critical care, but not in another, such as psychiatric nursing, just as a highly expert obstetrician may be less than proficient in managing an adult with neurological problems.

The levels of experience and expertise of nursing staff have not been well measured. Experience is typically assessed using a proxy measure—the number of years an individual has been employed in nursing. This measure may capture exposure to opportunities for experience and the gaining of expertise, but as noted above, such exposure is not always a guarantee of expertise. Using years of nursing work as a proxy measure, however, experience has been associated with better patient care. In an analysis of data from two studies (involving 42 inpatient units in one large tertiary-care hospital and 39 patient care units in 11 other hospitals), nursing units whose nurses had more years of experience were found to have lower rates of medication errors and patient falls (Blegen et al., 2001). Likewise, a 1996–1998 analysis of nurses and errors in a Japanese cardiology ward found that nurses with less than 3 years of experience made significantly more rule-based and skill-based errors than those with more than 3 years of experience (Narumi et al., 1999).

Further support for the beneficial effects of years of experience and expertise in providing nursing care to individuals with particular clinical conditions can be inferred from similar studies of physicians. Such studies have revealed better patient outcomes when clinical procedures are carried out by physicians who have performed greater numbers of those procedures and when care of patients with certain clinical conditions, such as AIDS, is rendered by physicians with more experience in treating those conditions. The Agency for Healthcare Research and Quality's (AHRQ) recent evidence-based report on the effect of health care working conditions on patient safety presents evidence that in a number of types of clinical care, greater experience of health professionals is associated with better patient outcomes (Hickam et al., 2003).

Currently, the experience level of nursing staff is threatened by high turnover rates in all health care delivery settings. Nationally in 2000, an estimated 21 percent of all acute care hospital nurses left the position in which they were practicing. Most hospitals reported turnover rates of 10 to 30 percent, but some experienced even higher rates (The HSM Group, 2002). The turnover rate is even higher in long-term care facilities. A 2001 national survey of the American Health Care Association (AHCA) revealed turnover rates of 78 percent for NAs, 56 percent for staff RNs, 54 percent for LPNs/LVNs, and 43–47 percent for directors of nursing and RNs with administrative duties (AHCA, 2002). If all these nursing personnel left their positions to take new positions in settings offering similar clinical services, the level of expertise of the nursing workforce would not be threatened.[3]

---

[3]Although safety would still be threatened by nurses' unfamiliarity with new HCO structures, policies, and practices.

However, NSSRN data show that a number of these nurses are leaving the field of nursing altogether. In 2000, 18.3 percent of licensed nurses were not working in the field of nursing. Evidence indicates that these are not just retired older nurses. Almost 3 percent of women and 2 percent of men graduating from nursing schools between 1988 and 1991 were not working in nursing within the first 4 years following graduation. By 9 to 12 years after graduation, 11 percent of women and 6 percent of men had departed from the profession. More recent graduating classes have higher departure rates. Among 1996–1999 graduates, 4.1 percent of women and 7.5 percent of men left the profession within 4 years of graduating (Sochalski, 2002). This loss of experienced nurses can represent a threat to patient safety.

Unique Demographic Characteristics of the Nursing Workforce

Most data on the nursing workforce are collected on RNs; less is known about LPNs/LVNs and NAs, who together make up 42.6 percent of nursing staff. It is known, however, that nursing staff overall are predominantly female and ethnically different from the workforce at large and those they serve. RNs are older than the total U.S. workforce and aging more rapidly. NAs are often poor and without health insurance—unable to receive the services they provide to others. A small portion of nursing staff are not employees of the health care organizations (HCOs) in which they work, but provide care to patients as "contingent" workers.

Predominance of Women

The RN workforce is predominantly female (94.6 percent), although the small proportion of male RNs rose from 2.7 percent in 1980 to 5.4 percent in 2000 (Spratley et al., 2000). The NA workforce is similarly largely female. Women are estimated to make up 79.6 percent, 90.9 percent, and 89.2 percent of hospital, nursing home, and home care aides, respectively (GAO, 2001b). Although data are unavailable on the gender of LPNs/LVNs, they are likely predominantly female as well.

The high proportion of women in the nursing workforce has a number of implications. Conflicts in nurse–physician relationships have been attributed in part to gender conflicts and inequalities in society at large (McMahan and Hoffman, 1994). In addition, responsibilities at home, such as caring for children or older family members and performing household chores, may contribute to the commission of errors in two ways. First, family obligations may add to the long hours worked by many nurses in their professional workplace and contribute to the sleep deficits and fatigue that are associated with the commission of errors. Of nurses employed in the field in 2000, 55 percent had children living at home (Spratley et al., 2000).

Nursing home and home health aides are also two to three times more likely than other workers to be unmarried and to have children at home (GAO, 2001b). Second, while research has shown that men and women both experience stress in balancing work and family obligations, multiple studies on the division of household tasks have found that women continue to perform far more chores than do men (Wentling, 1998).

An Older and More Rapidly Aging Nursing Workforce

The entire U.S. workforce is aging, largely as a result of the aging of baby boomers. As noted, however, the RN workforce is already older than the total U.S. workforce and is aging more rapidly. The average age of the RN workforce was 37.4 in 1983 (Buerhaus et al., 2000), but had increased to 45.2 years by 2000 (Spratley et al., 2000). In the 1980s, the majority of nurses were in their twenties and thirties; by 2000, this distribution had changed substantially, with four times more 40-year-old than 20-year-old nurses. The average age of RNs is projected to increase and peak at 45.5 years in 2010 (Buerhaus, et al., 2000). In contrast, the Department of Labor forecasts the age of the overall labor force to reach only 40.7 years by 2008 (Bureau of Labor Statistics, 1999).

The more rapid aging of the RN workforce is attributed to three factors. First, large cohorts of the existing RN workforce are in their fifties and sixties—a function of the baby boom. Only when RNs born in the 1950s reach retirement age in approximately 2020 is the age distribution of the RN workforce projected to shift back toward younger ages (Buerhaus et al., 2000). Also, fewer young people are choosing to become RNs, so the proportion of younger nurses among all RNs is declining (Buerhaus et al., 2000; Spratley et al., 2000). Finally, in recent years, new graduates of basic nursing programs have tended to be older, and thus the average age of entrants into the RN workforce has been higher (Spratley et al., 2000).[4]

This aging workforce has implications for nurses' work environments. The loss of strength and agility that often accompanies aging affects the ease with which nurses can perform patient care activities that require them to turn, lift, or provide weight-bearing support to patients. Focus groups of nurses have revealed that among nurses who plan to stay in the field, many are concerned that they will be unable to do so as they age because of the heavy physical demands of the job (Kimball and O'Neil, 2002). Ergonomic

---

[4]In contrast, NAs are younger than RNs, and their age distribution has remained comparatively stable. From the late 1980s to the late 1990s, the mean age of NAs working in hospitals, nursing homes, and home health care changed from 36.3 to 38.0 years, 36.6 to 36.4 years, and 46.7 to 42.8 years, respectively (Yamada, 2002).

patient and staff furniture and work tools will be needed to decrease the risk of injuries to patients (and nurses as well). Changes in hearing and vision also have implications for the design of work and technology used in patient care—for example, the need for increased lighting and larger size of print material (Curtin, 2002). There could be implications as well for shift lengths and rotations. Research has shown that adapting to shift work is more difficult for workers over age 40. A recent study of the effect of age on performance found that older individuals (mean age 43.9) had less ability to maintain performance on standard neurobiological tests across a 12-hour shift compared with younger individuals (mean age 21.2) (Reid and Dawson, 2001).

A Workforce That Does Not Yet Fully Reflect the Racial and Ethnic Diversity of the U.S. Population

The U.S. population is becoming more racially and ethnically diverse. At the beginning of the 1900s, one of every eight Americans identified himself or herself as a race other than "white." At the end of the century, one of four did so, as the white population had grown more slowly than every other racial/ethnic group. This increase in diversity accelerated in the latter half of the century. From 1970 to 2000, the population of races other than "white" or "black" grew considerably, and by 2000 was comparable in size to the black population. The black population represented a slightly smaller share of the total U.S. population in 1970 than in 1900, while the Hispanic population more than doubled from 1980 to 2000. In the 2000 census, 36 percent of the population reported belonging to "two or more" races (the 2000 census was the first to include this reporting category). The racial/ethnic composition of the U.S. population according to the 2000 census was as follows: 75.1 percent white, 12.3 percent black, 3.8 percent Asian or Pacific Islander, 0.9 percent American Indian or Alaska Native, 2.4 percent claiming two or more races, and 5.5 percent claiming a race other than those already cited. Individuals (of any race) claiming Hispanic origin constituted 12.5 percent of the U.S. population (Hobbs and Stoops, 2002).

The nursing workforce does not yet fully reflect this diversity. In 2000, a higher proportion of RNs (88 percent) than the general U.S. population (75.1 percent) was white; however, the 12 percent of racial/ethnic minority RNs was an increase from the 5 percent of 1980. Significantly, the increase in the overall RN population between 1996 and 2000 is attributed largely to the growth in the numbers of RNs from racial/ethnic minorities (Spratley et al., 2000). In contrast, the NA workforce has a higher proportion of such minorities than the U.S. population overall. Approximately 40–50 percent of NAs working in hospitals, long-term care facilities, and home health care are nonwhite racial/ethnic minorities (GAO, 2001b).

This phenomenon is not unique to nursing. Differences in the racial/ethnic and cultural composition of the health care workforce and the patient population have been a source of concern across all health professions. Such differences can be obstacles to fully understanding patient care needs. Language differences, in particular, can be a major barrier to care delivery. If nursing staff cannot communicate with patients effectively, health assessment, explanations of alternative treatments, informed consent, health education, involvement of patients in self-care, and discharge instructions are all compromised. Patients cannot be full partners in monitoring for threats to their safety if they do not understand the interventions being applied on their behalf. Other implications of racial/ethnic and cultural differences include, for example, limited understanding of the use of alternative therapies and other health- and illness-related practices of patients and their families, and the effects of those practices on planned care. In a previous study, the Institute of Medicine (IOM) found that greater racial and ethnic diversity in the health professions strengthens patient–provider relationships. The benefits of this diversity are believed to accrue broadly to the health professions and help expand their ability to conceptualize and respond to the health needs of the increasingly diverse U.S. population (IOM, 2003).

Hospital RN Salaries Might Be Increasing; Many NAs Live at or Below Poverty Level

The U.S. Department of Labor characterizes the earnings of licensed nurses as "above average" (Bureau of Labor Statistics, 2003). Although there is documentation of the need or desire of some RNs for higher salaries (Kimball and O'Neil, 2002), other studies of RNs find a lack of substantial dissatisfaction with their salaries (GAO, 2001a). Of 13,471 RNs surveyed in Pennsylvania, 57 percent reported their salaries were adequate (Aiken et al., 2001b). Only 26 percent of a national random sample of nurses identified "not making enough money" as a great concern when reflecting on their own experience (Kaiser Family Foundation and Harvard School of Public Health, 1999). The average annual salary in 2000 for RNs employed full time in their principal position was $46,782, although this figure varied by setting of care and position. RNs working full-time in hospitals[5] earned on average about $47,759 per year, while those working in nursing homes earned less—about $43,779 per year. In contrast to nurses working in administrative, research, or educational positions, staff nurses providing di-

---

[5]This included nurses in administrative positions as well as nurses providing direct patient care.

rect care to patients (the majority of employed nurses) earned an average of $42,133 annually in 2000 (Spratley et al. 2000). These salaries, when adjusted for inflation, have not changed greatly since the 1980s (Health Resources and Services Administration, 2002). However, recent data indicate that hospital nurses received base salary increases of approximately 8 percent in 2002 (Bolster and Hawthorne, 2003). LPNs/LVNs are paid, on average, about two-thirds of what RNs in staff positions earn (Bureau of Labor Statistics, undated).

Many NAs, in contrast, are among the working poor. In particular, NAs working in nursing homes and home care are much more likely than other workers to live below the poverty level, to be uninsured, and to receive public benefits such as food stamps and Medicaid. A U.S. General Accounting Office (GAO) analysis of 1998, 1999, and 2000 data from the Current Population Survey (CPS) of the U.S. Census Bureau and the Bureau of Labor Statistics found that the average wages of full-time, full-year NAs in hospitals, nursing homes, and home health care agencies ranged from $19,216 to $21,432. These wages place 17.8 percent, 18.8 percent, and 8.1 percent of NAs working in nursing homes, home health care, and hospitals, respectively, at or below the federal poverty level. Additionally, 13.5 percent, 14.8 percent, and 5.3 percent, respectively, receive food stamps, while 25.0, 32.1, and 14.2 percent, respectively, are uninsured (GAO, 2001b). The stresses and distractions caused by their poverty, insurance status, and related conditions undoubtedly have an adverse effect on these workers' ability to provide maximal attention to work requirements and adapt to new workplace practices.

RNs Employed as "Contingent Workers"

"Contingent workers" are those who provide their services to an organization on a short-term or periodic basis. They include temporary staff, independent contractors, and seasonal hires (Rousseau and Libuser, 1997). In 2000, only 2 percent of RNs working in their principal nursing position did so through a temporary employment service; most were employed by the organization in which they worked. However, this 2 percent represented a 36 percent increase over that reported in 1996 and reversed a declining trend observed between 1988 and 1996. Further, in 2000 an additional 71,490 RNs reported working through temporary service agencies in positions that were in addition to their principal positions. Taken together, the total number of nurses employed through a temporary employment service was 110,994—a 65.6 percent increase over 1996 and considerably higher than 1988 and 1992 estimates (Spratley et al., 2000).

It is not clear whether this one-time measurement indicates a trend in nursing; the proportion is close to that observed nationally across all industries, where contingent workers constitute 3 percent of the workforce. The national use of contingent workers in all employment settings has remained relatively stable since the mid-1990s (Employment Policy Foundation, 2000). However, a 2001 survey of nurse executives in 693 acute care U.S. hospitals found that temporary staff or travelers were used by 54 percent of the respondents to fill vacancies (The HSM Group, 2002). Moreover, a 1997 survey of 187 employers of nurses in the District of Columbia found that 9.6 percent of hospital nursing staff were not hospital employees, but secured through nurse staffing agencies (Mailey et al., 2000). If the present high rate of vacancies in nursing positions (discussed below) continues, use of contingent workers may persist or even increase. Furthermore, the proportion of NAs who are employed by temporary agencies may be higher than the corresponding proportion of RNs: 35 percent of NAs report working in positions other than hospitals, home health agencies, and nursing homes; this large category of "other" includes temporary staffing agencies (GAO, 2001b).

Although use of temporary employees can increase the number of nurses available to care for patients, it can also represent a threat to patient safety because these temporary staff are unfamiliar with a nursing unit and an HCO's overall structure, policies, and practices. Temporary employees are less familiar with an organization's information systems, patient care technology, facility layout, critical pathways, interdependency among work components, ways of coordinating and managing its work, and other work elements. Permanent nursing staff in hospitals and nursing homes describe the use of agency nurses as hindering continuity of care and reducing quality of care (Anderson et al., 1996; Bowers et al., 2000).

These subjective impressions are supported by some objective analyses of patient safety indicators. Medication errors have been shown to increase with the number of shifts worked by temporary nursing staff and to decrease when permanent staff work overtime to ensure adequate staffing (Roseman and Booker, 1995). An observational cohort study in eight hospital intensive care units (ICUs) participating in the Centers for Disease Control and Prevention's National Nosocomial Infections Surveillance System found that, after controlling for other risk factors, care by a "float" RN for more than 60 percent of central line days was independently associated with an increased risk for central line–associated blood-stream infections, and the risk increased in proportion to "float" days of care (Jackson et al., 2002). These observations in health care are consistent with those made regarding the use of contingent workers in other industries. The latter studies have found that increased use of contingent workers results in higher accident rates due to decreasing familiarity with on-site personnel and equipment, undercuts teamwork, and impairs communication. It also is associated with poor labor–management relations when contingent workers are used in an attempt to bypass labor–management conflicts (Rousseau and Libuser, 1997). The International Atomic Energy Agency cites use of contract personnel to replace traditionally hired employees as a symptom of incipient weakness in an organization's safety culture. While hiring contract personnel has some benefits to the employer, it often comes at the expense of safety—either directly as a result of lower contractor standards or indirectly as a result of effects on permanent employees (Carnino, undated).

WHERE NURSES WORK[6]

RNs, LPNs/LVNs, and NAs are employed in a wide variety of inpatient, home health, and ambulatory HCOs. Many of these organizations have undergone turbulent changes in response to the rapid evolution of the U.S. health care system over the last 20 years. The relationships between these organizations and their nurse employees have been turbulent as well. Many of these HCOs report large vacancies in nursing positions and serious difficulties in securing enough nursing staff to care for patients.

Wide Variety of Health Care Settings for Nursing Staff

While RNs are employed primarily in hospitals (see Table 3-1), LPNs/LVNs are about equally employed in hospitals and nursing homes (28 and 29 percent, respectively). Another 14 percent of LPNs/LVNs work in physicians' offices and clinics (Bureau of Labor Statistics, undated). Nursing homes employ the largest proportion of NAs (see Table 3-2). The populations served in these settings have some differences in their health care needs. These differences, changes in the U.S. health care system, and changes in the ways nursing care is delivered have shaped all nurses' work environments, but especially hospitals, nursing homes, home care and community-based organizations, and public health agencies.

Hospitals

Hospitals have historically been the largest employer of the nursing workforce and continue to be so today, although there has been a decline in

---

[6]Licensed nurses function in a variety of capacities in a diverse array of locations, including serving as educators, researchers, managers, lawyers, public policy analysts, and government officials. In this section and the next, we do not describe all nursing roles, but focus on those nurses who provide direct clinical care to patients within HCOs (often referred to as "staff nurses") and their supervisors. Chapter 4 addresses some aspects of the work of nurse managers and nurse executives in HCOs.

TABLE 3-1 Primary Employment Settings of RNs Employed in Nursing, 2000

Location	Percent of RNs Employed
Hospital	59.1
Community/public health setting	12.8
Ambulatory care	9.5
Nursing home/extended care facility	6.9
Student health service	3.8
Insurance/claims/benefits	2.3
Nursing education	2.1
Occupational health	1.7
Other	0.8
Planning/licensing agency	0.5
Unknown	0.4
TOTAL	99.9[a]

[a]Total not equal to 100 percent because of rounding.
SOURCE: Spratley et al. (2000).

the last two decades. The proportion of the RN workforce employed in hospitals peaked in 1984 at approximately 68 percent. By 2000 the proportion had declined to 59 percent as the result of a shift in care and nurse employment to noninstitutional settings (Spratley et al., 2000). Most hospital nurses work on inpatient units; 53.7 percent of hospital RNs work in ICUs, step-down/transitional units, or general/specialty bed units (see Table 3-3) (Spratley et al., 2000). The deployment of nurses by hospitals has changed dramatically over the least two decades as hospitals themselves have changed.

TABLE 3-2 Employment Settings of NAs, 1999

Location	Percent of NAs Employed
Nursing home	32
Hospital	18
Home health	16
Other[a]	35

[a]Includes a range of employment settings, such as residential care, social services, and temporary staffing agencies.
SOURCE: GAO (2001b).

TABLE 3-3   Types of Work Units in Which Hospital-Employed RNs
Spend More Than Half of Their Direct Patient Care Time

Type of Work Unit	Percent of RNs Employed
General/specialty bed unit	30.9
Intensive care unit (ICU)	16.9
Operating room	9.0
Labor/delivery	8.2
Emergency department	7.9
Step-down/transition from ICU	5.9
Outpatient department	5.8
Post-anesthesia recovery room	3.1
Other area	2.5
No specific area	1.8
Not known	8.0
TOTAL	100

SOURCE: Spratley et al. (2000).

Fewer hospitals, fewer inpatient beds, and fewer (but more acutely ill) inpatients   In the last two decades, hospitals have been under tremendous pressure to remain financially solvent in the face of a widely acknowledged oversupply of hospital beds, cost-containment measures resulting in changes in reimbursement from public and private payors, and demands for greater accountability for the quality of the care they provide. Between 1980 and 2000, the number of hospitals in the United States declined by 17 percent, the number of hospital beds by 28 percent, the number of hospital admissions by 10 percent, and the average length of patients' hospital stays from 7.6 to 5.8 days (American Hospital Association, 2002).[7] Over about the same period, outpatient visits increased by more than 150 percent. By 1999, outpatient surgery constituted 50 percent of all hospital-based surgery—an increase from 16 percent in 1980 (American Hospital Association and The Lewin Group, 2001). As a result of this downsizing and technological advances in care, patients admitted to the hospital today are more acutely ill than was the case in the previous decade (Medicare Payment Advisory Commission, 2001).

---

[7]In 1999 and 2000, hospital days of care increased. It is not yet known whether this increase signals the beginning of a predicted increase in hospital utilization accompanying the aging of the U.S. population or is just a temporary phenomenon (American Hospital Association and The Lewin Group, 2001).

During this same period, the number of RNs working in hospitals increased substantially,[8] although this increase was not uniform across all hospitals (Unruh, 2002), and not all of it should be assumed to represent an increase in RNs providing direct patient care. Data also indicate that many of the above downsizing initiatives were accompanied by reductions in unlicensed support staff, such as NAs (Aiken et al., 1996). These changes were accompanied by changes in the ways nurses deliver care to patients and have been perceived as leading to an increased workload for nurses (as discussed further below).

Changes in approaches to care delivery   As described in Chapter 1, many hospitals attempting to respond to the pressures of the last two decades have undertaken efforts to reengineer or redesign patient care processes to make them more efficient. Because nurses are the largest category of hospital workers, these reengineering efforts have often involved changing the ways in which nursing care is provided—typically through personnel reductions; cross-training of personnel to perform additional duties; changes in the mix of nursing staff (RNs, LPNs/LVNs, NAs); reassignment of support services (e.g., laboratory, radiology) to nursing units; redistribution of patients across nursing units; redesign of patient care processes; use of clinical pathways; and other changes in organization structure, decision-making processes, and responsibilities of management and patient care staff (Aiken et al., 2000b; Norrish and Rundall, 2001; Ritter-Teitel, 2002; Walston et al., 2000; Walston and Kimberly, 1997).

In addition, redesign and reengineering have changed the way nursing staff are organized to provide patient care. Restructuring initiatives often have been marked by a departure from primary nursing and a return to variants of team nursing (Norrish and Rundall, 2001). As initially conceptualized, the latter approach involved a team of RNs, LPNs/LVNs, and NAs, with an RN serving as the team leader. The RN team leader determined assignments for team members consistent with their abilities and performed activities for which other team members were not qualified. At a daily team conference led by the team leader, patient care plans were reviewed. Ideally, the same team was assigned to care for the same group of patients each day. In practice, however, teams might include only a single RN. While team nursing was designed in part to make the most efficient use

---

[8]According to the 1980 National Sample Survey of RNs, 835,647 RNs were working in hospitals (information provided verbally by Marshall Fritz, HRSA, DHHS, May 16, 2003). The corresponding figure in the 2000 survey was 1,300,323 (Spratley et al., 2000)—a 56 percent increase.

of RNs, it was criticized both for being overly task oriented and for resulting in fragmentation of care (Mark, 2002).[9]

Partly in response to this fragmentation of care, primary nursing became popular in the 1970s. This model of care delivery is characterized by the establishment of a direct relationship between an RN and a patient (Pontin, 1999). The patient's primary nurse is responsible for all aspects of the patient's care, 24 hours a day, during the entire course of the hospitalization. This is achieved through a 24-hour plan of care created and implemented by the primary nurse, along with the use of associate nurses who care for the patient according to the plan in the absence of the primary nurse. Although primary nursing was not intended to require an all-RN staff, it was often interpreted in this way. The approach was viewed favorably by nursing staff because it emphasized the nurse–patient relationship and was perceived as most consistent with the practice of professional nursing (Norrish and Rundall, 2001).

Primary nursing still is often cited as the best way of organizing nursing care, although research on the effects of primary nursing has been hindered by the lack of a clear conceptual model (Pontin, 1999), and studies to date comparing team and primary nursing have had significant methodological weaknesses and yielded only equivocal results (Mark, 2002). Moreover, some now assert that the question of which model is best is moot. Because levels of nursing expertise, support personnel, patient acuity and needs, and resources vary across nursing units, it is likely that the best nursing model in one unit is not the best for another. For example, a nursing unit with a high proportion of novice nurses is more likely to require a care delivery model that affords higher levels of clinical nursing supervision, such as a modified team approach, than a unit whose staff is stable and possesses higher levels of expertise. According to this view, care delivery models tailored to each nursing unit's structures, processes, and resources are most desirable (Deutschendorf, 2003).

Changes in workload   Nurses in hospitals also report increasing workload as a result of the above changes (Aiken et al., 2001b; Hurley, 2000), and some have linked this increased workload to diminished patient safety (Kimball and O'Neil, 2002; Service Employees International Union, 2001; Sochalski, 2001). Nurses' workload is discussed most often in terms of the number of patients assigned to each nurse (see also the discussion of staffing levels in Chapter 5). In numerous surveys, nurses report inadequate

---

[9]Team nursing was preceded by "functional nursing," popular in the 1940s. Under the latter approach, patient care was organized like an assembly line; that is, one nurse was assigned to give baths, another to administer medications, another to do dressings and treatments, and so on (Mark, 2002).

numbers of nursing staff to accomplish their work (Kaiser Family Foundation and Harvard School of Public Health, 1999) and provide high-quality care (Aiken et al., 2001b). Although evidence indicates that nurses' perceptions of staffing adequacy can be influenced by structural characteristics of hospitals and units, such as the number of beds in a nursing unit and higher levels of patient technology (Mark et al., 2002), the hospital industry itself reports difficulties in securing the number of RNs it needs to care for patients (AHA Commission on Workforce for Hospitals and Health Systems, 2002; American Organization of Nurse Executives, 2000; JCAHO, 2002). Emergency room diversions, closures of nursing units, cancellation of elective surgeries, and other restrictions on service delivery have been documented as resulting from insufficient nurse staffing (First Consulting Group, 2001; Kimball and O'Neil, 2002; The HSM Group, 2002).

Staffing levels have been shown to vary considerably by hospital (Unruh, 2002). This variation is illustrated by data for 1998–2000 from the California Nursing Outcomes Coalition, which maintains a statewide database of nurse staffing levels from California hospitals. Although these data constitute a convenience sample of 52 California hospitals voluntarily contributing staffing data, the data are useful because they were collected at the level of the nursing unit (as opposed to the aggregate hospital level), because common data definitions and reporting were used, and because ongoing verification was performed to ensure the data's accuracy. Data reported on 330 critical care, step-down, and medical–surgical units in these hospitals across nine calendar quarters revealed that RNs provided 92 percent of the care in ICUs, 87 percent of the care in step-down units, and 57 percent of the care in medical–surgical units. The RN–patient ratios across these facilities were as follows:

- ICUs—a range of 0.5–5.3 patients for each RN (average 1.6)
- Step-down units—a range of 1.5–11.6 patients for each RN (average 4.2)
- Medical–surgical units—a range of 2.7–13.8 patients for each RN (average 5.9)

These findings did not vary over the nine quarters or by the size of the hospital (Donaldson et al., 2001).

Data from a fiscal year 2002 national convenience sample survey of hospitals on staffing, scheduling, and workforce management of nursing department employees further document this variation in staffing levels. The 135 hospitals responding showed variation in nurse staffing levels even with the shift and type of patient care unit being held constant. Although the average RN-to-patient ratio in medical–surgical units on the day shift was 1:6, the range was from 1:3 to 1:12. Twenty-three percent of hospitals reported that nurses in their medical–surgical units on the day shift were each responsible for caring for between 7 and 12 patients. On the night shift, 7 patients on average were assigned to each nurse, but 34 percent of hospitals reported between 8 and 12 patients assigned to each nurse. For critical care units, the average number of patients assigned to each nurse was 2 for both the day and the night shifts, but 7.4 percent of hospitals reported having nurses care for 3 or 4 ICU patients during the day shift, and 11 percent reported nurses caring for 3 or 4 ICU patients during the night shift (Cavouras and Suby, 2003).

In addition to staffing levels, work environment factors that have been identified as affecting nurse workload include RN expertise, patient acuity, patient turnover, physician availability, work intensity, unit physical layout, degree of teamwork, and available support staff (Pinkerton and Rivers, 2001; Salyer, 1995; Seago, 2002). Many of these factors also have been affected by hospital reengineering and redesign initiatives. Workload factors for which there is a strong evidence base with regard to their effects on patient safety, as well as strategies for modifying the work environment to address these factors, are examined in the succeeding chapters of this report.

Nursing Homes

As patients move more quickly through acute inpatient settings or undergo complex procedures in outpatient settings, their needs for long-term care follow-up escalate. Further, as older adults increasingly constitute a larger proportion of the U.S. population, there is a concomitant increased demand for services for older patients who have higher dependency needs. As a result, nursing homes (sometimes called long-term care or nursing facilities) and the populations they serve have changed significantly in recent years.

Like hospitals, nursing homes are seeing an increase in the dependency and acuity levels of their residents (as described in Chapter 1) and an expansion of the nursing facility workforce. In contrast to hospitals, however, there has been an increase in the number of nursing homes and nursing home beds. Between 1987 and 1996, the number of nursing home beds in the United States increased by 19 percent, from 1.48 to 1.76 million, reflecting in part a 20 percent increase in the number of nursing homes nationwide (from 14,050 to 16,480) (CMS, 2000, 2002). During this period, the percentage of nursing home patients whose care was paid for by Medicare increased from 3 to 9 percent, and the proportion of nursing homes certified to receive Medicare reimbursement increased from 28 to 73 percent, indicating that the number of nursing facilities planning to take residents with more acute illness or more complex needs rose substantially.

Concurrently, the number of nursing home residents over age 85 increased from 49 to 56 percent for women and from 29 to 33 percent for men (Rhoades and Krauss, 2001).

Caring for individuals in nursing homes also involves some other special safety considerations. For many nursing home residents, the nursing facility is the home where they live as well as where they receive services. Patient safety in these facilities therefore requires consideration of patients' long-term living environment, as well as their clinical care needs. Further, many long-term care clients have some degree of cognitive impairment. Data from the 1996 Nursing Home Component of the Medical Expenditure Panel Survey (MEPS) revealed that nearly three-quarters (70.8 percent) of nursing home residents had some form of memory loss. About the same proportion had problems with orientation, such as knowing where they were or the identity of staff members. Many residents (80.6 percent) had difficulties in making daily decisions, and almost one-third (30.2 percent) exhibited at least one form of inappropriate or dangerous behavior—including wandering off or resisting care (12.5 percent). Overall, nearly half of all nursing home residents had some type of dementia. These conditions make residents less able to participate in increasing their own safety, and in fact can cause behaviors that create their own threats to safety. Forgetfulness and disorientation in particular can be dangerous problems, requiring 24-hour supervision to provide for an individual's safety and well-being (Krauss and Altman, 1998).

This increase in resident dependency and acuity has important implications for staffing, oversight, work complexity, workload, and the overall nature of the work in nursing facilities. For example, the staff time required to meet basic needs of residents (such as feeding, toileting, and ambulation) increases with the overall dependency levels of residents (CMS, 2002). Further, since Medicare residents often have complex health conditions or are recovering from serious health events, a more sophisticated knowledge base is required to care for these residents, as are higher levels of vigilance and monitoring and of professional staffing. Consistent with this observation, a higher ratio of RN staff to residents in nursing homes has been demonstrated to reduce adverse health care events for residents (CMS, 2000, 2002).

Along with the growth in the number of nursing homes, nursing home beds, and patient acuity has come a significant expansion of the nursing home workforce. There has been not only an overall increase in the total number of workers to care for the increased population of residents, but also an increase in the ratio of all categories of nursing staff to residents (CMS, 2000). This increase is attributable in large part to the passage of the Nursing Home Reform Act in 1987, which mandated coverage by at least one RN for 8 hours a day, 7 days a week for all nursing homes accepting

Medicare or Medicaid reimbursement. Additional legislation required facilities to have a licensed nurse (RN or LPN/LVN) on duty at all times. As discussed in Chapter 5, however, evidence indicates that levels of staffing above these minimums are necessary to ensure an adequate level of patient safety.

NAs make up 60–70 percent of the total nursing staff in nursing facilities. They spend the most time with residents and provide 80–90 percent of direct patient care, working under the supervision of RNs and LPNs/LVNs (CMS, 2000; GAO, 2001a). LPNs/LVNs constitute approximately 25–30 percent of all nursing staff and approximately two-thirds of licensed nursing staff. RNs represent the smallest proportion—10–15 percent—of nursing staff in nursing facilities (CMS, 2000). In contrast to the hospital setting, physicians are less frequently on site in nursing homes.

There has also been an increase in the percentage of nursing homes that are large for-profit chains or networks of not-for-profit facilities, as opposed to being individually owned. The significance of this shift is unclear. However, a 1998 national study of 13,693 nursing homes[10] comparing those owned by investors with nonprofit and public nursing facilities found higher rates of deficiencies in the quality of care provided and lower staffing levels among the former. Chain ownership also was found to be associated with higher rates of deficiencies in quality of care. In both instances, the analysis adjusted for case mix, location, percentage of patients covered by Medicaid, whether the facility was hospital based, and whether it served only Medicare residents (Harrington et al., 2001, 2002).

Home Care and Community-Based Organizations

Home care and community-based organizations encompass a wide variety of noninstitutional long-term care settings, ranging from an individual's own home to various types of congregate living arrangements. The boundaries between institutional and noninstitutional care settings are blurring, however. Many assisted-living "board and care" facilities are large buildings that resemble nursing facilities. Other residential care sites are small and homey. In contrast to nursing homes, which are licensed and regulated by the federal government as a condition of Medicare and Medicaid reimbursement, residential care facilities are generally licensed and regulated by states and local jurisdictions. Consequently, there is no single definition of "residential care" or tally of the number of such facilities nationwide. A 1999 national study counted 11,472 assisted-living facilities

---

[10]Of the 15,401 facilities in the federal database of nursing facilities, the study excluded those with fewer than 16 beds, those reporting implausible staffing levels, and those with duplicate records.

with approximately 650,500 beds. Other community-based long term-care settings include adult day care programs, in which disabled elderly individuals receive supervision, personal care, and social integration in a group setting, usually during the work week and normal work hours (Stone and Wiener, 2001).

Home health care was the fastest-growing employment setting for all nursing personnel throughout the 1980s and 1990s (Buerhaus and Staiger, 1999). As of 2001, there were more than 20,000 home care agencies, approximately 7,000 of which were Medicare-certified. Free-standing, for-profit agencies represented 40 percent of that total and experienced the greatest growth. Hospital-based agencies made up another 30 percent of the total.

These free-standing and facility-based (usually hospital-based) Medicare-certified agencies, home care aide organizations, and hospices employ licensed nursing staff (as well as physical, occupational, and speech therapists) to provide such skilled services as illness management, medication management, infusion therapy, wound care, ostomy instruction, and end-of-life care to clients in their homes and other locations. Licensed home care nurses also supervise home care aides who provide such personal care services as assistance with bathing, eating, and ambulation, as well as monitoring of vital signs and patient status. NAs make up 54 percent of the nursing personnel working in home health care (GAO, 2001b).

The home care industry has experienced substantial turbulence. Since the 1960s, the National Association for Home Care (the home care industry association) has documented periods of rapid expansion and decline in the numbers of home care agencies (National Association for Home Care, 2001). In particular, the Balanced Budget Act of 1997 changed the way the Medicare program pays Medicare-certified home health agencies from a cost-based method to a prospective payment system of fixed, predetermined rates. Subsequently, the number of Medicare-certified home health agencies decreased by 32 percent—from 10,556 in 1997 to 7,715 in 2000 (Office of Inspector General, 2001). As with nursing home care, however, demands for home health services are expected to continue to grow because of reduced lengths of stay in acute care hospitals, advances in technology, and the aging of the U.S. population.

Public Health Agencies

Public health agencies comprise state, county, and local health departments that provide such health care services as immunizations, health education, case management for frail elders, and community assessment. All states have a public health structure and staff at the state level; some also have such a structure and staff in all counties or regions. Although many cities still have local health departments, the trend is toward decreasing duplication and cost by merging city and county units (Martin, 2002). RNs employed in public health and community health settings increased by 155 percent between 1980 and 2000 (Spratley et al., 2000).

During the 1990s, various factors, such as substance abuse and its impact on high-risk pregnancies and newborns and the incidence of HIV/AIDS, stimulated growth in the public health sector and caused these agencies to reassess their mission and purpose. An earlier IOM study found that the public health system was in disarray and incapable of fulfilling the fundamental core functions of assessment, policy development, and assurance (IOM, 1988). Following the events of September 11, 2001, and associated concerns about bioterrorism, the public health infrastructure began receiving additional attention.

Problems with Recruitment and Retention of Nursing Staff Across Clinical Settings

Hospitals, nursing homes, home health agencies, and other community-based long-term care organizations all report difficulties in securing enough RNs and NAs to provide needed patient care (AHA Commission on Workforce for Hospitals and Health Systems, 2002; GAO, 2001b; Stone and Wiener, 2001). For 2001, the American Organization of Nurse Executives (AONE) reported nationwide hospital RN vacancy rates[11] of 10.2 percent, with the highest rates being in critical (14.6 percent), medical–surgical (14.1 percent), and emergency room (11.7 percent) care (The HSM Group, 2002). Similarly, an AHCA national survey of long-term care facilities found vacancy rates of 18.5 percent for staff RNs, 14.6 percent for LPNs/LVNs, and 12 percent for NAs (AHCA, 2002). Some have expressed the view that this inability to attract and retain a sufficient number of nurses is the result of inhospitable working conditions. Others assert that, while work conditions may not be favorable, recruitment problems are due to an underlying shortage of nursing personnel. Evidence indicates that both factors are at work.

A Nationwide Nursing Shortage

The national employment of RNs per capita and the national unemployment rate for RNs have both declined. The national unemployment rate for RNs in 2000 (1.0 percent) was at its lowest level in more than a decade. At the same time, total employment of RNs declined by 2 percent

---

[11]The vacancy rate is calculated as the average number of vacant full-time equivalent (FTE) positions divided by the average number of budgeted FTE positions.

between 1996 and 2000, reversing steady increases since 1980 (GAO, 2001a). Data provided by the Health Resources and Services Administration (HRSA), the federal agency responsible for providing information and analysis on the supply of and demand for health professionals, show that this decline reflects a present and growing discrepancy between the supply of and demand for RN services. HRSA estimates that a 6 percent undersupply (110,000) of nurses existed in 2000 and projects a growing shortfall in nursing personnel, up to a 29 percent deficit by 2020. This undersupply of RNs is more the result of a growing demand for nursing than of a decreasing supply of RNs (HRSA, 2002).

Although the supply of RNs will grow, this growth will be limited by the aging of the RN workforce discussed previously and declining enrollments in nursing schools. Since 1973 there has been an approximately 40 percent drop in the percentage of college freshman who indicate that nursing is among their top career choices. The most prominent factor contributing to this decline appears to be the expansion of opportunities for women in formerly male-dominated professions, such as medicine, law, and business (Staiger et al., 2000). For example, in 1971–1972, women comprised 13.7 percent of the entering class of U.S. medical schools; in 2001–2002, they comprised 47.8 percent (Barzansky and Etzel, 2002).

The higher demand for nurses will be fueled by a projected 18 percent growth in the U.S. population between 2000 and 2020 and a 65 percent growth in those over age 65, who require a disproportionately larger share of health care services (HRSA, 2002). This workforce deficit is not unique to the United States; similar data from other countries indicate a global shortage of nurses (Buchan, 2002).

A similar shortage of NAs also has been documented (GAO, 2001b; Stone and Wiener, 2001), and the demographic changes cited above are predicted to worsen that shortage. With the aging of the population, the demand for NAs is predicted to increase greatly; however, the available supply is expected to increase much less. Between 2000 and 2030, the number of persons over age 85—those most in need of NA services—will more than double from 4.3 million to 8.9 million. At the same time, the population of women aged 20–54—the traditional pool of NAs—will increase by only 9 percent. The ratio of women aged 20–54 to the population aged 85 and older (sometimes referred to as the "elderly support ratio") will decline from 16.1 in 2000 to 8.5 in 2030 (GAO, 2001b).

Working Conditions That Discourage Nursing Staff from Remaining in the Workforce

The difficulties HCOs are having in attracting and retaining nursing staff are also linked to those individuals' dissatisfaction with their work environment. According to GAO (2001a:13), "Efforts undertaken to improve the workplace environment may both reduce the likelihood of nurses leaving the field and encourage more young people to enter the nursing profession."

Numerous surveys indicate the dissatisfaction of nursing staff with their work conditions (Aiken et al., 2001b; ANA, 2001; Spratley et al., 2000). Sources of that dissatisfaction include inadequate staffing to perform the work, heavy workloads, increased overtime, lack of sufficient support staff (GAO, 2001a), and the resulting stress (ANA, 2001). In the 2000 NSSRN, just 69.5 percent of all RNs reported being satisfied in their current position. Satisfaction levels varied by place of employment. Nurses working in hospitals and nursing homes reported the lowest levels of satisfaction—67 and 65 percent, respectively. Staff nurses (as opposed to nurses in administrative or management positions) consistently reported the lowest levels of satisfaction across hospital, nursing home, ambulatory care, and public/ community health settings. This level of satisfaction is significantly lower than that seen in the general employed U.S. population. Data from the General Social Survey of the National Opinion Research Center indicate that from 1986 through 1996, 85 percent of workers in general and 90 percent of professional workers expressed satisfaction with their job (as cited by Spratley et al., 2000).

This dissatisfaction is linked to the departure of RNs from the nursing workforce. In an Internet survey of RNs conducted by the American Nurses Association (ANA) in 2001, 75.8 percent of 4,826 self-selected nurse respondents stated that concerns about their personal health and safety resulting from their work environment affected their decisions about the kind of nursing work they did and their continued practice as nurses (ANA, 2001). In a survey of 50 percent of RNs working in acute care hospitals in Pennsylvania between 1998 and 1999, 41 percent reported being dissatisfied with their jobs. Only 33–34 percent of nurses reported that there were enough RNs to provide quality care and enough staff to get the work done; only 29 percent reported that their administration listened and responded to nurses' concerns; and a minority of 43 percent reported having enough support services. Not surprisingly, 43 percent also had high scores on a well-validated and widely used tool for measuring levels of employee burnout, and 22.7 percent reported plans to leave their job within the next year. Of nurses younger than age 30, 33 percent stated their intent to leave their present job within the year (Aiken et al., 2001b).

The work environment of NAs also is highly stressful. NAs' work is physically demanding, often requiring them to provide partial weight-bearing support to help feeble individuals turn in bed, sit, transfer from bed to chair, stand, and walk. They spend long hours on their feet and bathing, dressing, feeding, and toileting patients who may be disoriented or otherwise cognitively impaired and uncooperative in their own care. In 1999, the occupational injury rate for nursing home employees was 13 injuries per 100 employees, compared with 8 injuries per 100 employees for construction workers (GAO, 2001b). Heavy workloads, poor supervision, low wages and benefits, lack of involvement in work-related decisions, and a job that society holds in low regard cause significant stress among the NA workforce and contribute to difficulties in recruitment and retention of NAs in nursing homes, home health care agencies, and other long-term care settings (Parsons et al., 2003; Stone and Wiener, 2001). Evidence indicates that such stress contributes to errors in health care delivery (Campbell and Cornett, 2002).

WHAT NURSES DO

The work of direct-care nursing staff includes both visible and invisible activities (Star and Strauss, 1999). The visible activities are those physical actions observable by patients and others and often portrayed in the media, such as assisting a patient to walk, administering medications and treatments, and educating patients about their disease and therapies. The invisible or cognitive work incorporates knowledge learned from formal education and subsequently acquired expertise. It includes such processes as assessing a patient's health condition, monitoring and detecting when a change in therapy is needed, and integrating an individual patient's health care needs with the interventions of a variety of different health care providers to formulate a plan of care tailored to the particular patient. While certain assessment, monitoring, and care planning actions may be visible (e.g., a nurse watching a cardiac monitor or listening to a patient's chest), these cognitive processes are not. Often when a nurse appears to be carrying out a visible activity, such as bathing a patient, he or she is actually performing numerous invisible tasks, such as assessing the patient's skin color for evidence of poor oxygenation, evaluating skin integrity for signs of skin breakdown, engaging the patient in conversation to assess mental status, or educating the patient about his or her disease and its management.

These visible and invisible nursing activities are performed by all RNs, LPNs/LVNs, and NAs in all settings of care. The specific activities performed by a particular nurse depend on patient needs, the nurse's education and expertise, the setting of care in which the nurse practices, how nursing care services are organized and delivered within that setting of care, and the nurse's licensure status and scope of permitted practice as delineated in state licensure laws.

There is not always agreement across HCOs and even across nursing units within an HCO about whether less complex activities, such as bathing a patient or taking vital signs, should be performed by RNs or NAs (McCloskey et al., 1996; Pedersen, 1997). While NAs are clearly trained and competent to perform these activities, removing RNs from performing them may diminish the RNs' opportunities to simultaneously monitor other aspects of patient status, such as color, character of breathing, mental status, and manifestations of pain. Use of NAs to perform these less complex activities has been cited as creating opportunities for gaps and discontinuities in care (Cook et al., 2000). Available evidence is unclear as to whether assigning routine tasks to lower-skilled nursing staff enhances patient safety by allowing RNs to concentrate on tasks requiring more knowledge, or separating the RN from the patient while routine tasks are being performed results in greater opportunities for critical changes in patient condition to go unnoticed, unreported, or addressed less effectively.

There is agreement, however, that the preponderance of critical thinking and other cognitively complex work is in the domain of the RN. These cognitive processes are taught to every RN student in nursing school, using as a template the six components of clinical nursing practice: assessing, diagnosing, identifying outcomes, planning, implementing, and evaluating. This cyclical, interactive method of thinking forms the foundation for clinical decision making by RNs (ANA, 1998).

Variety of Ways in Which Direct-Care Nursing Staff Provide Patient Care[12]

Direct-care nursing staff (i.e., those nurses providing hands-on patient care as opposed to nurses in administrative or educational positions) perform a variety of interventions when delivering patient care. These interventions are used to monitor patient status, administer physiologic therapies, help patients compensate for loss of function, provide emotional

---

[12]Information on the exact type and volume of activities and procedures performed by nurses and the frequency with which nurses perform them across different setting of care is limited. Although each patient's medical diagnoses and procedures performed by physicians are recorded and aggregated for all inpatient and outpatient visits and admissions through the standardized Health Care Financing Administration 1500 and UB 92 reimbursement claim forms, similar data on nursing care are not collected on these reimbursement forms or through other mechanisms. The information presented in this section on what nurses do was synthesized from theoretical descriptions of the art and science of nursing, surveys of nursing personnel (such as the national Council of State Boards of Nursing's triannual surveys of newly licensed nurses and interim annual surveys of newly licensed nurses and other parties), observational studies, health services research that includes descriptions of nursing work as part of its methodology, work sampling studies conducted within individual nursing units, and a prominent initiative to develop a comprehensive standardized classification of interventions performed by nurses—the Nursing Intervention Classification project.

support, and educate patients and families. Nursing staff perform these basic functions in all care delivery settings in which they practice. While some of these direct patient care activities implement treatments ordered by physicians, a substantial amount of nursing care is not provided in response to a physician's treatment order, but is performed independently by nurses based on nursing's professional practice standards and the nurse's clinical judgment. In addition, nursing staff perform a variety of indirect-care functions, such as documenting patient care, integrating care across settings and providers (discussed further below), and supervising other nursing staff.

RNs also are frequently required to carry out a variety of non-nursing activities, such as performing clerical tasks (e.g., transcribing physician orders); transporting blood products and laboratory specimens; and locating and retrieving patient care supplies, such as bed linens and medical equipment when these are not at hand. Time spent in these non-nursing activities prevents RNs from providing patient care.

Monitoring of Patient Status (Surveillance)

Monitoring of patient status (also called patient surveillance) encompasses the first four of the six components of the nursing process noted above: assessing the health condition of the patient, diagnosing patient needs, identifying desired outcomes, and planning for necessary remedial or enhancing therapeutic interventions. Surveillance differs from assessment in that an assessment is typically performed at a single point in time; for example, an initial assessment of health is often made upon hospital admission or at the time of first contact with a practitioner. In contrast, surveillance is defined as the "purposeful and *ongoing* acquisition, interpretation, and synthesis of patient data for clinical decision-making [emphasis added]" (McCloskey and Bulechek, 2000:629). While novice and other less experienced nurses may understand and rely upon the performance of assessment, diagnosis, outcome identification, and planning as sequential activities, nurses with greater expertise perform these cognitive processes concurrently, repeatedly, and in a back-and-forth manner as they size up a situation (Benner et al., 1999).

The goal of surveillance is the early identification and prevention of potential problems, which requires both behavioral and cognitive skills. When RNs perform surveillance, they typically use a variety of means to gather patient data, including direct inspection, palpation, percussion, and auscultation of the patient. They also use noninvasive and invasive patient monitoring devices to measure such patient status indicators as temperature, pulse, blood pressure, respiration, tissue oxygenation, blood electrolytes, cardiac function, intracranial pressure, and neurologic status. These monitoring devices, such as those for invasive hemodynamic monitoring, are becoming progressively more sophisticated and complex. As new and more powerful monitoring devices are invented, nurses are the personnel primarily responsible for their use in patient care.

The cognitive aspect of surveillance involves studying, interpreting, analyzing, and evaluating the data and information produced by the above methods. These cognitive processes require a high level of knowledge (Dougherty, 1999). When done well, surveillance leads to recognizing problems early, initiating actions to intervene, and preventing complications (see Box 3-1) (Benner et al., 1999). When surveillance is not done or done poorly, changes are not recognized early, complications or adverse events

---

BOX 3-1   The Benefits of RN Surveillance: A Case Example

The following excerpt from Benner et al. (1999:92–95) illustrates the vital role played by RNs' surveillance of patients in recognizing problems and preventing them from causing complications:

Rita was an unsuspecting patron at a local restaurant one evening. As she was leaving . . . a stranger ran after her . . . and stabbed her. . . . The blade passed through the left ventricle of her heart.

The restaurant was about four blocks from the hospital . . . and . . . was a gathering place for paramedics, firefighters, and police officers. . . . Rita got to our trauma center emergency department within about two minutes. . . . A few minutes later Rita was being wheeled down the hall toward the operating room, with three units of blood running, her chest already open and Dr. R doing open heart massage. . . . Rita survived the surgery and was in the intensive care unit the next afternoon when I arrived at work. My orientee (Anna) and I were assigned to care for Rita

. . . I . . . [took] hold of Rita's foot. It was warm. Her heart rate, rhythm, and blood pressure looked good. The ventilator gave her each breath with ease. A few drops of light red fluid trickled through the tube that drained her chest. There was clear light yellow urine in her drainage bag. "Well, Anna," I said, "Things are looking pretty good here."

Anna and I spent the first couple of hours tracking down each line and tube from end to end . . . taking note of what was running in and what was coming out. We checked each IV bag, and I explained what effects the different drugs were supposed to have and how to calculate the doses and IV rates. We zeroed and calibrated the pressure transducers, and I explained how to recognize the waveforms on the monitor, and how to make sure that the measurements we took were accurate. We evaluated the physical findings—lung sounds, heart sounds, pulses, skin color, and temperature, etc. When I looked at the monitor tracings

develop or progress, and the patient's health status is adversely affected—a phenomenon described as "failure to rescue" (see Chapter 1) (Silber et al., 1992).

As the case example in Box 3-1 shows and as physicians in the American College of Critical Care Medicine note:

Critical care nurses do the majority of patient assessment, evaluation, and care in the ICU . . . critical care nursing staff . . . spend several hours per patient per shift collecting and integrating information and incorporating it into meaningful patient care. Through their caring practices, they improve the ICU experi-

and the chest tube drainings, I could see that her heart was OK. The pericardium was not filling up with blood and there were no signs of tamponade. . . .

A short time later, while I was out of the room at the nurses desk, the ventilator alarm began to sound. I reached her bedside immediately and could see that all that was calm moments ago was in chaos now. "What's going on?" I thought. "Is she seizing?" Her head was lifted off the pillow with convulsive coughing. The needle on the pressure gauge was hitting the red zone and the high-pressure valve was venting with loud hiss with each breath the ventilator tried to give. But the motions were not really seizure-like. My mind was racing. . . . Is the ET tube blocked? No. Has the ET tube moved? Can't tell. What do the lungs sound like? Right side OK, LEFT SIDE NOTHING!! What's going on here?" . . . As I was taking her off the vent and connecting the Ambu bag I'm thinking, "No breath sounds on the left . . . could be the ET tube is in the right main stem." . . . It took both hands on the Ambu bag to force a breath through the ET tube. Rita was dusky and tachycardic and her neck looked funny. I reached over and palpated, her trachea was shifted way over to the right. . . .

I gave the Ambu bag to a respiratory therapist that had come in and said, "Anna . . . go get a Pleur-Evac, a couple of sizes of chest tubes, and a bottle of sterile water." I beeped . . . the resident on call. "Come to ICU stat." Dr T. called me back. . . . I said, "Get down here now. This lady with stab wound through her heart has no breath sounds on the left, we can hardly bag her, her trachea is deviated to the right, she's turning blue. . . ."

Dr T. arrived and . . . took the 18 gauge needle and stuck it in Rita's chest wall. . . . The Pleur-Evac was ready and Dr. T put the chest tube in. I listened to her lungs, "breath sounds both sides now." Rita's breathing was calmer, and we could put her back on the vent. . . . Things went smoothly for the rest of the evening.

ence for both patients and their families, and through their critical thinking skills, experienced nurses readily recognize clinical changes to prevent further deterioration on these patients. They are familiar with the complications that may be seen in these patients and attempt to prevent them (Brilli et al., 2001:2011).

A competent RN is able to assess and monitor a given patient's health status as compared to age-appropriate norms, baseline health status, and the expected effects of treatments using a variety of techniques and instruments in a systematic and ongoing manner (ANA, 1998). Newly licensed RNs report that they spend the greatest amount of time in patient assessment and evaluation (Smith and Crawford, 2003). A skilled NA, while not educated to assess normative health status across multiple dimensions of health using a variety of assessment tools and skills, is trained to monitor health status using basic devices that measure a more limited number of indicators, such as temperature, heart rate, and blood pressure. NAs also assess patient status based on their ongoing knowledge of the patient's "normal" health status. In this way, they serve as the foundation for the monitoring and surveillance system in nursing homes, and nurses are dependent upon NAs to bring abnormal findings to their attention. The low proportions of RN and LPN/LVN staff in most nursing homes means that NAs are the nursing staff in most frequent contact with patients and that they often possess information not available to anyone else in the nursing home (Henderson, 1994).

The one resource required by all types of nursing staff to perform patient monitoring is time (Dougherty, 1999). This also is the resource that many nursing staff identify as dangerously low, as a result of the high numbers of patients assigned to individual nursing staff.

Physiologic Therapy

Licensed nurses perform a wide array of interventions on patients to treat the physiological effects and mitigate the health consequences associated with a disease. The very broad spectrum of such therapies includes such interventions as managing the patency and functioning of artificial airways; changing dressings on traumatic wounds or surgical incision sites; providing care to women during childbirth; providing surgical assistance; participating in resuscitation activities during cardiac or respiratory failure; inserting intravenous, urinary, gastric, or other body catheters or tubes; providing bodily care to comatose patients, such as mouth care and range-of-motion exercise to prevent the formation of contractures; peritoneal dialysis; mechanical ventilation and weaning; and administration of medications and blood products (McCloskey and Bulechek, 2000).

As explained earlier, the exact types and frequency of interventions performed by nurses across different setting of care have not been quantified. However, it is consistently observed that administration of medication—oral, enteral, intrapleural, parenteral, topical, or through a ventricular reservoir (McCloskey and Bulechek, 2000)—is the most frequently performed physiologic therapeutic intervention (Bulechek et al., 1994).

Helping Patients Compensate for Loss of Functioning

Illness is accompanied by a loss of functioning with a variety of manifestations and with varying degrees of debilitation. Loss of functioning and resulting dependency can range from mild temporary weakness and malaise that accompanies the flu; to a temporary acute loss of strength and capacity to perform activities of daily living (ADLs) (i.e., bathing, dressing, eating, or other personal care activities) after major surgery; to a temporary inability to perform essential life functions, such as breathing, eating, or moving, as a result of more serious illnesses or injuries; to permanent disabilities, such as paralysis of extremities.

Most of the services provided by nursing staff in long-term care organizations (both institutional and home and community based) are designed to minimize, rehabilitate, or compensate for the loss of independent physical or mental functioning, and include assistance with basic ADLs (Stone and Wiener, 2001). An ethnographic report by an investigator who worked for 13 months as an NA to obtain an insider's view of NAs' work experiences found that NAs' day shift tasks can be categorized as follows: (1) getting patients in and out of bed; (2) providing food services, especially feeding; (3) checking patients for incontinence and making and cleaning beds; (4) shaving patients; (5) walking to and from the linen closet; (6) helping patients shower; and (7) performing miscellaneous tasks, such as rinsing dirty linen and fixing sinks. NAs spent the most time helping patients shower; followed closely by providing food services, and checking, making, and cleaning beds (Henderson, 1994).

More telling than the official tasks performed by NAs, however, is their unofficial work. For example, Henderson (1994) found that each aide knew a great deal about the personal habits of the residents, which allowed care to be individualized and rendered more efficiently. These details included such things as removing a napkin from the tray of a resident who could feed herself but was known to eat paper, or placing a juice glass on the left side of a tray to make the glass more visible and accessible to a stroke patient (Henderson, 1994).

RNs also perform these types of activities, as well as activities intended to prevent further deterioration (e.g., fall prevention)—typically when they are providing care to a hospitalized patient who has more acute health care needs. The extent to which these activities should be performed by RNs has been the subject of much discussion and has not been resolved in the health care literature (Kovner, 2001). Under the primary model of nursing care delivery discussed earlier in this chapter, an RN assigned to a patient provides total care for that patient, including bathing and ambulatory support. Under a team or functional nursing care approach, a mix of RNs and NAs coordinates their skill set in the provision of care to the patient.

Providing Emotional Support

Providing emotional support is recognized by nursing staff and patients as an essential part of nursing practice. Quality hospital nursing care has been described by patients as "accepting, empathetic, compassionate . . . and respectful," as well as technically competent (Miller, 1995:31). A survey of individual nurses in clinical practice conducted in 1992 to validate the content of the Nursing Interventions Classification (NIC) system and determine the frequency with which nurses performed each of 336 nursing interventions identified provision of emotional support as one of the six most frequently used nursing interventions and the one reported most often by nurses as being used in their patient care activities (Bulechek et al., 1994). Rather than a vague, intangible attitude, caring—showing kindness, preserving dignity, explaining with empathy, and being patient—is recognized as requiring actions that impose their own time requirements as illustrated in the case of Ana in Box 3-2.

Emotional support is a key feature of the care provided by NAs in a variety of long-term care settings (Stone and Wiener, 2001). Providing such support necessitates establishing, nurturing, and sustaining relationships with residents, as well as responding to and effectively managing disruptive, aggressive, or uncooperative resident behavior. Indeed, responding to aggressive residents has increasingly become an aspect of CNAs' work. In studies describing the epidemiology of workplace violence, NAs in long-term care facilities have been found to represent the occupation most at risk of workplace assault. NAs frequently are subjected to residents' hitting, scratching, pinching, biting, pulling hair, twisting wrists, spitting, and throwing objects. Verbal assaults include threats of physical harm, cursing, racial slurs, demeaning remarks, screaming, and yelling. In focus groups with NAs and nursing directors at six nursing homes, NAs reported such physical and verbal incidents as occurring on a daily basis, resulting in their feeling "hurt, angry, frustrated, resentful, sad, . . . violated . . . fearful" (Gates et al., 1999:17). Unless a physical attack requires medical attention, most violent incidents are not reported for several reasons, including the acceptance of such violence as part of the job; a lack of receptivity and follow-up on the part of administration; and, in five of the six nursing homes, a requirement that individuals involved in an incident report submit to drug testing. NAs generally reported little training or support from management in dealing with such incidents. Separate focus groups with nursing directors from the six nursing homes confirmed that many incidents likely are not reported and that there is little support for NAs after such incidents occur. Directors of nursing cited resistance to drug testing and fear of job loss as reasons for failure to report incidents. Violence by residents against NAs was not viewed as a priority by administrators (Gates et al., 1999).

The increased workloads associated with hospital reorganization and redesign initiatives, as discussed earlier, and hierarchical and bureaucratic management styles that overemphasize efficiency also have been identified as creating obstacles to the provision of emotional support (Miller, 1995). "Physical tasks can be recorded in medical records, used for reimbursement purposes, and easily quantified. Caring for patients' psychological needs, which is not charted or paid for as a special service item, is missing from the usual litany of tasks and activities for which aides are responsible" (Foner, 1995:231), as was illustrated in Box 3-2.

Educating Patients and Families

Education of patient and families is another of the primary responsibilities of RNs. This education is aimed at providing patients and families with appropriate information so they can make informed decisions about their health care and treatments, and develop the knowledge, skills, and abilities needed to perform self-care (ANA, 1998, 2001). Surveys of individual nurses in clinical practice conducted in 1992 to validate the content of the NIC system and determine the frequency with which nurses performed each of the 336 nursing interventions identified teaching patients as an intervention used by more than 90 percent of nurses (Bulechek et al., 1994). However, shorter hospital stays challenge nurses to find the time to provide effective patient education. In a survey of 50 percent of RNs living in Pennsylvania and working in acute care hospitals between 1998 and 1999, 27.9 percent of respondents stated that they had left necessary patient or family teaching undone (Aiken et al., 2001a).

Additional Activities Related to Hands-on Patient Care

Integrating care The increasing complexity of health care often requires that patients be cared for by multiple providers with specialized expertise in diverse roles for a single or across multiple episodes of care (Shortell et al., 2000b). A patient may also be cared for by multiple HCOs or units within one organization, such as ICU, step-down unit, general medical–surgical unit, skilled nursing facility, and home health agency. The coordination of

**BOX 3-2   Time Required for Emotional Support:
A Case Example**

Foner (1995:232–235) describes the following example of a situation in which the time needed to provide emotional support to patients is undervalued relative to speed and efficiency in accomplishing the physical tasks of nursing:

Gloria James and Ana Rivera (pseudonyms) were exact opposites. Ms. James . . . was mean and verbally abusive of patients. . . . Ana was gentle, considerate and kind. Yet Gloria was the nurses' favorite, while Ana was constantly criticized by the nursing coordinator in charge of the floor. . . .

Why was Ms. James so favored by the nurses? Mainly for being quick, efficient, and neat. . . . Ms. James' rooms . . . were immaculate. By lunchtime the beds were neatly made . . . items in the drawers were properly in place and neatly folded. The yellow trays by the sink were sparkling, lined with paper towels to keep toothbrushes and other toilet articles clean. Ms. James was typically the first nursing aide in the day room at lunchtime getting residents ready to eat. She was a fast worker. She . . . was punctilious about getting her paperwork done neatly and on time. . . .

Ms. James' attitude toward dressing, bathing, and feeding patients was much the same as her attitude toward her other chores. She was determined to get them done quickly whether patients liked it or not. . . . She had no tolerance for patients' resistance which slowed her down. Besides, she could get in trouble if, for example, their nails were not cut or their weights not done. . . . Ms. James' behavior to patients was far from gentle . . . she bullied and taunted them; she badgered and yelled. . . . Ms. James humiliated and verbally abused patients . . . in front of nurses, administrators, doctors and visitors. Yet she received the best evaluation on the floor and had privileges denied other aides . . . when the two nurses were away from the floor, it was Ms. James whom they left in charge.

Ana is an expert in . . . the emotional work of caring: holding, cuddling, calming, and grieving. My first view of Ana was typical. . . . Ana

patient care services across these people, functions, activities, and sites over time is referred to as "clinical integration" (Shortell et al., 2000a).

RNs spend a large amount of time integrating patient care as part of planning for patients' discharge from hospitals or other health care facilities to enable continued care in the home, school, or long-term care facility; educating the patient and family about the patient's disease, course of quietly fed a frail and weak resident, cradling her with one arm and gently calling her "Mama" as she coaxed her to eat. . . . One of her residents, Ms. Calhoun, was a witty, sarcastic woman with Parkinson's disease whose mental status, as the problem book noted, fluctuated from alert and oriented to disruptive and verbally abusive. One afternoon she went out of control, screaming and shaking when a new rehabilitation aide mistakenly put a restraint on her chair. Ana gently removed the restraint and gently stroked Ms. Calhoun's head for several minutes as she calmed her down. "She [the rehabilitation aide] didn't know, its her first time," she tried to explain to Ms. Calhoun. "Calm down now, calm down. You're better now."

With completely disoriented and unresponsive patients, Ana assumed a maternal air; with the alert, she chatted and joked as an equal, asking them what they wanted to wear, explaining the tasks she was doing or was about to do, and trying to reassure them about the anxieties they had. . . . Ana empathized with the residents' situation and was aware of their family and personal histories. "It's not just a job," she explained. "Some of them are lonely. They have nobody; they need love and understanding." Beyond emotional work, Ana was fastidious about keeping residents clean. She was careful about the way she gave baths and made sure to wash and lubricate residents before changing their undergarments.

But . . . her efforts were unappreciated by the coordinating nurse. . . . One day she was berated for not doing tasks in the right order; another for not having a resident dressed on time for lunch. . . . Slowness was part of the problem. Though Ana maintained a steady even pace throughout the day, she was sometimes late in completing her tasks . . . sometimes behind schedule weighing patients; and she did not always have her paperwork finished on time. Sometimes she ended up staying late just to complete her basic chores. . . .

Ana's trouble, paradoxically, was that she had the misfortune to work on what the administration then judged to be the best floor, under the best registered nurse in the facility. . . . At every level of the nursing department, from aides to registered nurses, efficiency and organization were valued over compassion to residents.

therapy, medications, self-care activities, and other areas of concern to the patient; and preventing gaps in care delivery, or discontinuities in care that can result in a loss of information relevant to patient care or interruptions in care. Patient transfers—e.g., from unit to unit, facility to facility, or hospital to home—are a common occurrence resulting in a high potential for gaps in care. Gaps also occur from shift to shift or from provider to provider (Cook et al., 2000b).

Integrating activities to prevent these gaps requires that nursing staff communicate and coordinate with a wide variety of health care workers who participate in a patient's health care, including multiple physicians, other nursing personnel, pharmacists, social workers, nutritionists, housekeeping and maintenance personnel, and community care providers. Communication, collaboration, and interactions between physicians and nurses have been shown to result in better patient care (Knaus et al., 1986; Mitchell and Shortell, 1997; Shortell et al., 1994).

The activities that RNs perform in integrating and coordinating patient care have sometimes been classified as "indirect" patient care[13] (McCloskey et al., 1996), and the amount of time nurses spend integrating or coordinating care is indicated, in part, by the amount of time they spend on indirect as opposed to direct patient care. Although the location of some indirect-care activities may be shifting to the bedside (as is the case with automated patient records), the numerous work sampling studies of hospital nursing care that have been performed (with varying degrees of divergence from the standard definitions of "direct" and "indirect" care), have found that RNs spend as much as 25–45 percent of their time in indirect-care activities (Hendrickson et al., 1990; Prescott et al., 1991).

Documentation Documenting nursing work and other activities to meet facility, insurance, private accreditation, state, and federal requirements, as well as to furnish information needed by other providers, is uniformly cited across all care delivery settings as imposing a heavy demand on nurses' time. See Chapters 1 and 6 for a discussion of the demands placed on nursing staff by various documentation requirements.

Supervision RNs also supervise other nursing personnel—LPNs/LVNs and NAs, as well as other RNs. Supervision activities include assigning and scheduling work, collaborating with staff to make patient care decisions, overseeing nursing staff performance and patient care quality, resolving problems, and evaluating performance. In addition, as non-nursing patient care services have been decentralized and located at the nursing unit as part

---

[13]Direct patient care activities are activities carried out in the presence of the patient and family, such as performing a physical examination of the patient, administering medications, and performing treatments and procedures. Indirect-care activities are those that are performed away from, but on behalf of, the patient, such as documenting care, communicating with other health care providers, seeking consultations, and preparing medications (Division of Nursing, 1978).

of hospital reengineering initiatives, nurses have taken on responsibility for supervising non-nursing personnel (McCloskey et al., 1996).

Effective supervision is associated with nurses' satisfaction, recruitment, and retention (Aiken et al., 2001b), as well as with patient care quality. The impact of supervision is particularly clear in studies of nursing homes, where, as discussed earlier, NAs provide most of the care. Poor supervision is often a source of work dissatisfaction among NAs and associated with NA staff turnover (Parsons et al., 2003).

Workplace Characteristics That Hinder Safe Nursing Care

It has long been documented that, in addition to providing nursing care, RNs spend a significant portion of their time performing non-nursing activities. In 1954, the first work sampling study of nursing in three general hospitals in Michigan documented that 11–22 percent of nursing time was spent on activities typically the responsibility of other departments, such as housekeeping, dietary functions, and errands off the unit (Abdellah and Levine, 1954). Subsequent work sampling studies and surveys of nurses have documented the continuation of this phenomenon. Large proportions of nurses continue to spend substantial amounts of time performing non-nursing activities, including delivering and retrieving food trays; performing housekeeping duties, such as cleaning patients' rooms; transcribing physicians' orders; transporting patients; and ordering, coordinating, or performing ancillary services, such as delivery of medical equipment or supplies, blood products, or laboratory specimens (Aiken et al., 2001a). These tasks often prevent nurses from performing the patient care activities detailed above (Aiken et al., 2001b; Prescott et al., 1991; Upenieks, 1998). Other characteristics of the work environments of nurses have been documented as creating obstacles for their provision of appropriate patient care. These characteristics include low staffing levels, poor collaboration across health professions, inadequate decision support, poorly designed work and workspaces, and organizational cultures that inhibit nurses and other health care workers from raising patient safety concerns to management and creating mechanisms to prevent health care errors and adverse events. These problems and recommendations for their resolution are described in Chapters 4 through 7.

REFERENCES

Abdellah F, Levine E. 1954. Work-sampling applied to the study of nursing personnel. *Nursing Research* 3(1):11–16.

AHA (American Hospital Association). 2002. *Hospital Statistics 2002.* Chicago, IL: Health Forum LLC, an affiliate of AHA.

AHA Commission on Workforce for Hospitals and Health Systems. 2002. *In Our Hands: How Hospital Leaders Can Build a Thriving Workforce*. Chicago, IL: AHA.

AHA, The Lewin Group. 2001. Forces driving inpatient utilization. *TrendWatch* 3(3):1–8.

AHCA (American Health Care Association). 2002. *Results of the 2001 AHCA Nursing Position Vacancy and Turnover Survey*. Washington, DC: AHCA.

Aiken L, Sochalski J, Anderson G. 1996. Downsizing the hospital nursing workforce. *Health Affairs* 15(4):88–92.

Aiken L, Havens D, Sloane D. 2000a. The magnet nursing services recognition program: A comparison of two groups of magnet hospitals. *American Journal of Nursing* 100(3):26–36.

Aiken L, Clarke S, Sloane D. 2000b. Hospital restructuring: Does it adversely affect care and outcomes? *Journal of Nursing Administration* 20(10):457–465.

Aiken L, Clarke S, Sloane D, Sochalski J, Busse R, Clarke H, Giovannetti P, Hunt J, Rafferty A, Shamian J. 2001a. Nurses' reports on hospital care in five countries. *Health Affairs* 20(3):43–53.

Aiken L, Clarke S, Sloane D. 2001b. An international perspective on hospital nurses' work environments: The case for reform. *Policy, Politics, & Nursing Practice* 2(4):255–263.

American Organization of Nurse Executives. 2000. *Perspectives on the Nursing Shortage: A Blueprint for Action*. Washington, DC: American Organization of Nurse Executives.

ANA (American Nurses Association). 1998. *Standards of Clinical Nursing Practice*. Washington, DC: ANA.

ANA. 2001. *NursingWorld.org Health and Safety Survey*. [Online]. Available: http://www.nursingworld.org/surveys/hssurvey.pdf [accessed May 25, 2003].

Anderson F, Maloney J, Knight C, Jennings B. 1996. Utilization of supplemental agency nurses in an Army medical center. *Military Medicine* 161(1):48–53.

Barzansky B, Etzel S. 2002. Educational programs in U.S. medical schools, 2001–2002. *Journal of the American Medical Association* 288(9):1067–1072.

Benner P. 1984. *From Novice to Expert: Excellence and Power in Clinical Nursing Practice*. Menlo Park, CA: Addison-Wesley Publishing Company.

Benner P, Hooper-Kyriakidis P, Stannard D. 1999. *Clinical Wisdom and Interventions in Critical Care: A Thinking-In-Action Approach*. Philadelphia, PA: W.B. Saunders Company.

Blegen M, Vaughn T, Goode C. 2001. Nurse experience and education: Effect on quality of care. *Journal of Nursing Administration* 31(1):33–39.

Bolster C, Hawthorne G. 2003. *Big Raises All Around: Hospitals and Health Networks*. [Online]. Available: http://www.hospitalconnect.com/hhnmag/jsp/articledisplay.jsp?dcrpath=AHA/NewsStory-Article/data/hhn0902Coverstory-salary&domain=HHNmag [accessed October 4, 2003].

Bowers B, Esmond S, Jacobson N. 2000. The relationship between staffing and quality in long-term care facilities: Exploring the views of nurse aides. *Journal of Nursing Care Quality* 14(4):55–64.

Brilli R, Spevetz A, Branson R, Campbell G, Cohen H, Dasta J, Harvey M, Kelley M, Kelley K, Rudis M, St. Andre A, Stone J, Teres D, Weled B, Peruzzi W, the members of the American College of Critical Care Medicine Task Force on Models of Critical Care Delivery, the members of the American College of Critical Care Medicine Guidelines for the Definition of an Intensivist, and the Practice of Critical Care Medicine. 2001. Critical care delivery in the intensive care unit: Defining clinical roles and the best practice model. *Critical Care Medicine* 29(10):2007–2019.

Buchan J. 2002. Global nursing shortages. *British Medical Journal* 3:751–752.

Buerhaus P, Staiger D. 1999. Trouble in the nurse labor market? Recent trends and future outlook. *Health Affairs* 18(1):214–222.

Buerhaus P, Staiger D, Auerbach D. 2000. Implications of an aging registered nurse workforce. *Journal of the American Medical Association* 283(22):2948–2954.

Bulechek G, McCloskey J, Titler M, Denehey J. 1994. Report on the NIC project: Nursing interventions used in practice. *American Journal of Nursing* 94(10):59–62, 64, 66.

Bureau of Labor Statistics. Undated. *Licensed Practical and Licensed Vocational Nurses.* Occupational Outlook Handbook, 2002–2003 Edition. [Online]. Available: http://www.bls.gov/oco/ocos102.htm [accessed May 14, 2003].

Bureau of Labor Statistics. 2003. *Registered Nurses.* Occupational Outlook Handbook. [Online]. Available: www.bls.gov/oco/ocos083.htm [accessed May 14, 2003].

Bureau of Labor Statistics, U.S. Department of Labor. Undated. *2001 National Occupational Employment Statistics.* [Online]. Available: http://stats.bls.gov/oesdate [accessed December 13, 2002].

Bureau of Labor Statistics, U.S. Department of Labor. 1999. *Millenial Themes: Age, Education, Services.* Originally published December 1, 1999 as *MLR: The Editors Desk.* [Online]. Available: http:www.bls.gov/opub/ted/1999/nov/wk5/art03.htm [accessed October 4, 2003].

Campbell D, Cornett P. 2002. How stress and burnout produce medical mistakes. In: Rosenthal M, Sutcliffe K, eds. *Medical Error.* San Francisco, CA: Jossey-Bass. Pp. 37–57.

Carnino A, Director, Division of Nuclear Installation Safety, International Atomic Energy Agency. Undated. *Management of Safety, Safety Culture and Self Assessment: International Atomic Energy Agency.* [Online]. Available: http://www.iaea.org/ns/nusafe/publish/papers/mng_safe.htm [accessed January 15, 2003].

Cavouras C, Suby C. 2003. *2003 Survey of Hours Report: Direct and Total Hours per Patient Day (HPPD) by Patient Care Units.* Phoenix, AZ: Labor Management Institute.

CMS (Centers for Medicare and Medicaid Services). 2000. *Report to Congress: Appropriateness of Minimum Nurse Staffing Ratios in Nursing Homes—Phase I Report: U.S. Department of Health and Human Services.* [Online]. Available: www.cms.gov/medicaid [accessed April 22, 2002].

CMS. 2002. *Report to Congress: Appropriateness of Minimum Nurse Staffing Ratios in Nursing Homes—Phase II Final Report: U.S. Department of Health and Human Services.* [Online]. "last modified on Wednesday, June 12, 2002" Available: www.cms.gov/medicaid/reports/rp1201home.asp [accessed June 25, 2002].

Cook R, Render M, Woods D. 2000. Gaps in the continuity of care and progress on patient safety. *British Medical Journal* 320(7237):791–794.

Cooper M. 2000. Towards a model of safety culture. *Safety Science* 36:111–136.

Curtin L. 2002. Adjusting to an aging workforce. Paper presented at the conference on *Solving the Nursing Shortage: Strategies for the Workplace and the Profession.* Washington, DC: JCAHO.

Deutschendorf A. 2003. From past paradigms to future frontiers: Unique care delivery models to facilitate nursing work and quality outcomes. *Journal of Nursing Administration* 33(1):52–59.

Division of Nursing. 1978. *Methods for Studying Nurse Staffing in a Patient Unit.* DHEW Publication No. HRA 78-3. Washington, DC: U.S. Government Printing Office.

Donaldson N, Brown D, Aydin C, Bolton L. 2001. Nurse staffing in California hospitals 1998–2000: Findings from the California Nursing Outcomes Coalition Database Project. *Policy, Politics, & Nursing Practice* 2(1):19–28.

Dougherty C. 1999. Surveillance. In: Bulechek G, McCloskey J, eds. *Nursing Interventions: Effective Nursing Treatments, 3rd Edition.* Philadelphia, PA: W.B. Saunders Company.

Dreyfus H, Dreyfus S. 1986. *Mind over Machine.* New York: The Free Press, A Division of Macmillan, Inc.

Employment Policy Foundation. 2000. *Temporary Workers: No Longer Growing.* [Online]. Available: http://www.epf.org/research/newsletters/2000/et02feb2000.asp [accessed May 18, 2003].

First Consulting Group. 2001. *The Healthcare Workforce Shortage and Its Implications for America's Hospitals: First Consulting Group.* [Online]. Available: http://www.fcg.com/webfiles/pdfs/FCGWorkforceReport.pdf [accessed May 19, 2003].

Foner N. 1995. The hidden injuries of bureaucracy: Work in an American nursing home. *Human Organization* 54(3):229-237.

GAO (General Accounting Office). 2001a. *Nursing Workforce: Emerging Nurses Shortages Due to Multiple Factors.* GAO-01-944. Washington, DC: GAO.

GAO. 2001b. *Nursing Workforce: Recruitment and Retention of Nurses and Nurse Aides is a Growing Concern.* GAO-01-750T. Testimony before the Committee on Health, Education, Labor and Pensions, U.S. Senate, Washington, DC: GAO.

Gates D, Fitzwater E, Meyer U. 1999. Violence against caregivers in nursing homes: Expected, tolerated, and accepted. *Journal of Gerontological Nursing* 25(4):12–22.

Harrington C, Woolhandler S, Mullan J, Carrillo H, Himmelstein D. 2001. Does investor-ownership of nursing homes compromise the quality of care? *American Journal of Public Health* 91(9):1452–1455.

Harrington C, Woolhandler S, Mullan J, Carrillo H, Himmelstein D. 2002. Does investor-ownership of nursing homes compromise the quality of care? *International Journal of Health Services* 32(2):315–325.

Henderson J. 1994. Bed, body, and soul: The job of the nursing home aide. *Generations.* Fall:20–22.

Hendrickson G, Doddato T, Kovner C. 1990. How do nurses use their time? *Journal of Nursing Administration* 20(3):31–37.

Hickam D, Severance S, Feldstein A, Ray L, Gorman P, Schuldheis S, Hersh W, Krages K, Helfand M. 2003. *The Effect of Health Care Working Conditions on Patient Safety.* Evidence Report/Technology Assessment Number 74. (Prepared by Oregon Health & Science University under Contract No. 290-97-0018) AHRQ Publication No. 03-E031. Rockville, MD: AHRQ.

Hobbs F, Stoops N, Census Bureau, U.S. Department of Commerce. 2002. *Demographic Trends in the 20th Century.* Washington, DC: U.S. Government Printing Office. Census 2000 Special Reports. Series CENSR-4. [Online]. Available: http://landview.census.gov/prod/2002pubs/censr-4.pdf [accessed October 4, 2003].

HRSA. 2002. *Projected Supply, Demand, and Shortages of Registered Nurses: 2000–2020.* [Online]. Available: ftp://ftp.hrsa.gov/bhpr/national center/rnproject.pdf [accessed May 18, 2003].

Hurley M. 2000. Workload, UAPs, and you. *RN* 63(12):47–49.

IOM (Institute of Medicine). 1988. *The Future of Public Health.* Washington, DC: National Academy Press.

IOM. 2003. *Unequal Treatment: Confronting Racial and Ethnic Disparities in Health Care.* Smedley B, Stith A, Nelson A, eds. Washington, DC: The National Academies Press.

Jackson M, Chiarello L, Gaynes R, Gerberding J. 2002. Nurse staffing and health care-associated infections: Proceedings from a working group meeting. *AJIC: American Journal of Infection Control* 30(4):199–206.

JCAHO (Joint Commission on Accreditation of Healthcare Organizations). 2002. *Health Care at the Crossroads: Strategies for Addressing the Evolving Nursing Crisis.* JCAHO.

Kaiser Family Foundation and Harvard University School of Public Health. 1999. *1999 Survey of Physicians and Nurses.* [Online]. Available: http:/www.kff.org/content/1999/1503/PhysiciansNursesSurveyChartpack.PDF [accessed October 4, 2003].

Kimball B, O'Neil E. 2002. *Health Care's Human Crisis: The American Nursing Shortage.* [Online]. Available: www.rwjf.org/publications/publicationsPdfs/nursing_report.pdf [accessed October 4, 2003].

Knaus W, Draper E, Wagner D, Zimmerman J. 1986. An evaluation of outcome from intensive care in major medical centers. *Annals of Internal Medicine* 104(3):410–418.

Kovner C. 2001. The impact of staffing and organization of work on patient outcomes and health care workers in health care organizations. *The Joint Commission Journal on Quality Improvement* 27(9):458–468.

Krauss N, Altman B. 1998. *Characteristics of Nursing Home Residents—1996.* AHCPR Publication No. 99-0006. MEPS Research Findings No.5. Rockville, MD: Agency for Health Care Policy and Research (subsequently renamed Agency for Healthcare Research and Quality [AHRQ]).

Mailey S, Charles J, Piper S, Hunt-McCool J, Wilborne-Davis P, Baigis J. 2000. Analysis of the nursing work force compared with national trends. *Journal of Nursing Administration* 30(10):482–489.

Mark B. 2002. *The Work of Registered Nurses, Licensed Practical Nurses, and Nurses Aides in Acute Care Hospitals.* Paper commissioned by the Institute of Medicine Committee on the Work Environment for Nurses and Patient Safety and presented to the Committee on September 24, 2002.

Mark B, Salyer J, Harless D. 2002. What explains nurses' perceptions of staffing adequacy? *Journal of Nursing Administration* 32(5):234–242.

Martin K. 2002 (September 24). *The Work of Nurses and Nursing Assistants in Home Care: Public Health, and Other Community Settings.* Paper commissioned by the Institute of Medicine Committee on the Work Environment for Nurses and Patient Safety and presented to the Committee.

McCloskey J, Bulechek G, eds. 2000. *Nursing Interventions Classification (NIC), 3rd Edition.* St. Louis, MO: Mosby, Inc.

McCloskey J, Bulechek G, Moorhead S, Daley J. 1996. Nurses' use and delegation of indirect care interventions. *Nursing Economics* 14(1):22–33.

McMahan E, Hoffman K. 1994. Physician–nurse relationships in clinical settings: A review and critique of the literature, 1966–1992. *Medical Care Review* 51(1):83–112.

Medicare Payment Advisory Commission. 2001. *Report to the Congress: Medicare Payment Policy.* [Online]. Available: www.medpac.gov/publications/congressional_reports/Mar01 %Entire%20report.pdf [accessed February 24, 2003].

Miller K. 1995. Keeping the care in nursing care: Our biggest challenge. *Journal of Nursing Administration* 25(11):29–32.

Mitchell P, Shortell S. 1997. Adverse outcomes and variations in organization of care delivery. *Medical Care* 35(Supplement 11):NS19-32.

Narumi J, Miyazawa S, Miyata H, Suzuki A, Kohsaka S, Kosugi H. 1999. Analysis of human error in nursing care. *Accident Analysis and Prevention* 31:625–629.

National Association for Home Care. 2001. *Basic Statistics about Home Care.* [Online]. Available: http://www.nahc.org/Consumer/hcstats.htm [accessed May 17, 2003].

Norrish B, Rundall T. 2001. Hospital restructuring and the work of registered nurses. *Milbank Quarterly* 79(1):55.

Office of Inspector General, DHHS. 2001. *Access to Home Health Care after Hospital Discharge.* OEI-02-01-00180. [Online]. Available: http://oig.hhs.gov/oei/reports/oei-02-01-00180.pdf [accessed October 4, 2003].

Parsons S, Simmons W, Penn K, Furlough M. 2003. Determinants of satisfaction and turnover among nursing assistants: The results of a statewide survey. *Journal of Gerontological Nursing* 29(3):51–58.

Pedersen A. 1997. A data-driven approach to work redesign in nursing units. *Journal of Nursing Administration* 27(4):49–54.

Pinkerton S, Rivers R. 2001. Integrated delivery systems: Factors influencing staffing needs. *Nursing Economics* 19(5):208, 236–237.

Pontin D. 1999. Primary nursing: A mode of care or a philosophy of nursing? *Journal of Advanced Nursing* 29(3):584–591.

Prescott P, Phillips C, Ryan J, Thompson K. 1991. Changing how nurses spend their time. *Image* 23(1):23–28.

Reid K, Dawson D. 2001. Comparing performance on a simulated 12 hour shift rotation in young and older subjects. *Occupational & Environmental Medicine* 58(1):58–62.

Rhoades J, Krauss N. 2001. *Chartbook #3: Nursing Home Trends, 1987 and 1996.* [Online]. Agency for Healthcare Research and Quality. Available: http://www.meps.ahrq.gov/papers/cb3_99-0032/cb3.htm [accessed October 4, 2003].

Ritter-Teitel J. 2002. The impact of restructuring on professional nursing practice. *The Journal of Nursing Administration* 32(1):31–41.

Roseman C, Booker J. 1995. Workload and environmental factors in hospital medication errors. *Nursing Research* 44(4):226–230.

Rousseau D, Libuser C. 1997. Contingent workers in high risk environments. *California Management Review* 39(2):103–123.

Salyer J. 1995. Environmental turbulence: Impact on nurse performance. *Journal of Nursing Administration* 25(4):12–20.

Seago J. 2002. The California experiment: Alternatives for minimum nurse-to-patient ratios. *Journal of Nursing Administration* 32(1):48–58.

Service Employees International Union. 2001. *The Shortage of Care: A Study by the SEIU Nurse Alliance.* Washington, DC: Service Employees International Union, AFL-CIO, CLC.

Sexton J, Thomas E, Helmreich R. 2000. Error, stress, and teamwork in medicine and aviation: Cross sectional surveys. *British Medical Journal* 320:745–749.

Shortell S, Zimmerman J, Rousseau D, Gillies R, Wagner D, Draper E, Knaus W, Duffy J. 1994. The performance of intensive care units: Does good management make a difference? *Medical Care* 32(5):508–525.

Shortell S, Gillies R, Anderson D. 2000a. *Remaking Health Care in America, 2nd Edition.* San Francisco, CA: Jossey-Bass.

Shortell S, Jones R, Rademaker A, Gillies R, Dranove D, Hughes E, Budetti P, Reynolds K, Huang C. 2000b. Assessing the impact of total quality management and organizational culture on multiple outcomes of care for coronary artery bypass graft surgery patients. *Medical Care* 38(2):207–217.

Silber J, Williams S, Krakauer H, Schwartz J. 1992. Hospital and patient characteristics associated with death after surgery: A study of adverse occurrence and failure to rescue. *Medical Care* 30(7):615–629.

Smith J, Crawford L. 2003. *Report of Findings from the 2002 RN Practice Analysis.* NCSBN Research Brief. 9. Chicago, IL: National Council of State Boards of Nursing, Inc.

Sochalski J. 2001. Quality of care, nurse staffing, and patient outcomes. *Policy, Politics, & Nursing Practice* 2(1):9–18.

Sochalski J. 2002. Nursing shortage redux: Turning the corner on an enduring problem. *Health Affairs* 21(5):157–164.

Spratley E, Johnson A, Sochalski J, Fritz M, Spencer W. 2000. *The Registered Nurse Population: Findings from the National Sample Survey of Registered Nurses.* DHHS: Health Resources and Services Administration. [Online]. Available: http://bhpr.hrsa.gov/healthworkforce/rnsurvey/rnss1.htm [accessed October 4, 2003].

Staiger D, Auerbach D, Buerhaus P. 2000. Expanding career opportunities for women and the declining interest in nursing as a career. *Nursing Economics* 18(5):230–236.

Star S, Strauss A. 1999. Layers of silence, arenas of voice: The ecology of visible and invisible work. *Computer Supported Cooperative Work* 8:9–30.

Stone R, Wiener J. 2001. *Who Will Care for Us? Addressing the Long Term Care Workforce Crisis.* The Urban Institute and the American Association of Homes and Services for the Aging.

The HSM Group. 2002. *Acute Care Hospital Survey of RN Vacancy and Turnover Rates.* Chicago, IL: American Organization of Nurse Executives.

Unruh L. 2002. Nursing staff reductions in Pennsylvania hospitals: Exploring the discrepancy between perceptions and data. *Medical Care Research and Review* 59(2):197–214.

Upenieks V. 1998. Work sampling: Assessing nursing efficiency. *Nursing Management* 29(4):27–29.

Walston S, Kimberly J. 1997. Reengineering hospitals: Evidence from the field. *Hospital and Health Services Administration* 42(2):143–163.

Walston S, Burns J, Kimberley J. 2000. Does reengineering really work? An examination of the context and outcomes of hospital reengineering initiatives. *Health Services Research* 34(6):1363–1388.

Ward D, Berkowitz B. 2002. Arching the flood: How to bridge the gap between nursing schools and hospitals. *Health Affairs* 21(5):42–52.

Wentling R. 1998. Work and family issues: Their impact on women's career development. *New Directions for Adult and Continuing Education* (80):15–24.

Yamada Y. 2002. Profile of home care aides, nursing home aides, and hospital aides: Historical changes and data recommendations. *Gerontologist* 42(2):199.

4

Transformational Leadership and Evidence-Based Management

Creating work environments for nurses that are most conducive to patient safety will require fundamental changes throughout many health care organizations (HCOs)—in the ways work is designed and personnel are deployed, and how the very culture of the organization understands and acts on the science of safety. These changes require leadership capable of transforming not just a physical environment, but also the beliefs and practices of nurses and other health care workers providing care in that environment and those in the HCO who establish the policies and practices that shape the environment—the individuals who constitute the management of the organization.

Behavioral and organizational research on work and workforce effectiveness, health services research, studies of organizational disasters and their evolution, and studies of high-reliability organizations (see Chapter 1) have identified management practices that are consistently associated with successful implementation of change initiatives and achievement of safety in spite of high risk for error. These practices include (1) balancing the tension between production efficiency and reliability (safety), (2) creating and sustaining trust throughout the organization, (3) actively managing the process of change, (4) involving workers in decision making pertaining to work design and work flow, and (5) using knowledge management practices to establish the organization as a "learning organization." These five management practices, which are essential to keeping patients safe, are not applied consistently in the work environments of nurses.

The committee concludes that transformational leadership and action by each organization's board of directors and senior and midlevel management are needed to fully secure the advantages of these five management practices. Because HCOs vary in the extent to which they currently employ these practices, as well as in their available resources, collaborations with other HCOs can facilitate more widespread adoption of these practices.

This chapter takes a detailed look at the crucial role of transformational leadership and evidence-based management in accomplishing the changes required in nurses' work environments to improve patient safety. We first discuss transformational leadership as the essential precursor to any change initiative. We then review in turn the five management practices enumerated above and describe their uneven application in nurses' work environments. Next, we present several models for evidence-based management in nurses' work environments. Finally, we examine how evidence-based management collaboratives can be used to stimulate the uptake of health care quality improvement practices. During the course of the discussion, we offer four recommendations (highlighted in bold print) for addressing the deficiencies in nurses' work environments through enhanced leadership and management practices.

TRANSFORMATIONAL LEADERSHIP: THE ESSENTIAL PRECURSOR

The central function of leadership is to achieve a collective purpose (Burns, 1978). Not surprisingly, leadership has been observed to be the essential precursor to achieving safety in a variety of industries (Carnino, undated), a critical factor in the success of major change initiatives (Baldridge National Quality Program, 2003; Davenport et al., 1998; Heifetz and Laurie, 2001), and key to an organization's competitive cost position after a change initiative. In a study of hospital reengineering initiatives in U.S. acute care hospitals from 1996 to 1997, only the chief executive officer's (CEO) involvement in core clinical changes had a statistically significant positive effect on the cost outcomes of reengineering (Walston et al., 2000). The exercise of leadership has also been associated with increased job satisfaction, productivity, and organizational commitment among nurses and other workers in HCOs (Fox et al., 1999; McNeese-Smith, 1995).

In his Pulitzer Prize–winning, seminal study on leadership, James Burns identifies the essential characteristics of leadership (as distinct from the wielding of power) and distinguishes "transactional" leadership from the more potent "transformational" leadership (Burns, 1978). He stresses that leadership, like the exercise of power, is based foremost on a relationship between the leader and follower(s). In contrast to power, however, leadership identifies and responds to—in fact, is inseparable from—the needs and goals of followers as well as those of the leader. Leadership is exercised by engaging and inducing followers to act to further certain goals and purposes "that represent the values and motivations, the wants and needs, the aspirations and expectations of both leaders and followers" (Burns, 1978: 19). The genius of leadership lies in the manner in which leaders see, act on, and satisfy followers' values and motivations as well as their own.

Leadership therefore can be either transaction-based or transformational. Transactional leadership typifies most leader–follower relationships. It involves a "you scratch my back; I'll scratch yours" exchange of economic, political, or psychological items of value. Each party to the bargain is conscious of the power and attitudes of the other. Their purposes are related and advanced only as long as both parties perceive their individual interests to be furthered by the relationship. The bargainers have no enduring relationship that holds them together; as soon as an item of value is perceived to be at risk, the relationship may break apart (Burns, 1978). This point is illustrated by labor strikes resulting from a change in the terms of work. The compliance of labor with management is based on an acceptable set of transactions; when the transactions are changed, the relationship may not have much to hold it together. Burns notes that in such cases, a leadership act takes place, but it is not one that "binds leader and follower together in a mutual and continuing pursuit of a higher purpose" (Burns, 1978:20). Transactional leadership is not a joint effort of persons with common aims acting for a collective purpose, but "a bargain to aid the individual interests of persons or groups going their separate ways" (Burns, 1978:425).

In contrast, transformational leadership occurs when leaders engage with their followers in pursuit of jointly held goals. Their purposes, which may have started out as separate but related (as in the case of transactional leadership), become fused. Such leadership is sometimes described as "elevating" or "inspiring." Those who are led feel "elevated by it and often become more active themselves, thereby creating new cadres of leaders" (Burns, 1978:20). Transformational leadership is in essence a relationship of mutual stimulation and elevation that raises the level of human conduct as well as the aspirations of both the leader and those led, and thereby has a transforming effect on both (Burns, 1978).

Transformational leadership is achieved by the specific actions of leaders. First, leaders take the initiative in establishing and making a commitment to relationships with followers. This effort includes the creation of formal, ongoing mechanisms that promote two-way communication and the exchange of information and ideas. On an ongoing basis, leaders play the major role in maintaining and nurturing the relationship with their followers. Burns notes that, most important, leaders seek to gratify followers' wants, needs, and other motivations as well as their own. Understanding of followers' wants, needs, and motivations can be secured only through ongoing communication and exchange of information and ideas. Leaders change and elevate the motives, values, and goals of followers by addressing their followers' needs and teaching them about their commonly held goals. Doing so may require that leaders modify their own leadership in recognition of followers' preferences; in anticipation of followers' responses; or in pursuit of their common motives, values, and goals.

Although a transforming leader plays the major role in achieving the combined purpose of leader and followers, transformational leadership recognizes that leaders and followers are engaged in a common enterprise and thus are dependent on each other. The premise of transformational leadership is that, regardless of the separate interests people may hold, they are presently or potentially united in the pursuit of higher goals. This point is evidenced by the achievement of significant change through the collective or pooled interests of leaders and followers. The effectiveness of leaders and leadership is measured by the extent to which intended change is actually accomplished and human needs and expectations are satisfied (Burns, 1978).

Burns offers reassurance that transformational leadership is far more common than might be thought, given the above discussion. He notes that acts of transformational leadership are not restricted to (and often are not found in) governmental organizations, but are widespread in day-to-day events, such as whenever parents, teachers, politicians, or managers tap into the motivations of children, students, the electorate, or employees in the achievement of a needed change.

In acute care hospitals, individuals in potential transformational leadership roles range from board-level chairmen and directors; to chief executive, operating, nursing, and medical officers; through the hierarchy to unit managers. In nursing homes, such leadership can come from a facility's owners, administrator, director of nursing, and unit managers. Leadership by these senior organization managers and oversight boards is essential to accomplishing the breadth of organizational change needed to achieve higher levels of patient safety—changes in management practices, workforce deployment, work design and flow, and the safety culture of the organization (see Chapter 1).

However, if these individuals rely solely on a traditional, transactional approach to leadership, such substantive changes are likely to be difficult to achieve and sustain, as leaders will need to conduct frequent, ongoing, possibly contradictory renegotiations with workers in response to rapidly changing external forces. In contrast, transformational leadership seeks to engage individuals in the recognition and pursuit of a commonly held goal— in this case, patient safety. For example, individual nurses may desire wide variation in the number of hours they would like to work on a 24-hour or weekly basis. Attempting to secure their commitment to the organization by accommodating all such requests (transactional leadership) despite evidence that extended work hours may be detrimental to patient safety would likely be both time-intensive and unsuccessful. Instead, transformational leadership would engage nursing staff in a discussion of patient safety and worker fatigue and seek to develop work hour policies and scheduling that would put patient safety first and respond to individual scheduling needs within that construct. Such a discussion could have a transforming effect on both staff and management as knowledge was shared.

A leadership approach that aims to achieve a collective goal rather than a multitude of individual goals and aims to transform all workers—both managers and staff—in pursuit of the higher collective purpose can be the most efficient and effective means of achieving widespread and fundamental organizational change. In practicing transformational leadership, leaders need to engage managers and staff in an ongoing relationship based on the commonly held goal of patient safety, and communicate with and teach managers and staff about this higher collective purpose.

When teaching managers about the actions they can take to minimize threats to patient safety, HCO leaders should underscore the five management practices enumerated earlier that have been found to be consistently associated with successful implementation of change initiatives and with the achievement of safety in organizations with high risk for errors. These management practices also underlie all of the worker deployment, work design, and safety culture practices that are addressed in the remaining chapters of this report.

FIVE ESSENTIAL MANAGEMENT PRACTICES

"The more removed individuals are from . . . front-line activities . . . , the greater is their potential danger to the system" (Reason, 1990:174).

As discussed in Chapters 1 and 2, latent work conditions have been documented as posing the greatest risk of errors. Therefore, it should not be surprising that errors often have their primary origins in decisions made by fallible system designers and high-level managerial decision makers (Reason, 1990). The corollary to this statement is that these high-level managerial decision makers have a substantial role to play in error prevention—a role that deserves more attention and support.

The concept of evidence-based practice first emerged in clinical medicine and now suffuses the language, decision making, and standards of care of health care clinicians, managers, policy makers, and researchers throughout the world. Evidence-based clinical practice is defined as the conscientious, explicit, and judicious integration of current best evidence—obtained from systematic research—in making decisions about the care of individual patients (Sackett et al., 1996). The use of systematic research findings for evidence-based practice is also supported and applied in the fields of education, criminal justice, and social welfare through the efforts of the international Campbell Collaboration—a sibling of the Cochrane Collaboration that prepares and maintains evidence-based systemic reviews of the effects of health care interventions (The Campbell Collaboration, undated). Evidence-based *management*, however, is a newer concept—not yet as widely embraced, but just as important (Axelsson, 1998; Hewison, 1997; Kovner et al., 2000; Walshe and Rundall, 2001).

Evidence-based management means that managers, like their clinical practitioner counterparts, should search for, appraise, and apply empirical evidence from management research in their practice. Managers also must be prepared to have their own decisions and actions systematically recorded and evaluated in a way that will further add to the evidence base for effective management practices (Axelsson, 1998).

While health care practitioners have been encouraged and supported in the adoption of evidence-based practice, the same support and encouragement has not been widely available to health care managers for multiple reasons:

- Organizational research is sometimes esoteric and does not consistently address practical management questions (Axelsson, 1998). Further, research conducted on health care management is limited compared with management research in other industries. The main funders of research in health care (government agencies and private foundations) have historically not funded management research. When large health systems have funded such research, its findings have often been considered proprietary and the results not widely published. As a result, little empirical evidence has been generated about best health care management practices (Kovner et al., 2000).

- The empirical evidence on effective management practices that does exist is difficult to locate. Management literature is poorly indexed for practical applications and is not easily reviewed and synthesized (Walshe and Rundall, 2001).

- Many managers are not trained or experienced in the use of such evidence in making management decisions (Kovner et al., 2000). While physicians are trained in a strongly professional model with fairly uniform educational preparation, managers come from a variety of very different professional backgrounds and training. Some management training comes more from long-term practical experience in the workplace, as opposed to formal professional education (Axelsson, 1998; Walshe and Rundall, 2001).

- Although many health systems spend millions of dollars on consultants for strategic recommendations based on data, they typically underfund their own data systems designed to support decision making and internal management research (Kovner et al., 2000). A study of 14 U.S. hospitals implementing reengineering initiatives in the 1990s found that existing operating budgets often were used to measure progress in meeting reengineering goals, but did not contain baseline statistics managers could use for comparative purposes or identification of causes and effects (Walston and Kimberly, 1997).

- Some HCOs lack sufficient size and resources to conduct and evaluate applied research (Kovner et al., 2000).
- Managers' decision-making practices are often quite different from those of health care practitioners. While practitioners' decisions are many in number and made independently, management decisions are often few, large, and made by groups, involving negotiation or compromise and many organizational constraints (Walshe and Rundall, 2001).

For the above reasons, in health care, often "the weapons are ahead of the tactics"—a description used by historian Shelby Foote to characterize military leadership during the U.S. Civil War (Ward et al., 1990). In the case of American health care, the sophisticated medical technology (the weaponry) outclasses the tactics (management) used to organize work and implement change.

Despite the limitations discussed above in the supply of and access to empirical information to guide managerial decision making, there is strong evidence that the management practices enumerated at the beginning of this chapter play a critical role in achieving organizational goals and successfully implementing change within an organization. These five practices are discussed in turn below.

Balancing the Tension Between Efficiency and Reliability

The health care cost-containment pressures of the last two decades (see Chapter 1) have forced HCOs to examine their work processes and undertake work redesign initiatives to deliver care more efficiently. Efficiency frequently calls for conducting production activities in as cost-effective and time-efficient a manner as possible. Organizations in many industries often try to accomplish efficiency by downsizing, outsourcing, and cutting costs. Such efficiency measures can be at odds with safety (Carnino, undated; Cooper, 2000; Spath, 2000). For example, when system failures associated with four large-scale disasters (Three-Mile Island, Chernobyl, the Challenger space shuttle, and the Bhopal chemical plant) were compared, subordination of safety to other performance goals was one of 11 common attributes found (Petersen, 1996). HCOs are not immune to these pressures. Concerns have been raised that HCOs, in responding to production and efficiency pressures, may adopt practices that threaten patient safety (Schiff, 2000; SEIU Nurse Alliance, 2001; Thomas et al., 2000).

For example, one of the practices used by high-reliability organizations to increase safety is to consciously incorporate personnel and equipment redundancy into some aspects of work design. This redundancy creates some slack in the system such that if one component in the work production process fails, a replacement will be available to perform the function. Air traffic controllers, for example, are assigned to radar screening in groups of two. While their job functions are somewhat different, each controller acts as a check on the other (Roberts, 1990). This redundancy and other practices characteristic of high-reliability organizations—such as promoting inter- and intragroup communication, cross-training personnel, and attending to the interdependencies of work production processes—might be viewed by other organizations as "frills" (Roberts and Bea, 2001b) and a hindrance to efficient production. In high-reliability organizations, however, performance reliability (safety) rivals productivity as a dominant organizational goal, and such work components are viewed as essentials rather than frills (Roberts, 1990). Organizations can achieve balance between production efficiency and reliability by balancing and aligning their organizational goals; accountability mechanisms; and reward, incentive, and compensation mechanisms (Roberts and Bea, 2001a).

Creating and Sustaining Trust

Creating and sustaining trust is the second of the five management practices essential to patient safety. Trust has been defined as the willingness to be vulnerable to the intentions of another (Mayer et al., 1995; Rousseau et al., 1998) and is strongest when parties believe each other to be competent and to have one another's interests at heart. When trust links people and groups to organizations, it generally makes workers willing to contribute their efforts without expecting an immediate payoff, and increases the extent to which leaders can rely on workers to have the organization's interests at heart (and vice versa). Workers' trust in organizational leaders has been found to be directly related to positive business outcomes, such as increased sales and profitability, and inversely related to employee turnover (Mayer et al., 1995).

Trust has the added advantage of increasing workers' capacity for change by reducing the uncertainty and discomfort with change that otherwise impair individual and group adaptability (Coff and Rousseau, 2000; Rousseau, 1995) and increasing workers' willingness to take risks associated with change (Mayer et al., 1995). Honest and open communication, necessary for successful organizational change, depends on the development of trust throughout the organization (Carnino, undated; DeLong and Fahey, 2000), in part because the level of trust that exists between the organization and its employees greatly influences the amount of knowledge that flows among individuals and from individuals into organization databases, archives, and other records (DeLong and Fahey, 2000). Further, when trust is lacking, participants are less likely to believe what leaders say and to contribute the extra effort, engagement, and knowledge needed to make change successful. It is easier to share information, downplay differences, and cooperate when those involved in a change trust each other.

Trust flows two ways—up and down the hierarchies of organizations. Top-down trust is based largely on competence (Rousseau et al., 1998). Leaders are more willing to entrust subordinates with complete information and with the authority to make decisions when they believe those subordinates to be competent and capable of making and carrying out appropriate decisions. It is well established that leaders manage subordinates differently depending on the employees' perceived competence (Graen et al., 1982; Lowin and Craig, 1968). This is because when hiring, employers put themselves at risk, depending on those they hire to act in ways that help rather than hinder the organization. Employees are hired to act for their employers by making decisions and carrying out responsibilities on the employers' behalf (Pearce, 2000). Employers cope with this vulnerability by attempting to hire employees they can trust and by managing those they hire in ways that sustain that trust. Top-down trust is reinforced whenever leaders have positive exchanges with their employees. Such exchanges are more likely to occur in long-standing relationships in which both parties have made investments in each other, for example, when leaders have developed subordinates who in turn have worked to understand the leader's goals and preferred ways of managing and adjusted their behavior accordingly (Huselid, 1995; Miles and Snow, 1984).

Bottom-up trust, on the other hand, is based in part on workers' perceptions of a manager's or organization's ability, benevolence, and integrity (Mayer et al., 1995). An organization's ability comprises its collective skills, competencies, and expertise. Trust can be fostered by an organization's strong reputation for competence and capabilities, as well as by members' ability to directly access the expertise of others within the organization, the collective capabilities of members, their shared knowledge of each other's expertise, and recognition of "who knows what" based on a history of shared experience (Coff and Rousseau, 2000). Conversely, trust can be damaged by disclosure of failures in competence or by workers' direct observation of instances in which competence falls short of prior expectations.

Bottom-up trust is also based on benevolence, that is, the extent to which managers and organizations are understood by workers to want to do good (aside from a self-concerned or profit motive) for the person who trusts the entity (the trustor). Benevolence gives rise to an attachment between the entity being trusted (the trustee) and the trustor. An example of such a benevolent relationship is that between a mentor and a protégé. The mentor wants to be helpful to the protégé, even though there is no extrinsic reward to the mentor for doing so. Benevolence also has been associated with a trustee's motivation to speak truthfully (Mayer et al., 1995).

The relationship between integrity and trust involves the trustor's perception that the trustee adheres to a set of principles that the trustor finds acceptable (Mayer et al., 1995). In health care organizations, where many workers have strong professional identifications, trust of leadership by subordinates often reflects the extent to which leadership is committed to the values inherent in the professions of medicine and nursing (Bunderson, 2001; Thompson and Bunderson, in press). Conversely, evidence indicates that change initiatives targeting quality improvement are far less likely to generate support when clinical caregivers believe those changes are motivated by either economic or political considerations (Rousseau and Tijoriwala, 1999). Integrity is assessed by the consistency of a party's past actions, credible communication about the trustee from other parties, the belief that the party has a strong sense of justice, and the extent to which the party's actions are consistent with his or her word.

Trust between workers and the organizations in which they work therefore results from the workers' perceptions of the interplay among the organization's ability, benevolence, and integrity. Each of these factors exists to a varying degree along a continuum. Although in the best case, high degrees of trust result from high levels of all three factors, meaningful trust can exist with lesser levels of a combination of the three. The degree of trust between parties also is dynamic and evolves over time as the parties interact. The outcomes that result when a trustor takes a risk and places his or her trust in the trustee affect the degree of trust that exists for subsequent potential interactions (Mayer et al., 1995). Mutual trust is enhanced by positive exchanges that have occurred in the past and are expected to continue in the future (Zucker, 1986). Therefore, trust in organizations also depends to a certain extent on the extent of stability in the relationships that make up the organization (e.g., worker to manager, manager to senior executive). In organizations with high turnover, mutual trust is difficult to achieve (Bryman et al., 1987). In firms in which promotions tend to be internal and the employee development system builds organization-specific capabilities, both workers and managers are more likely to possess common knowledge and similar points of view, and managers are more likely to trust workers (Miles and Snow, 1984). Such bases for trust are less common in many contemporary firms, where external mobility and reduced opportunities for within-firm development mean that organization members, leaders, and workers have fewer shared experiences and frames of reference (Leana and Rousseau, 2000).

It is widely evident that over the course of the twentieth century, senior managers in many industries have come to place greater trust in workers

(Miles and Creed, 1995). Employees increasingly have experienced greater discretion and reduced standardization in the way they accomplish their work, coordinated more of their interactions with coworkers and other departments, and reduced their dependence on supervisors for problem solving. At the same time that modern organizational practices presume a higher degree of trustworthiness among workers, however, workers' trust in management remains highly variable (Freeman and Rogers, 1999). In a large-scale survey of the American workforce, Freeman and Rogers found that workers generally reported levels of loyalty to their employer greater than the degree of trust they placed in their employer to keep its promises to them or other workers. This low level of trust is connected to a widespread sense on the part of American workers that they have little influence over workplace decisions. Where workers exercise greater influence over workplace decisions, they are more likely to trust their managers and act in ways that ease implementation of those decisions. With respect to nursing, higher levels of nurse autonomy and control over nursing practice have been associated with greater trust in management among nurses and greater commitment to their employing HCO (Laschinger et al., 2000, 2001b).

Actively Managing the Process of Change

Actively managing the process of change is essential to patient safety because all organizations have difficulty in navigating major organizational change (Kimberly and Quinn, 1984). HCOs are no exception. Despite their vast experience with introducing new medical technologies, HCOs have a history of ineffective attempts at organizational change and remain prone to poor change implementation (Mintzberg, 1997). A large body of research and other published work offers frameworks, models, and guidance for undertaking change (Baer and Frese, 2003; Goodman, 2001; Parker, 1998; Rousseau and Tijoriwala, 1999; Walston et al., 2000). This work consistently calls attention to five predominantly human resource management practices[1] as particularly important for successful change implementation: ongoing communication; training; use of mechanisms for measurement, feedback, and redesign; sustained attention; and worker involvement.

Ongoing Communication

Frequent, ongoing communication through multiple media is a key ingredient of successful organizational change initiatives (Ingersoll et al.,

---

[1]The human resource side of change tends to be undermanaged as compared with management of the implementation of technological changes (Kimberly and Quinn, 1984).

2001). Such communication is a powerful facilitator of change, whereas poor communication creates significant problems (Rousseau and Tijoriwala, 1999). In its work with more than 200 managers from 32 different countries, the Change Program at the International Institute for Management Development in Lausanne, Switzerland, identified employee acceptance of the need for and nature of a change and its effect on their "personal compact" with the organization as a critical determinant of whether change will be successful (Strebel, 1996).

In the present context, it is essential to have ongoing communication with employees about the goals and mission of the HCO, the reasons for change (including contributing economic and policy factors), and the nature of the change (including changes in employee roles and responsibilities). Soliciting feedback about the change throughout its planning, implementation, and continuance is also necessary (Heifetz and Laurie, 2001; Ingersoll et al., 2001). Studies of HCO redesign, reengineering, and reorganization initiatives identify role conflict and ambiguity as consistent issues in change initiatives; nurses who view their roles as ambiguous have lower job commitment (Ingersoll et al., 2001). Clear communication about changes in employee roles and responsibilities can reduce such ambiguity. Even discussions about how the HCO is financed are recommended. In one study, nurses expressed concern about money being available for construction of new buildings even as staff was being admonished to conserve resources. This is a sentiment commonly expressed by those unfamiliar with the multiple sources and allocations of revenue that can exist within an institution (Ingersoll et al., 2001).

When nurse managers in one 700-plus bed hospital undergoing organizational change were asked to rank the behaviors of health care executives in terms of how supportive those behaviors were to the change management process, respondents ranked frequent communication about the goals and progress of organizational change as the most important behavior (Knox and Irving, 1997). Communication between nurses and nurse managers also has been shown to increase nurses' commitment to the organization (McNeese-Smith, 1997), which is essential to weathering the stresses of organizational change.

Training

Because change often requires employees to adopt new roles and responsibilities, training is essential to successful change. This need is not always appreciated, however. A study of 14 U.S. hospitals implementing reengineering initiatives in the 1990s found that needs for new knowledge were often underestimated; the result was periods of deteriorated quality and inefficiency (Walston and Kimberly, 1997). Training is especially needed in such specialized topics as work redesign, knowledge management, error prevention and detection (Spear and Bowen, 1999), and change management itself (Strebel, 1996). In a 1995 survey of nurse leaders in VHA Inc. HCOs and nurse executives and managers belonging to the American Organization of Nurse Executives (AONE), expertise in change management was one of five learning needs reported by the nurse leaders (Gelinas and Manthey, 1997).

Mechanisms for Feedback, Measurement, and Redesign

Few changes in complex organizations work perfectly when first introduced. Virtually all changes require modification over time to achieve optimum results. It is not unusual for organizations, departments, or plants that have implemented innovations most recently to perform worse than those that implemented comparable innovations a year or two before (Macduffie and Pil, 1996). New practices often initially undermine existing routines and competencies and require ongoing learning adjustment, redesign of the change, and supportive efforts to capture the intended benefits of the innovation. Ongoing monitoring, feedback, and redesign are needed to create and sustain effective change (Goodman, 2001; Walston and Kimberly, 1997).

Sustained Attention

Effective organizational transformations require long periods of time and constant effort. Macduffie and Pil (1996) point out that in the auto industry, plants in the first year following adoption of a new work system struggle with the right mix of incentives, managerial supports, and training needs, and experience coordination difficulties with other units. Those that sustain the change into the second year begin to see cost and quality improvements. The above-cited study of 14 U.S. hospitals implementing reengineering initiatives in the 1990s found that 2 to 3 years into their reengineering efforts, many had yet to implement a number of their initial plans. Although difficulties arose during the long implementations, the transition from implementation to a sustained, institutionalized process was even more problematic. While most study participants perceived reengineering to be an ongoing change process, and managers realized that continual effort was needed to move reengineering forward, many ended their efforts or decreased them after initial implementation. Without continued attention, the change was not sustained. The hospitals that were able to sustain a change were those that embedded the new initiative within ongoing operations, such as a continuous quality improvement or total quality management process, or established specific, measurable goals and mechanisms to track their progress. In two cases in which tracking measures were employed, the "established goals and feedback monitors appeared to galvanize the organization to make and maintain changes in these areas" (Walston and Kimberly, 1997:158).

Codifying a change to ensure consistency of application and direction through implementation manuals, guidelines for decision making, and provision of budgetary support has been identified as a critical ingredient in successful and sustained implementation (Walston et al., 2000). Credible commitment to stay with the change over time in the face of personnel changes or economic factors is especially important in organizations with a history of dysfunctional labor–management relations and ineffective change management (Heller, 2003). Such commitment can take the form of public statements and written documents articulating the agreement.

Worker Involvement

Evidence from multiple studies indicates that change is typically turbulent and difficult for staff members (Ingersoll et al., 2001; Strebel, 1996). Changes often affect worker roles and responsibilities, work group relationships, and resource availability and use. Consequently, a natural human response is to react negatively to the challenges created by change. This negativity can be overcome by actively involving workers in the planning and design of a change and providing them with information about the progress being made in achieving the goals of the redesign (Walston and Kimberly, 1997). The importance of such worker involvement is discussed in greater detail below.

Involving Workers in Work Design and Work Flow Decision Making

Evidence indicates that a highly bureaucratic structure, so useful in organizations into the early twentieth century, is inappropriate to many organizations today (Ciborra, 1996; Ilinitch et al., 1996) because both human potential and technology have matured since the beginning of the Industrial Revolution. Organizational structures that are strongly hierarchical in design with resultant hierarchical decision making are hampered in their ability to respond to situations with high variability (Moorman and Miner, 1998; Quinn, 1992) and are associated with reduced safety (Roberts and Bea, 2001b). Since the 1980s, a worldwide evolution has taken place in the organizing principals of manufacturing, as the mass production system (which itself replaced the old craft system in the early twentieth century) was transformed at the end of the 1900s into the flexible production system (Macduffie and Pil, 1996). This flexible production system was enabled and reinforced by two related forces: managers' expanded trust in their workers and an ever-greater reliance on workers as the basis for organizational success (Miles and Creed, 1995).

The relationship between greater reliance on workers and organizational success is being documented across a variety of industries and types of research. Studies of high-reliability organizations show that effective decision making is flexible decision making, pushed to the lowest level commensurate with available knowledge (Bigley and Roberts, 2001; Roberts et al., 1994; Weick and Roberts, 1993). For example, any level of military personnel on an aircraft carrier can call a halt to a flight operation if he or she sees what looks like a dangerous situation (Roberts, 1990). Health services research supports these findings. The above-cited study of 14 U.S. hospitals implementing reengineering initiatives in the 1990s found that involving the total organization in the reengineering process was frequently mentioned as an important factor in success and, conversely, that inconsistent involvement was a barrier (Walston and Kimberly, 1997). Nurses working in organizations whose work culture emphasized decentralized decision making reported significantly higher commitment to the organization, empowerment, and job satisfaction and significantly lower intent to leave (Gifford et al., 2002).

Such high-involvement work systems have been described across a number of industries. They are characterized by shifting more decisions down the organization's hierarchy to the level of individual workers or teams of workers, increasing worker responsibility for quality control (monitoring safety and taking action to prevent risks to safety or quality), and broadening the knowledge workers possess about the activities of other work groups (e.g., through cross-functional teams). Such work systems promote greater contributions on the part of workers to the value of the organization by releasing underutilized worker competence (Edmondson, 1999; Frese et al., 1999; Ho et al., 1999; MacDuffie, 1995; Parker, 1998). Preconditions for implementing such systems include a relationship of trust between senior leadership and workers (Rousseau and Tijoriwala, 1999) and credible commitment on the part of leadership to persist with implementing high-involvement work systems over time.

In nursing research, this involvement in decision making has been studied under a number of constructs, including shared governance, nursing empowerment, control over nursing practice, and clinical autonomy. These constructs have certain common elements.

Shared governance—"a decentralized approach which gives nurses greater authority and *control over their practice* and work environment [emphasis added]" (O'May and Buchan, 1999:281)—began to be incorporated into nurse work environments in the late 1970s. The results of these efforts are uncertain because of the lack of a uniform definitional construct, wide variation in implementation models, infrequent evaluations, and poorly designed evaluation methodologies. "As a result, studies to evaluate shared governance tend to yield mixed results, leave questions as to what has been evaluated, and often produce little opportunity for cross-comparison of results" (O'May and Buchan, 1999:292).

Nursing research on empowerment similarly has not generally included a uniform operational definition of this construct, but has described empowerment in terms of its goal (i.e., "empower nurses to exercise more *control over the content and context of their practice*" [emphasis added]) and in terms of the resources needed to achieve it (i.e., "the ability to access and mobilize support, information, resources, and opportunities from one's position in the organization") (Laschinger and Havens, 1996:27–28). Conger and Kanungo (1988:474) define empowerment as "a process of enhancing feelings of self-efficacy among organizational members through the identification of conditions that foster powerlessness and through their removal by both formal organizational practices and informal techniques of providing efficacy information." A series of studies of nurses employed at individual Canadian and U.S. hospitals found that perceived empowerment is strongly related to perceptions of autonomy and control over nursing practice (Laschinger and Havens, 1996; Sabiston and Laschinger, 1995). Additional studies in this series found higher levels of organizational trust among nurses reporting greater workplace empowerment (Laschinger et al., 2000, 2001a). Evidence also indicates that organizational structures that foster nurses' empowerment (combined with strong managers) may be important factors in increasing the organizational commitment of nurses working in nursing facilities (Beaulieu et al., 1997).

Studies of shared governance and empowerment highlight nurses' control over their practice as a key element. The construct of control of nursing practice has been addressed more explicitly and fully in studies seeking to determine the attributes of hospitals that are rated by their nurses as making them "good place to work" and that do not experience difficulties in attracting and retaining nurses. These hospitals (referred to as "magnet hospitals") have been the subject of multiple studies. A distinction is made in these studies between control over nursing practice and clinical autonomy. Clinical autonomy refers to nurses' ability to assess *individual* patient needs and practice nursing care appropriate to those needs, that is, their ability to make independent clinical decisions and define the scope of practice in relationship to patients in their care (Kramer and Schmalenberg, 2003; McClure et al., 1983; Scott et al., 1999). Autonomy is a characteristic commonly identified by staff nurses, nurse managers, and chief nurse executives (CNEs) as important to a magnet hospital (Aiken, 2002; McClure et al., 1983). Control over nursing practice is defined as nurses' ability to shape not just the care of an individual, but also the organizational policies and practices to be followed within nursing units and the HCO overall that affect nursing care, as well as to control the resources need to provide that care (Hinshaw, 2002). Control over nursing practice represents an organization-level (as opposed to patient-level) autonomy, in which staff nurses, nurse managers, and CNEs take part in hospital policy and decision making about professional practice and patient care (Scott et al., 1999). A review of studies conducted on magnet hospitals reveals that both autonomy and control over nursing practice are consistently identified as magnet characteristics (Scott et al., 1999). Other research suggests that nurses' autonomy and control over their practice environment are positively associated with their trust in management (Laschinger et al., 2001b).

Creating a Learning Organization

The final evidence-based management practice calls for all HCOs to become learning organizations. The ongoing acquisition and management of knowledge has been identified as one of the intrinsic characteristics of high-performing organizations in postindustrial societies (Quinn, 1992). Economists and business strategists point to how an organization manages its knowledge assets as more important to its competitive advantage in today's economy than how it manages bureaucratic control of its capital resources (Blackler, 1995; DeLong and Fahey, 2000). Continuous organizational learning also has been documented as playing a central role in the development and maintenance of safety in organizations (Carnino, undated). This point is particularly salient to a high-tech industry such as health care, which is characterized by rapidly accelerating scientific and technologic advances. The Institute of Medicine (IOM) report *Crossing the Quality Chasm: A New Health System for the 21st Century* (IOM, 2001), cites this growth in health care knowledge, drugs, medical devices, and technologies as one of the four defining attributes of the U.S. health system affecting health care quality.

A learning organization is an organization "skilled at creating, acquiring, and transferring knowledge, and at modifying its behavior to reflect new knowledge and insight" (Garvin, 1993:80). Learning organizations do not passively wait for knowledge to present itself, but actively manage the learning process by taking advantage of all sources of knowledge, using systematic experimentation to generate new knowledge internally, and transferring knowledge quickly and efficiently throughout the organization (Garvin, 1993). These processes are used to create better work tools, processes, systems, and structures in order to improve the organization's production processes (DeLong and Fahey, 2000).

Actively Managing the Learning Process

Taking advantage of all sources of knowledge   Learning organizations know that knowledge can come from many sources, including internal flashes of creativity or insight, knowledgeable experts within the organization, external experts, the best practices of other organizations, and other sources. They learn from their own and others' experiences by reviewing past organizational successes and failures, assessing them systematically, and recording them in a format that employees can easily access (Garvin, 1993). Learning from the experiences and best practices of others is a major factor in the success and sizable cost savings of a number of organizations' reengineering initiatives (Stewart, 1999), although knowledge gained from failures can often be the most helpful (DeLong and Fahey, 2000). However, knowledge from these sources serves as a starting point only; organizations are expected to test and improve upon it through continual experimentation (DeLong and Fahey, 2000).

Using systematic experimentation to generate new knowledge internally Experimentation is widely recognized as a cornerstone of a learning organization. Experimentation involves the systematic searching for and testing of new knowledge using the scientific method through an ongoing series of small experiments, designed to produce incremental gains in knowledge access (Garvin, 1993). It can be undertaken on existing programs or on planned new demonstration projects. This application of the scientific method in a continuing series of controlled experiments has been identified as the hallmark of the Toyota Production System, which has been widely hailed as a benchmark work system (see Box 4-1). Toyota teaches the scientific method to workers at every level of the organization, thereby creating a "community of scientists" (Spear and Bowen, 1999).

Other knowledge management organizations, while perhaps not using the scientific method as rigorously as the Toyota System, employ similar methods associated with continuous quality improvement or total quality management. These methods include employing the "plan–do–check–act" cycle; insisting on data, rather than assumptions, for decision making; and using simple statistical analysis tools, such as histograms, pareto charts, and tests of correlations, to organize data and raw inferences. These methods help the organization and its employees become more disciplined in their thinking and more attentive to details of work processes and production (Garvin, 1993).

Transferring knowledge quickly and efficiently throughout the organization Learning organizations spread knowledge quickly and efficiently throughout the organization. They know that ideas have the greatest im-

BOX 4-1   The Toyota Production System

The Toyota Production System (TPS) has long been hailed as the reason for the Toyota Company's outstanding performance and has been used as a model by many other organizations around the world. In essence, the TPS creates a learning organization by forming a community of scientists among its workers. In the TPS, work processes are studied so intensely that each activity is defined by an exacting set of specifications. This approach allows workers to vary a work process and test the effects of the change on production efficiency and reliability. Toyota's work specifications thereby serve as sets of hypotheses that can be tested. When making a change, workers use a rigorous problem-solving process that is, in effect, an experimental test of the proposed change using the scientific method. This learning environment is enabled by four signature TPS practices:

- **How people work**—All work processes are conducted following exacting specifications as to content, sequence, timing, and outcome. Even complex activities, such as training new workers, are conducted according to specifications. While on the surface this may appear to represent organizational rigidity, it actually affords workers and the organization flexibility and adaptability. The use of work specifications enables workers to identify needed changes to work processes more easily and allows for controlled trials of new work processes.
- **How workers connect**—Worker interactions across all levels also are characterized by standardization and directness. This approach minimizes ambiguity, decreases the number of problems that fall through the cracks, and maximizes accountability. When workers encounter a problem, they are expected to ask for help at once, instead of trying to solve problems on their own. In this way, work flow problems become apparent and are not left to fester as latent error–producing situations. When a request for help is made, assistance is expected to be given immediately and the problem resolved within a certain time. This expectation fosters trust across workers.
- **How work is constructed**—Work is designed to maximize reliability. Production lines are set up according to a specified pathway that does not change unless the production line is specifically redesigned. This approach also facilitates redesign through experimentation.

pact when they are shared broadly rather than tightly held by a few individuals, and that knowledge must be transferred through multiple, reinforcing channels to create synergy and enhance its absorption and application. A variety of knowledge dissemination mechanisms can promote this transfer, including written, oral, and visual reports; site visits and tours; person-

- **How work is improved and errors reduced**—The preceding three work practices are designed to identify production problems. This last practice creates a learning environment in which improvement is an ongoing activity, and errors are continually reduced. To this end, Toyota first teaches all employees how to change, specifying that any improvement to production activities must be made in accordance with the scientific method, under the guidance of a teacher, and at the lowest possible organizational level. To accomplish this, Toyota teaches the scientific method to workers at every level of the organization. Workers are taught how to effect change and who is responsible for making changes; they are not expected to learn directly from their on-the-job personal experiences. The scientific method is thereby ingrained in the organization, which becomes a learning organization.

An extensive 4-year study of the TPS in more than 40 organizations found that the successful implementation of the above four principles in each organization is guided by a strong, shared vision of the ideal product the company desires to produce and the ideal production system to create that product. This shared vision motivates all employees to make improvements beyond what would be necessary merely to meet current customer needs. This notion of the ideal is not abstract. For Toyota workers, it is one in which the product is defect free; can be delivered one request at a time; can be supplied on demand in the version requested; can be delivered immediately; can be produced without wasting any materials, labor, energy, or other resources; and can be produced in a work environment that is safe physically, emotionally, and professionally for every employee.

To reinforce the learning and improvement process, each plant and major business unit in the Toyota Group employs a number of TPS consultants to help senior managers move their organization toward the ideal. Many of these individuals have received intensive training at Toyota's Operations Management Consulting Division or the Toyota Supplier Support Center in the United States. Although most companies are auto suppliers, participants also come from other industries, universities, government organizations, and industry associations.

SOURCE: Spear and Bowen (1999).

nel rotations; and education and training programs. Each of these mechanisms, however, can be a cumbersome way to transfer knowledge. Active experience in performing a new activity is much more effective (Garvin, 1993); some research indicates that knowledge is exchanged in direct proportion to the level of face-to-face contact (Davenport et al., 1998). For this reason, personnel rotations have been identified as one of the most powerful methods of transferring knowledge (Garvin, 1993). It is important to note that such face-to-face knowledge transfers depend on a stable organizational workforce. A relatively stable workforce permits members to hold common understandings of important organizational priorities and processes and adequate information regarding the people and places in the organization where specific knowledge resides (Coff and Rousseau, 2000).

Knowledge management and organizational learning also are found to be more successful when they are supported by information technology (Davenport et al., 1998; Hansen et al., 1999). However, the type and extent of information technology needed vary according to the predominant knowledge management strategy in use. In a study of knowledge management practices at management consulting firms, HCOs, and computer manufacturers, researchers found that organizations that produced relatively standardized products to meet fairly standard needs relied heavily on codified knowledge stored in databases where it could easily be used by anyone in the company (Stewart, 1999). This capability required a heavy investment in information technology. Alternatively, organizations that provided more customized services to address unique problems tended to rely more on person-to-person sharing of knowledge and used information technology primarily to help people communicate (Hansen et al., 1999).

HCOs are likely to provide both standardized and customized services, and must adapt their knowledge management strategies to their settings and particular needs. In all cases, it can be important to avoid overreliance on information technology at the expense of shared personal knowledge through face-to-face contact (Goodman and Darr, 1996).

Time Required to Create a Learning Organization

The creation of a learning organization first requires an organizational commitment to learning through the establishment of a culture conducive to knowledge creation, sharing, and use—a knowledge-friendly culture (DeLong and Fahey, 2000; Garvin, 1993). Yet research on more than 50 companies pursuing knowledge management projects revealed that organizational culture was the major barrier to creating a learning organization (DeLong and Fahey, 2000). This situation will not be remedied overnight; most successful organizational learning and knowledge initiatives are the product of carefully cultivated attitudes, commitments, and management processes that have been built up slowly and steadily over time. The Toyota Production System, discussed earlier (see Box 4-1), is the product of decades of work (Spear and Bowen, 1999).

On the other hand, some changes can be made immediately to foster an environment conducive to learning. These include assessing the existing knowledge culture within an organization; freeing up employee time for thinking, learning, and training; and aligning incentives to reinforce and facilitate uptake of knowledge management practices.

Assessing the existing knowledge culture within the organization   Companies whose cultures are most effective at creating new knowledge and integrating it into the organization have norms and practices that demand broad participation in knowledge gathering and distribution (DeLong and Fahey, 2000). Some organizations, however, favor individual knowledge over group or organizational knowledge. In these organizations, individual knowledge is associated with power, control, and security of one's position in the organization. When employees believe that sharing what they know poses personal risk and decreases power, the free exchange of knowledge is impeded (Davenport et al., 1998). Before undertaking a knowledge management initiative, therefore, management should assess the culture of its organization to determine existing attitudes toward ownership of knowledge and how those attitudes would be altered by the initiative. Depending on the results of that assessment, management might also need to adopt new behaviors to communicate a shift from valuing individual over collective knowledge. It is necessary as well to make explicit what practices need to change to promote more collaborative use of knowledge (DeLong and Fahey, 2000).

In addition, organizations should examine their internal communication patterns. Communication patterns that make executives accessible and approachable and encourage open and frank dialogue are an essential element of a learning organization. Questioning fundamental beliefs and existing ways of working is difficult for organizational leadership, but is usually a key step in creating new knowledge for the organization. Intense debate on key strategic issues, drawing on extensive and intensive internal and external inputs—sometimes called "constructive confrontation" or "ferocious arguing with one another while remaining friends"—is identified as a key characteristic of cultures that are relatively effective at creating and integrating new knowledge. Learning organizations must identify norms and practices that are barriers to discussing sensitive topics, find and evaluate evidence about the extent to which senior management is perceived as accessible and approachable, and identify the norms and practices within the organization that encourage high frequency of interaction and the expectation of collaborative problem solving. Although the senior executive ultimately must make a decision not everyone will like, the process for engaging and listening to many views on an issue increases the likelihood of a better decision and broader acceptance of the decision once made (DeLong and Fahey, 2000).

Shared information is enhanced by familiarity, that is, where people know each other and the conditions under which they work. Familiarity can be compromised by status or other differences that suppress interaction (Goodman and Garber, 1988; Goodman and Leyden, 1991). As a result, people from different parts of the organization and different status levels often find it difficult to share knowledge. Such boundaries inhibit the flow of information; they keep individuals and groups isolated and reinforce preconceptions. A solution to this problem is to break down boundaries and stimulate the exchange of ideas between individuals at multiple levels of the organization through formal and informal practices that bring people together for this purpose (DeLong and Fahey, 2000). Conferences, meetings, and project teams that cut across organizational levels promote a fresh flow of ideas and the chance to consider competing perspectives (Garvin, 1993).

Providing time for thinking, learning, and training   For knowledge to be created and adopted, employees must have sufficient time for reflection and analysis to assess current work systems and devise new work processes. Such learning is difficult when employees are harried or rushed; it tends to be displaced by the pressures of the moment. Only if top management explicitly frees up employee time for this purpose does learning occur with any regularity.

Further, employees must posses the skills to use learning productively. To perform and evaluate experiments, managers and staff members need skills in such areas as statistical methods and experiment design in order to perform and evaluate experiments. These skills are seldom intuitive and must be learned. Such training is often most effective when intact work groups participate in the training together. Training in brainstorming, problem solving, evaluation of experiments, and other core learning skills is essential (Garvin, 1993). All of the organizations managed according to the Toyota Production System, for example, share an overarching belief that people are the most significant corporate asset and that investments in their knowledge and skills are necessary to build competitiveness. They invest heavily in training and in creating among coworkers shared understandings of problem solving and innovation processes (Spear and Bowen, 1999).

Organizations need to create formal programs or events with explicit learning goals in mind. These programs can take a variety of forms, including strategic reviews that examine the changing external environment and the organization's services, technology, and market position; systems audits that review the performance of the large processes and delivery systems in the organization; internal benchmark reports that compare the organization's performance with that of other best-practice organizations; the results of "study missions" in which individuals are dispatched to leading external organizations to better understand their performance and distinctive skills; and symposiums that bring customers, suppliers, outside experts, and internal groups together to share ideas and learn from one another. Each of these activities fosters learning by requiring employees to grapple with new knowledge and consider its implications for the organization (Garvin, 1993).

Aligning incentives to reinforce and facilitate uptake of knowledge management practices Knowledge has been described as being "intimately and inextricably bound with people's egos and occupations" and therefore as not flowing easily across roles or functional boundaries (Davenport et al., 1998:53). Knowledge is more likely to be transferred effectively when the right incentives are in place (Garvin, 1993). In a study of 31 knowledge management projects at 24 corporations, the motivation to create, share, and use knowledge was found to be a critical success factor for the projects. The researchers concluded that incentives to contribute should be long-term and should be linked to both the general evaluation and compensation structure of the organization (Davenport et al., 1998). Some organizations have used the extent to which employees contribute to the organization's knowledge repository as a component of employee evaluations and compensation decisions (Davenport et al., 1998). The U.S. Army is one of a growing number of organizations that formally consider knowledge-sharing capabilities when identifying candidates for promotion (DeLong and Fahey, 2000).

UNEVEN APPLICATION OF EVIDENCE-BASED MANAGEMENT PRACTICES IN NURSES' WORK ENVIRONMENTS

While some nurses have had firsthand experience with the successful application of the above evidence-based management practices in their workplace, this has not consistently been the case. Concerns about changes in nursing leadership, increased emphasis on production efficiency in response to cost-containment pressures, weakened trust, poor change management, limited involvement in decision making pertaining to work design and work flow, and limited knowledge management are all found in nurses' work environments. Each of these barriers to the application of evidence-based management practices in nurses' work environments is discussed in turn below.

Concerns About Changes in Nursing Leadership

Nursing leadership in hospitals and other HCOs has a key role with respect to the deployment of the nurse workforce in these institutions and overall patient care. This role, however, at least in hospitals, is changing. Evidence suggests that these changes may diminish the ability of hospital nursing leadership to (1) represent nursing staff and management to each other and facilitate their mutual trust, (2) facilitate the input of direct-care nursing staff into decision making on the design of work processes and work flow, and (3) provide clinical leadership in support of knowledge acquisition and uptake by nursing staff.

The senior nurse leadership position in hospitals has not always been an executive-level position. A 1983 national Commission of Nursing report and publications of the American Hospital Association recommended to hospitals that chief nursing officers (CNOs) be regarded as a key component of a hospital's executive management team.[2] Prior to this time, CNOs typically were not involved in strategic planning for the hospital overall; many did not participate in the development of the budget for their own department. Recommendations that nurses be involved in policy development and decision making throughout the organization were important in bringing the CNO position to the executive management team in many hospitals (Clifford, 1998).

This view of the CNO position is consistent with both old and new management concepts. Florence Nightingale, the founder of modern nursing, made major improvements in the education and training of nurses in the latter part of the nineteenth century. She proposed an administrative system for hospitals that included a triad of lay administrator, physician leader, and senior nursing leader. Her model was an important contributor to the development of hospital management systems and was responsible for the introduction of the position of superintendent of nurses to U.S. hospitals. Nightingale asserted that only those trained as nurses were qualified to govern other nurses (Clifford, 1998). This view also is consistent with the more recent management philosophy embodied in the Toyota Production System, which requires that all managers know how to perform the jobs of those they supervise (Spear and Bowen, 1999). Until recently, the CNO was the official leader of a hospital's nursing staff. Although other administrative responsibilities may have been involved, the primary role of the CNO was the administration and leadership of the nursing service (Clifford, 1998).

---

[2]Unlike the title of CEO or chief financial officer (CFO), the title of CNO is not used consistently across HCOs, nor is it always accompanied by executive-level functioning. The CNO designation can be found at all levels of an HCO (Clifford, 1998).

In the past two decades, the role of the CNO has continued to expand as a result of service integration and hospital reengineering initiatives. In surveys conducted in 1993 and 1995 of nurse leaders in VHA, Inc. (a nationwide network of community-owned health care systems) and nurse executives and managers who were members of the AONE, 80 percent of all respondents reported changes in their role. Nearly all of these respondents identified expanded responsibilities as a major feature of their role change. The proportion of respondents holding positions whose title included the word "nursing" (e.g., director of nursing or vice president of nursing) declined from 55 to 24 percent, while the proportion holding positions whose title did not explicitly mention nursing (e.g., vice president of patient care, vice president of operations, and chief operating officer) increased from 35 to 53 percent. The new, expanded roles of these hospital nurse leaders included responsibilities for radiology departments, surgery, emergency departments, cardiology, nursing homes, outpatient services, admitting, and infection control units (Gelinas and Manthey, 1997). A more recent, 1997–1998 study of hospital restructuring in 29 university teaching hospitals found that the CNE position had been transformed into a "patient care" executive position in 97 percent of the institutions surveyed (Sovie and Jawad, 2001).

Even as CNOs have increasingly assumed these expanded managerial duties, they also have retained responsibility for managing nursing services. Research is needed on whether the expanded role of the CNO has beneficial or adverse effects on patients (Clifford, 1998). Some assert that expanding the CNO role increases senior nurse executives' influence in desirable ways. Others express concern that the expansion of the CNO's areas of responsibility beyond those directly associated with clinical nursing takes attention away from nursing care and hinders the development of strong nursing leadership for nursing practice in the hospital. What is agreed upon is that as the roles of nurse leaders have expanded, so have the demands of balancing two, often competing, sets of responsibilities as senior administrative staff and leader of nursing staff. As senior executive, the CNO must help the hospital meet its strategic goals, which are often financially focused. As leader of nursing staff, the CNO is responsible for providing clinical leadership. Concern has also been expressed that the attempt to meet both sets of responsibilities has resulted in the potential loss of a common voice for nursing staff and a weakening of clinical leadership.

Potential Loss of a Common Voice for Nursing

A 1996 qualitative study of the changing role of hospital CNOs in the not-for-profit flagship hospitals of three urban integrated delivery systems chosen by a panel of experts as being "at the forefront of change" found that at these hospitals, the organizational boundaries of nurse leaders had shifted away from the traditional department of nursing to an organizational structure in which nursing services were unidentifiable and integrated. An expansion of management responsibilities appeared to be taking place in all nursing management roles, in one hospital resulting in the "dismantling of the nursing department." That is, an identifiable central nursing department was no longer visible in the restructured hospital, as was manifest in the absence of nursing as an organizational element on the hospital organization chart. Moreover, fewer nurse managers, directors, and assistant nurse managers were found at all levels of the hospitals (Clifford, 1998).

This phenomenon has been documented to occur on a more widespread basis. In the previously cited 1993 and 1995 surveys of nurse leaders in VHA, Inc. HCOs and AONE nurse executives and managers, nearly one-third of all respondents indicated that after their redesign initiatives, there would no longer be a separate department of nursing (Gelinas and Manthey, 1997). Hospital staff nurses further affirm these findings. An examination of changes in the work environments of nurses in 12 hospitals identified as having characteristics associated with high rates of nurse retention found that from 1986 to 1998, the percentage of nurses reporting "a chief nursing executive equal in power/authority to other top hospital officials" declined from 99 to 69 percent. Those reporting "a director of nursing highly visible and accessible to staff" fell from 89 to 41 percent (Aiken et al., 2000). A more recent, 1998–1999 survey of nurses working in acute care hospitals in Pennsylvania additionally found that 58.3 percent of nurses reported a decrease in the number of nurse managers, and 16.8 percent reported the loss of a CNO without replacement (Aiken et al., 2001). The potential loss of the ability of these nursing leaders to represent staff nurses is articulated in a report on the findings of interviews with executives of 13 VHA, Inc. HCOs conducted in 1992. The nurse authors of the report state:

> It was not uncommon to find nursing personnel reporting to non-nurse administrators, and former nurse executives responsible for non-clinical, non-patient care departments. . . . Nurse executives are fulfilling a variety of roles previously considered strictly administrative, including those of chief operating officer and CEO. In this capacity, it is inappropriate for them to be spokespersons for the nursing profession within their institution—they must be spokespersons for the broad function of patient care. Although this bodes well for improvements in patient care, it also dislocates the strongest voice for professional nursing issues. For the past 20 years or so, nurse executives have been spokespersons for the profession at the institutional, local, state, and national levels, both as individuals and through their organizations and associations. Because of the dramatic role changes underway, the ability of this group to effectively represent the nursing profession may be seriously compromised. The

nursing profession may be well-advised to find leaders from other settings—practice, education, or research. (Gelinas and Manthey, 1995:63)

Weakening of Clinical Leadership

Leadership for the clinical practice of nursing also has been identified as at risk. In the above-cited 1996 qualitative study of the changing role of hospital CNOs in three not-for-profit flagship hospitals, changes in the clinical leadership role of the CNO were found not to have kept pace with the growth and strength of the administrative responsibilities of that role. Similar changes were experienced down the line. The span of control of the midlevel director of nursing increased, and the incumbent had less time to spend with individual unit managers. Unit managers had less ready access to the midlevel director of nursing. They no longer had someone to whom they could readily turn to help them reflect on problems and issues requiring their attention. Similarly, the nurse unit managers' span of control had increased. Some nurse managers were now responsible for more than one patient care unit as the number of nurse managers in these three hospitals decreased (Clifford, 1998).

These findings echo those of interviews with executives of 13 VHA, Inc. HCOs beginning in 1992. These executives reported that in organizations that had retained a traditional nursing structure, the number of nursing directors and nurse managers had been reduced. Nurse managers were often assigned responsibility for two nursing units, with an expansion in the number of assistants or charge nurses reporting to them at the shift level (Gelinas and Manthey, 1995). These additional duties likely leave the nurse manager with less time to provide clinical supervision or teaching (Norrish and Rundall, 2001).

Interview data from all three flagship hospitals in the 1996 study suggest the need for an ongoing, central locus of clinical leadership within the HCO (Clifford, 1998). And in the 1997–1998 survey of 29 university teaching hospitals described above, researchers found that as the responsibilities of nurse executives were expanded, consolidation or downsizing of nursing departments occurred in 82 percent of hospitals. Further, nurse manager positions were reduced in 91 percent of the hospitals, and nurse managers' span of control was broadened to include more than one patient care unit. Nearly half of the nurse managers were also given additional responsibility for supervising personnel other than nursing staff (e.g., housekeepers, transportation staff, dietary aides). Assistant nurse manager positions were reduced in 68 percent of the hospitals. "The cumulative effect . . . was a reduction in the direct management support available to patient care staff" (Sovie and Jawad, 2001:591). This effect also is reported in other studies of HCO reorganization of nursing services (Ingersoll et al., 2001).

The committee finds that strong nursing leadership is needed in all HCOs in order to (1) represent nursing staff and management to each other and foster their mutual trust, (2) facilitate the input of direct-care nursing staff into decision making on the design of work processes and work flow, and (3) provide clinical leadership in support of knowledge acquisition and uptake by nursing staff. Recent changes in the responsibilities of senior nurse executives and nursing management in hospitals, in particular, may place these functions at risk. The committee therefore makes the following recommendation:

Recommendation 4-1.[3] HCOs should acquire nurse leaders for all levels of management (e.g., at the organization-wide and patient care unit levels) who will:

- **Participate in executive decisions within the HCO.**
- **Represent nursing staff to organization management and facilitate their mutual trust.**
- **Achieve effective communication between nursing and other clinical leadership.**
- **Facilitate input of direct-care nursing staff into operational decision making and the design of work processes and work flow.**
- **Be provided with organizational resources to support the acquisition, management, and dissemination to nursing staff of the knowledge needed to support their clinical decision making and actions.**

Although the committee did not find evidence supporting the use of one particular organizational structure for locating nursing leadership within any one type of HCO or across all HCOs, the intent of this recommendation is to institute (among other management practices) well-prepared clinical nursing leadership at the most senior level of management—e.g., CEO's direct reports—commensurate with physician leadership within the HCO.

Increased Emphasis on Production Efficiency

Many of the changes in nursing leadership described above were the result of organizational efforts to achieve greater efficiency (Sovie and Jawad, 2001). This increased emphasis on production efficiency (discussed also in Chapter 1) has been a hallmark of the hospital and health care reengineering initiatives of the last two decades (Bazzoli et al., 2002), par-

---

[3]For ease of reference, the committee's recommendations are numbered according to the chapter of the main text in which they appear.

ticularly with respect to the work of nurses (Norrish and Rundall, 2001). In the 1993 and 1995 surveys of nurse leaders discussed above, although fewer than 17 percent of respondents identified cost reduction as a primary reason for their hospital's redesign initiative, "reduction of costs" was the criterion employed most frequently to evaluate the outcomes of the initiative (reported by 90 percent of respondents) (Gelinas and Manthey, 1997). Concern that reorganization initiatives have focused on efficiency at the expense of patient quality also are commonly expressed by nursing staff involved in such initiatives (Barry-Walker, 2000; Ingersoll et al., 2001).

Experts in patient safety have identified safeguards that can be used by HCOs to defend against an overemphasis on efficiency at the expense of reliability (patient safety). First, HCO boards of directors should spend as much time overseeing an organization's patient safety performance as they do dealing with financial goals and performance (Appleby, 2002). They should know (1) how patient safety is addressed in the HCO's mission statement; (2) what mechanisms are used by the HCO to assess the safety of its patient care environment; and (3) what the HCO's overall plan or approach is for ensuring patient safety and whether it has defined objectives, senior-level leadership, and adequate personnel and financial resources. The board should also receive regular progress reports on patient safety (Mohr et al., 2002) and review all sentinel events and the organization's follow-up activities (Appleby, 2002). Further, a member of the HCO's senior leadership team (excluding risk management) should serve as chief quality and safety officer, comparable to the chief financial officer. Just as the latter individual is in charge of monitoring and strengthening the organization's financial performance, the chief safety officer should be responsible for patient safety measures and metrics (Appleby, 2002). This responsibility can be met by developing indicators of patient safety and quality that are collected and monitored before and after change initiatives are undertaken (Ingersoll et al., 2001).

Weakened Trust

Weakened trust has been widely observed by researchers studying and comparing hospitals as part of a national recognition program for hospitals that have achieved high levels of nurse retention (Kramer and Schmalenberg, 1993:62): "As we have visited and studied nursing departments all over the country, we have been struck by the amount of distrust perceived by nurses—not only from physicians but also from nurse managers and administrators." The researchers contrast this situation with the work environment observed at one hospital (Edward Hospital in suburban Chicago), where high levels of trust were present:

At EH we observed some of the most flagrant disregard for the "on paper" bureaucratic structure that we have ever seen. Repeatedly, when asked how they would handle a situation, nurses told us that it depended on the situation, but that they felt free to ignore the formal structure if the situation demanded it. The perception of openness and trust was almost unbelievable; there was absolutely no reticence to share anything with us—good or bad. "We can say what we think and feel; I know that nothing bad will happen to me if I do." Nurses talked openly and freely about failures, faults and mishaps, as well as about the positive things in the organization. Not a single nurse asked that any of our interview material be kept confidential. This open and trusting atmosphere is remarkable, especially because of its scarcity. (Kramer and Schmalenberg, 1993:62)

Loss of trust in administration by nursing staff is frequently reported in studies of HCO redesign and reorganization initiatives that have taken place in the last two decades (Decker et al., 2001; Ingersoll et al., 2001). The above-cited 1996 qualitative study of the changing role of hospital CNOs in the not-for-profit flagship hospitals of three urban integrated delivery systems found that loss of trust on the part of nursing staff was acutely felt and attributed to changes in the role of the CNO. These changes affected the relationships of CNOs with nurse managers, which were perceived as characterized by a growing distance. "Whether the change was actual or symbolic did not matter; the distancing was felt." The nurses needed to trust that someone who understood their practice was advocating at the highest levels of the organization for what they were doing on behalf of patients and families (Clifford, 1998:111).

Other reports of loss of trust during reengineering initiatives are frequently associated with poor communication practices. In a study of major reorganization at two acute care hospitals, loss of a trusting relationship with administration was reported as stemming from a perception (constant across hospitals and nursing units) that information was being withheld and that administrators were not aware of the circumstances that existed at the nursing unit level (Ingersoll et al., 2001). A study of reengineering efforts at 14 U.S. hospitals provides examples of poor communication patterns that reduced employees' trust in the administration:

Many hospitals promised that there would be no "sacred cows" or areas that would be exempt from reengineering examination. In reality, however, almost every hospital exempted certain areas. One major vendor was also a major donor to the hospital and was excluded. A specialized service area earned too much income to be disturbed and was declared off-limits. A physician was too powerful to be challenged. It seemed that every hospital had some idiosyncratic situation that prevented full participation. The promise of full participation, followed by selective exemptions, resulted in increased cynicism and damaged trust. (Walston and Kimberly, 1997:157)

> Honesty with communication is also important . . . executives would initially communicate through the planning process that quality and employees' jobs would be protected but, when implementation occurred, employees felt both were affected. One chief financial officer in the final stages of planning his reengineering project told us he did not think that they had been totally honest about what was going to happen as he anticipated a large layoff, but they had not been allowed to even use the words layoff or severance. (Walston and Kimberly, 1997:156)

As a result of these poor communication patterns, trust was low, and employees repeatedly disregarded information. Hospitals reported that employees would regularly discard internal communications and fail to attend informational meetings. Executives would then wonder why letters and speeches to employees were not helping to alleviate concerns and communicate the organization's direction. This distrust was found to result from the organization's own actions (Walston and Kimberly, 1997).

Countermeasures to diminished trust include frequent and ongoing communication, involvement of workers in the design and evaluation of change initiatives, and other change management practices as described in the next section. Moreover, regardless of whether an HCO is undertaking a formal redesign or reengineering process, involving nurses in work decisions and providing them with control over caregiving practices by empowering them to make clinical decisions have been linked to greater levels of organizational trust (Laschinger et al., 2000). This observation is discussed in greater detail in the section below on work design and work flow decision making.

Poor Change Management

Very little documentation exists about how HCOs have implemented reengineering and restructuring initiatives. One well-designed study involved intensive interviews with 60 executives, 121 midlevel managers, 31 physicians, 24 staff nurses, and 19 non-nurse staff members at 14 hospitals that had undertaken reengineering initiatives in the past 5 years (Walston and Kimberly, 1997). The hospitals were selected in collaboration with a consulting firm specializing in hospital reengineering. Although the researchers acknowledge that selecting hospitals that used the same consulting firm may have created bias, they note that they took great care in choosing a sample of hospitals that varied by size, geographic location, and organizational affiliation and ownership. The findings of this study and a few others indicate that the change management practices identified in the previous section (i.e., ongoing communication; worker training; use of mechanisms for measurement, feedback, and redesign; sustained attention; and worker involvement) are not consistently observed in the reorganization, redesign, and reengineering initiatives undertaken by hospitals. Often these failures are intertwined.

Inadequate Communication

Walston and Kimberly (1997) found that although all redesign initiatives began with planned communication strategies that included special newsletters, employee meetings, forums, and one-to-one meetings between managers and employees, communication was either discontinued or not updated to provide feedback on the status of the project after its initial stages. As communication efforts declined, employees fell back into old routines. Thus, these poor communication practices also reflected a lack of sustained attention to the change initiative. Poor communication from administration to staff throughout reengineering initiatives has also been reported by nurses (Barry-Walker, 2000; Ingersoll et al., 2001) and other workers (Decker et al., 2001) involved in other individual hospital reengineering initiatives.

Insufficient Worker Training

Walston and Kimberly (1997) found that, as result of reengineering projects, staff nurses and individual unit nurse managers were frequently assigned greater managerial responsibilities without additional training. Nurses commented that excellent clinical nurses frequently lacked the management skills necessary to direct and delegate responsibilities to a subordinate team, and that delegation and managerial skills were not routinely taught. At the same time, senior management did not appear to recognize that many of the necessary managerial skills are cognitively learned competencies and should be addressed prior to the assignment of new responsibilities.

This finding is echoed by hospital nurse executives involved in reengineering initiatives who reported needing the following additional knowledge to help them meet the new expectations set for them by their HCO (Gelinas and Manthey, 1997):

- Use of clinical pathways and other quality improvement tools to measure and manage outcomes
- Understanding of managed care
- Understanding of finance, including capitated environments and risk sharing
- Team-building skills
- Change management expertise

The need to train nurse managers in delegation and management skills, strategies for dealing with role change, and the economic and policy factors that contribute to changes has been documented in other studies as well (Ingersoll et al., 2001).

Walston and Kimberly (1997) also found that many hospitals that employed cross-training of non-nursing staff to perform patient care activities underestimated the amount of initial training and retraining that was needed. Researchers were told that often after initial, brief training periods (some as short as 3 days), new workers were assigned patient responsibilities, such as the performance of electrocardiograms and phlebotomies, only to function very inadequately. Much of the rework fell back on nursing staff. The researchers note that training costs are high when comprehensively addressed. One 500-bed hospital spent $700,000 on its training in the first 2 years of its reengineering initiative. This hospital also performed a gap analysis to identify those roles not being performed adequately and to evaluate what additional training was needed. The reviewers concluded that such continual evaluation of training needs is important to the effective implementation of new roles and responsibilities.

Lack of Measurement and Feedback

Walston and Kimberly (1997) observed a lack of measurement and feedback to staff on the progress of reengineering efforts. In many situations, feedback either was not provided at all or if provided, was not well understood. Both managers and employees frequently reported that they rarely heard about the results of reengineering efforts. Although every hospital developed some type of data tracking mechanism, employees typically either lacked access to the data or felt that the availability of the data was inadequate. This inability to record and display the progress of reengineering frequently caused a perception that the outcomes would not be sustained and resulted in diminished efforts to sustain the process.

Short-Lived Attention

Walston and Kimberly (1997:153) further found that effective organizational reengineering initiatives require long periods of time and constant effort. "Many hospitals that were two to three years into their engineering effort had yet to implement all of their initial plans. The most simplified plan of any of the hospitals demanded at least a year to analyze, plan, and implement." During this time, employees expressed concern that the engineering initiative "drifted" and lacked consistency. The transition from initial implementation to sustained operation of the reengineered processes was most at risk. "Although many hospitals perceived reengineering to be a continual change process that would reorient their organizations, many facilities ended their efforts at least temporarily, after the initial implementation. Without continued and constant efforts, the organizations drifted back to the status quo. A mid-manager from a large teaching hospital reported, 'The gains are now disappearing as people go back to their old ways of doing things'" (Walston and Kimberly, 1997:160).

Lack of sustained attention is, in part, a function of how an organization codifies a change through formal reporting structures, management tools, and policies and procedures. A 1996–1997 survey of CEOs of U.S. general medical–surgical hospitals located in urban areas and with more than 100 beds found that 40 percent of the 29.4 percent of responding CEOs had not formalized the change process through written manuals, guidelines, budgets, or some combination of the three (Walston et al., 2000).

Low Worker Involvement in Developing Change Initiatives

Walston and Kimberly (1997:157) also found a lack of uniform involvement by organizational departments in HCO reengineering efforts:

> Most of the hospitals had a single individual that was the "champion" of reengineering. This was generally a top executive—the chief nursing officer, the chief executive officer, the chief financial officer, or an associate administrator. . . . At one hospital where the chief nursing officer was the key patron of engineering, each department was directed to develop cost reduction recommendations. Nursing developed a patient-focused plan to incorporate many services, including respiratory therapy, into nursing units, which was projected to save substantial costs. When they presented their plan to the hospital's steering committee for approval, they were informed that they could proceed with their recommendation except for the respiratory therapy component. Respiratory therapy had previously obtained approval from the steering committee without nursing's knowledge for its own plan that called for laying off a number of part-time respiratory therapists, providing a fixed number of inpatient therapists, ranking all patients according to the severity of their need for respiratory therapy, and providing care to only the sickest patients as far as the fixed hours would allow. Nursing was both astonished and angry, for respiratory therapy was allowed to exempt itself from a *coordinated* reengineering process and its solution would pass a great amount of work back to nursing services. Variations of this problem occurred in many other hospitals causing inconsistent participation and ineffective implementation.

In addition, limited involvement of nurses (Barry-Walker, 2000) and other health care workers (Decker et al., 2001) has been reported in studies of individual HCO reengineering efforts.

Limited Involvement in Decision Making
Pertaining to Work Design and Work Flow

The involvement of nurses in decision making has varied over time and by the hierarchical level of the nurse within the HCO. In the 1970s and 1980s, under the primary care model of nursing practice, hospital nurses had responsibility for clinical nursing care decisions for assigned patients for the patients' entire hospital stay (see also Chapter 3). Moreover, as a result of some of the health care integration and reengineering initiatives of the 1980s and 1990s, nurses in charge of an 8-hour shift (often called shift "charge nurses") were elevated to the position of "nurse managers" who functioned—with responsibility 24 hours a day, 7 days a week—as the head of a nursing unit. These nurse managers often were made responsible for hiring personnel, allocating resources, evaluating performance, setting standards of practice, and disciplining staff who did not meet standards or competency expectations (Norrish and Rundall, 2001). This shift in responsibilities coincided with the promotion of "shared-governance" models of nursing practice that promised increased participation of nursing staff and management in operational and policy decision making. As described previously, however, descriptions of shared governance have shown wide variation in the specific decisions made or shared by nurses and managers, which staff are included in the shared-governance decision making, and whether nurses have authority for decisions individually or collectively. Thus, models of shared governance have ranged from minimal, ad hoc, informal participation by some nursing staff in a limited number of decisions to models in which the authority and accountability of professional nurses are codified within the organization, and formal decision-making structures and processes are in place that enable nurses to define and regulate nursing practice and share decisions with administrators regarding the management of resources (Maas and Specht, 2001).

Shared-governance practices waned in the 1990s as reengineering and integration initiatives modified the roles of nursing staff and management. The above-cited study of changes in the work environments of nurses in 12 hospitals identified as having characteristics associated with high rates of nurse retention found that from 1986 to 1998, the percentage of nurses reporting "the freedom to make important patient care and work decisions" declined from 98 to 80 percent (Aiken et al., 2000:463). In a 1998–1999 survey of nurses working in acute care hospitals in Pennsylvania, only 29 percent reported that their administration listened and responded to nurse concerns; 40.6 percent reported that nurses had the opportunity to participate in policy decisions; and 60.5 percent reported being able to participate in developing their own schedules (Aiken et al., 2001).

Limited Knowledge Management

As discussed earlier, learning organizations take advantage of all sources of knowledge, use systematic experimentation to generate new knowledge internally, and transfer knowledge quickly and efficiently throughout the organization. The little available evidence on knowledge management as practiced in nurses' work environments indicates very limited use of these practices. A search for "knowledge management" or "learning organization" in the Cumulative Index to Nursing and Allied Health Literature (CINAHL) for English-language publications, with no date limitations, yielded but a few articles. These articles are primarily exhortations for the adoption of knowledge management and learning organization practices, as opposed to descriptions of their application. This may be in part because these practices are catalogued under different labels, such as "decision support," "informatics," "continuous quality improvement," or "total quality management." Also, the use of knowledge management and learning organization principles does not apply solely to nursing, but to all health care providers, so it may not be described as a "nursing" practice. However, a similar MEDLINE search for the years 1971–2003 returned only 24 articles with these topics in the title.

Knowledge is available from multiple sources: from internal HCO sources such as total quality management, risk management, and patient and provider experiences with care delivery, as well as from external sources such as research, the professional literature, technology assessment reports, and authoritative practice guidelines. According to Donaldson and Rutledge (1998:6), however, organizational translation of new knowledge from external sources into language and operations familiar to potential users has been "largely ignored in nursing literature." Six large-scale multifaceted studies of the diffusion and utilization of nursing research undertaken over the past two decades have documented the need to build knowledge utilization infrastructures, expand the capacity of individual nurses to take up new knowledge, and expedite the transmission of new knowledge from external sources to nurses (Donaldson and Rutledge, 1998).

There is also evidence that HCOs do not learn well from internal sources of information. A Harvard Business School study of hospital nurses, their errors, and the extent to which they actively seek to prevent future occurrences of similar errors found that hospitals are not learning from the daily problems and errors encountered by their workers (Tucker and Edmondson, 2003). Twenty-six nurses at nine hospitals were observed for 239 hours, and interviews were conducted with 12 of the nurses at seven sites. Researchers purposely selected hospitals with a reputation for nursing excellence by asking nursing governing boards for referrals to such hospitals and by searching the nursing literature on magnet hospitals. Their goal was not to employ a representative sample of hospitals, but to assess how excellent nursing hospitals handle service failures. From these observations, common basic patterns of problem-solving behavior across the nine hospitals were identified.

Researchers distinguished two types of process failures: "errors" and "problems." "Errors" were defined as the execution of a task that was either unnecessary or carried out incorrectly. "Problems" were defined as disruptions of the nurse's ability to execute a prescribed task because a resource was unavailable at the needed time, location, or condition or in sufficient quantity (e.g., missing supplies, information, or medications), thus preventing the task from being implemented.

Of the 194 observed failures, 86 percent were problems rather than errors. This finding is significant to improving patient care for several reasons. Problems are relatively frequent and visible, and also carry fewer stigmas than errors; all of these features facilitate an HCO's taking action on a problem to improve patient care and safety. However, researchers found that nurses tended to practice "first-order" problem solving, that is, fixing the immediate problem without communicating that it occurred, investigating why it occurred, or seeking to change its cause. Thus the problem was isolated so that it did not become visible to the hospital as an opportunity to learn how to be more efficient or effective in patient care. Second-order problem solving, in contrast, occurs when a worker, in addition to fixing the problem so the task at hand can be completed, takes action to address the underlying cause. Researchers used lenient criteria—i.e., encompassing any behavior that called attention to the problem—to assess the extent to which second-order problem solving had occurred. Nonetheless, only 7 percent of nurse responses were second-order.

Researchers identified three human resource practices that explained why so few problems had received second-order attention that would have enabled the organization to learn from the problems and correct systemic weaknesses. First, instilling in nurses a strong sense of responsibility for individual vigilance can, as a side effect, encourage such a strong emphasis on independence and self-sufficiency that they see a failure not as a system problem, but as one that can be overcome or withstood through individual competence. The majority of the nurses interviewed commented that they believed their manager expected them to work through daily disruptions on their own. Speaking up about a problem or asking for help was likely to be viewed as a sign of incompetence. Second, staffing levels were so tight, with so little slack in the system, that nurses did not have the time to eliminate underlying causes of problems. Instead, they were "barely able to keep up with the required responsibilities and [were] in essence forced to quickly patch problems so they [could] complete their immediate responsibilities" (Tucker and Edmondson, 2003:9). Finally, removal of front-line managers and other personnel not involved in direct patient care from daily work activities left workers on their own to resolve problems. At hospitals characterized by second-order problem solving, either nurse managers were a strong presence on the floor, or there was a designated person available to provide guidance and support to nurses (Tucker and Edmondson, 2002). The researchers concluded that "reducing the degree to which managers are available to front-line staff can be a loss for improvement efforts, especially when workers are already overburdened by existing duties" (Tucker and Edmondson, 2003:10).

The researchers identified several countermeasures to first-order problem solving to enable organizational learning. First, managers must be available to staff nurses for at least a portion of all shifts. The researchers observed that the presence of managers increased the likelihood of their being informed of problems occurring on the unit, thus enabling them to investigate and intervene with systemic solutions. Managers also serve as role models for system-level thinking, encouraging nurses to think of second-order solutions. Second, management needs to create a "fair and just" work environment (discussed in Chapter 7) that encourages workers to feel secure in reporting both errors and problems so system performance can be enhanced (Tucker and Edmondson, 2003). Also, if workers are to engage in identification and elimination of systemic problems, this activity should be an explicit part of their job description (Tucker et al., 2002), and they should receive training in its application (Tucker and Edmondson, 2002). Finally, management needs to act on reported problems with second-order solutions so workers will have an incentive to continue to identify these opportunities for learning and improvement (Tucker and Edmondson, 2003).

Recommendations to Promote Evidence-Based Management Practices

To address the deficiencies discussed above in nurses' work environments with respect to the application of the five management practices introduced in this chapter, the committee offers the following two recommendations:

Recommendation 4-2. Leaders of HCOs should take action to identify and minimize the potential adverse effects of their decisions on patient safety by:

- **Educating board members and senior, midlevel, and line managers about the link between management practices and safety.**
- **Emphasizing safety to the same extent as productivity and financial goals in internal management planning and reports, and public reports to stakeholders.**

Recommendation 4-3. HCOs should employ management structures and processes throughout the organization that:

- Provide ongoing vigilance in balancing efficiency and safety.
- Demonstrate trust in workers and promote trust by workers.
- Actively manage the process of change.
- Engage workers in nonhierarchical decision making and in the design of work processes and work flow.
- Establish the organization as a "learning organization."

These recommendations are feasible. Indeed, they are currently practiced in a number of nursing work environments described in the next section.

MODELS OF EVIDENCE-BASED MANAGEMENT IN NURSES' WORK ENVIRONMENTS

The five evidence-based management practices described above have been employed successfully in a number of nurse work environments by HCOs acting alone or in collaboration with one another. Examples include magnet hospitals, the Pittsburgh Regional Healthcare Initiative, and the Wellspring model of long-term care.

Magnet Hospitals

In the early 1980s, during one of the cyclical nursing shortages, a task force of the American Academy of Nursing undertook a study to identify those hospitals—labeled "magnet hospitals" that had no difficulty in attracting and retaining nurses during such shortages (McClure et al., 1983). Through two decades of research, the characteristics of these magnet hospitals have been articulated and their relationship to nurse and patient outcomes studied.

In the original magnet hospital study, 165 organizations were identified across the country that fit three criteria: (1) nurses saw the hospital as a good place to work; (2) the hospital was able to recruit and retain nurses (as measured by a lower-than-usual turnover rate during a nursing shortage situation); and (3) the hospital was located in a market area that included other hospitals competing for its nurses. Based on a review of the hospitals' recruitment and retention records as well as other material, 41 organizations were selected as magnet hospitals (McClure et al., 2002). Systematic interviews with the CNE and a selected staff nurse from each organization provided the data for an analysis of the characteristics that attracted and retained nurses in these hospitals. Magnet characteristics were identified in the areas of administration, professional practice, and professional development. Many of the leadership and management practices cited previously (providing strong leadership, managing change, creating and sustaining trust throughout the organization, involving workers in decision making pertaining to work design and work flow, and establishing the organization as a learning organization) have been documented as present in magnet hospitals.[4]

In a series of six surveys between 1985 and 2001, Kramer and Schmalenberg refined the original set of magnet characteristics. Their studies included a subset of 16 of the original magnet hospitals, selected by geographic location. The surveys involved interviews of CNEs, staff nurses, nurse managers, and clinical experts (Kramer, 1990a,b; Kramer and Schmalenberg, 1988a,b, 1991, 1993; Kramer et al., 1989). In these surveys, eight essential characteristics associated with magnetism were again identified by two-thirds or more of the staff nurses interviewed. They included working with clinically competent nurses (an essential element of trust), nurse autonomy and accountability, having a supportive nurse manager/supervisor (a component of both leadership and trust), control over nursing practice, and educational support (Kramer and Schmalenberg, 2002).

Two studies have examined patient mortality rates in relation to magnet hospital status. In the late 1980s, 39 magnet hospitals were compared with 195 nonmagnet matched hospitals using Medicare mortality rates. Adjusting for differences in predicted mortality for Medicare patients, the magnet hospitals had a 4.6 percent lower mortality rate, which translates to 0.9 to 9.4 fewer deaths per 1,000 discharges (Aiken et al., 1994). In a second study, patients with AIDS in magnet hospitals and those with AIDS in nonmagnet hospitals with and without designated AIDS units were compared. Patients in the magnet hospitals had a lower chance of dying than those in the nonmagnet hospitals regardless of the existence of designated AIDS units (Aiken et al., 1999). In the early 1990s, the American Nurses' Association, through the American Nurses' Credentialing Center (ANCC), established a formal certification program through which hospitals and nursing homes may apply for "magnet status." The criteria for selection are based on the characteristics originally identified, as well as on specific standards of practice and administration.

Leadership

In the above studies, the major administrative determinant of magnetism was found to be the quality of leadership from the CNE (Kramer and

---

[4]The studies of magnet hospitals have also identified other important practices, such as maintaining adequate staffing levels and professional nurse–physician relationships. These other characteristics of magnet hospitals are discussed in the relevant chapters of this report.

Schmalenberg, 1988a,b; McClure et al., 2002). This individual was visible in the organization, took part in policy-level decision making, and set the stage for a decentralized organizational structure and participative management. His/her leadership style conveyed respect for the staff nurses and trust in their ability to provide high-quality patient care. In Kramer and Schmalenberg's 1989–1990 study comparing magnet and nonmagnet hospital nurses' perceptions of leadership–management values, staff nurses at magnet hospitals gave significantly more positive responses (p > 0.001) on such items as "Our nursing leaders are visionary, and they communicate and implement ideas, values and goals"; "Potential problems are anticipated and worked on before they become problems"; and "With stable expectations of what must be done to achieve goals, people here are free to experiment and try new things" (Kramer and Schmalenberg, 2002).

Presence of Trust

The presence of trust in the work environment of magnet hospitals was found to be facilitated by the nursing leadership, as discussed above, and also by strong clinical competence among nursing colleagues. Competence was revealed as one of the most essential characteristics of trust, as described earlier in this chapter. Indeed, the clinical competence of nurse colleagues has been identified consistently by staff nurses as a feature of magnet hospitals since 1986, when Kramer and Schmalenberg's first study surveyed 1,634 staff nurses in 16 of the originally designated magnet hospitals (Kramer and Schmalenberg, 1988a,b). Kramer and Hafner (1989), for example, report that working with clinically competent nurses was associated with positive relationships among coworkers, low turnover, effective nursing, and job retention. The investigators quote staff nurses as saying they could work with fewer staff if they had clinically competent nurses they knew and could trust.

Involving Workers in Decision Making

Autonomy and control over nursing practice recurrently have been identified as strong characteristics possessed by staff nurses, nurse managers, and CNEs in magnet hospitals (Aiken, 2002; Kramer and Schmalenberg, 2002; McClure et al., 1983; Scott et al., 1999). As discussed earlier, a distinction is made between autonomy and control over nursing practice. Autonomy refers to nurses' control over their work, that is, their ability to make independent clinical decisions and define the scope of practice in relationship to patients in their care (Kramer and Schmalenberg, 2002; McClure et al., 1983; Scott et al., 1999). Control over nursing practice is an organizational level of autonomy, in which staff nurses, nurse managers, and CNEs participate in all levels of hospital policy decisions about professional practice and patient care (Kramer and Schmalenberg, 2002; Scott et al., 1999). Magnet hospitals score higher on greater autonomy for nurses to act and greater nurse control over resources for patient care (Aiken et al., 1997).

A series of studies comparing the hospitals identified as having magnet characteristics in 1983 (the original magnet hospitals) with hospitals that subsequently received that designation from the ANCC found that the latter hospitals had significantly higher levels of nurse autonomy and control over practice. Staff nurses perceived the ANCC magnet hospitals as having greater resources available for patient care; increased time to discuss patient problems with other colleagues; greater involvement in decision making; and strong, visionary CNEs. Stronger magnet characteristics were also evident in the ANCC magnet hospitals when CNEs were interviewed. CNEs in ANCC magnet hospitals (n = 24) viewed autonomy and control over nursing practice as stronger than did CNEs in the original magnet hospitals (n = 24). Three differences among the hospitals were identified as explaining the higher rating of the ANCC hospitals: the latter hospitals had a department of nursing to which nurses were responsible; they were more apt to have a nurse-researcher providing data for decision making; and they regarded nursing as a distinct profession, making a highly valued contribution (Havens, 2001).

Knowledge Management

Professional development, including teaching students, is consistently cited as an important magnet characteristic in terms of continued learning and career development through formal and informal methods. In the original magnet hospital study (McClure et al., 1983), an essential characteristic identified was professional development, including continuing educational opportunities and support for career development through formal education. A high proportion (92.7 percent) of the directors of nursing held masters or doctoral degrees. In Kramer and Schmalenberg's 1986 study of a subset of the magnet hospitals, a median of 51 percent of the staff nurses had a BSN or had matriculated in BSN study, compared with a national average of 33–34 percent (Kramer and Schmalenberg, 1988a,b).

This magnet characteristic was identified more recently by Kramer and Schmalenberg as one of the most essential features of magnetism cited by staff nurses. Magnet hospitals use a number of strategies to provide support for education and continuing career development for staff nurses, such as tuition for degree programs, in-service programs, short-term courses, externships for student nurses, and internships for new graduates (Kramer and Schmalenberg, 2002).

Pittsburgh Regional Healthcare Initiative

The Pittsburgh Regional Healthcare Initiative (PRHI) is a coalition, begun in 2000, of 35 hospitals; four major insurers; more than 30 major and small-business health care purchasers; numerous corporate and civic leaders; organized labor; state and federal governments; and academic and research institutions, including Carnegie Mellon University, RAND Corporation, the University of Pittsburgh Center for Health Services Research, and Purdue University (Feinstein, 2002). PRHI adapted the principles of the Toyota Production System and implemented practices to manage change, involve workers in decision making about work design and work flow, and become a learning organization to achieve the goal of "perfecting patient care" (Feinstein et al., 2002). PRHI participants have as their goal "delivering patient care on demand, defect free, one by one, immediately, without waste or error, in an environment that is physically, emotionally, and professionally safe" (The Jewish Healthcare Foundation of Pittsburgh, 2002:12).

PRHI is spearheaded by a "leadership obligation group" comprising hospital and other corporate CEOs charged with keeping the initiative moving forward (Robinet, 2002). It focused initially on two patient safety goals: eliminating medication errors and hospital-acquired infections (Feinstein et al., 2002). Multidisciplinary advisory committees at each PRHI partner facility adopted and use the same incident-reporting system for hospital-acquired infections and medication errors. In a partnership with the U.S. Centers for Disease Control and Prevention (CDC), PRHI hospitals developed a common reporting tool based on CDC's national Nosocomial Infection Surveillance System—the oldest and most widely used surveillance system for hospital-acquired infections—and a similar standardized web-based error-reporting tool for medication errors. PRHI hospitals share their data with each other, as well as nationally. The data are translated into knowledge that front-line health care workers can use to protect patients (Feinstein, 2002).

PRHI collects data from all participating hospitals, maps them to patient outcomes, and correlates them with processes of care. Based on those findings, its members institute experimental changes in work design to improve patient safety. In this way, PRHI carries out the practice of becoming a learning organization. Groups of people actually performing the work determine the root cause of a problem, experiment with ways to solve the problem using scientific methods, and then measure the results and share what has been learned (Feinstein et al., 2002). PRHI partners empower health care workers to address problems. When a problem is detected, a team of workers designs a solution immediately, employing a set of pre-designed principles and scientific methods. Every worker is expected to become a scientist and to contribute to rapid, frequent improvements. PRHI also includes a Center for Shared Learning that coordinates all PRHI improvement efforts.

The Wellspring Alliance

Wellspring Innovative Solutions, Inc. (Wellspring) is a federation of 11 freestanding not-for-profit nursing homes in eastern Wisconsin. Fully operational since 1998, its two-fold purpose is to improve the clinical care provided to residents and to create a better work environment for employees. A 15-month evaluation of the Wellspring model found:

- Better patient surveillance by staff.
- Improved performance as measured by federal oversight surveyors.
- Better quality of life for patients and improved quality of staff–resident interactions.
- Lower staff turnover relative to comparable nursing homes in Wisconsin for the same time period.

In achieving these benefits, Wellspring has attended to the leadership of these organizations, trusted workers to make decisions about improvements to patient care, created structures and processes to sustain these changes, and instituted practices aimed at supporting members as learning organizations.

Leadership and management support is provided by a formal organizing superstructure (The Wellspring Alliance) that, in addition to carrying out several practical functions, such as joint purchasing, provides a forum for collaborative information sharing, education and training, and knowledge dissemination across the facilities. The Alliance functions on many levels, including CEOs; administrators; line staff; and a designated Wellspring coordinator in each facility, whom evaluators identified as arguably the single most important contributor to the successful implementation and sustained operation of the Wellspring model. Coordinators serve as both a formal link between the facility and the Alliance and an informal conduit of information across facilities. These individuals meet and interact at quarterly meetings and training events and help codify lessons learned.

Employee education and training are facilitated by a geriatric nurse practitioner who serves as a primary resource on clinical care, develops staff training modules, provides centralized clinical education and training to staff, and travels to member facilities on a quarterly basis to provide feedback to the facility and reinforce and sustain the adoption of the clinical practices taught in the various modules. Training is cross-disciplinary and targeted to employees as team members. Team members learn collaborative problem solving and share responsibility for resident outcomes. Wellspring uses this team training as a way of decreasing the hierarchical relationships that are typical in nursing home staff relationships.

Care resource teams are described as the "main engine" of the patient care improvement activities undertaken by the facilities. These teams are interdisciplinary, nonhierarchical (e.g., nursing assistants may lead a team), voluntary, and self-directing. Teams are expected to identify and develop new work strategies, monitor implementation success, and intervene when problems in implementation arise.

The Wellspring Alliance fosters the evolution of all its member facilities into learning organizations through several practices. One is the sharing of the geriatric nurse practitioner and the facility coordinators to disseminate and nurture the adoption of evidence-based best practices in the care of residents. Another strategy being pursued is having each member facility enter data (e.g., number of incontinent episodes, falls, and weight loss) into a common data set on a quarterly basis (although evaluators found this aspect of the Wellspring model to be most problematic and least well implemented). A data analyst aggregates the data, prepares analytic reports, and presents these reports at quarterly meetings. This practice facilitates the systematic transfer of knowledge across facilities and nursing units, through the clinical resource teams, to staff, and the application of that knowledge is sustained through regularly scheduled care resource team meetings in the facility (Stone et al., 2002).

USE OF EVIDENCE-BASED MANAGEMENT COLLABORATIVES TO STIMULATE FURTHER UPTAKE

The PRHI and Wellspring models described above are examples of learning collaboratives in which resources, knowledge, and experiential learning are shared to improve clinical practice. Collaborative approaches have also been used as mechanisms to facilitate the uptake of health care quality improvement practices (Institute for Healthcare Improvement, undated), technology assessment and dissemination (The Health Technology Center [HealthTech], 2003), and strategic marketplace assistance for HCOs (VHA, 2003).

Evidence-based management collaboratives (EBMCs) have been proposed as a means of bringing together managers, consultants, and researchers to improve health care management and thereby organizational performance (Kovner et al., 2000). These collaboratives would consist of a team of managers, researchers, and consultants from a variety of organizations whose aim would be to better understand problems in effective health care management and to develop more effective approaches to managing health systems. EBMCs would provide access to data and partners within an organization's network to permit pooling of data and resources for the conduct of research, demonstrations, and evaluations that no single organization could undertake. Estimates are that just 10 percent of the annual consulting budget for a large health system redirected to such a collaborative would be sufficient to finance this capacity. EBMCs could be implemented across several different health systems, in one health system, or both. Organizing across systems that are in competition in specific markets has been identified as difficult; thus, organizing noncompeting organizations and their existing alliances has been proposed as an initial approach.

EBMCs would require (1) a strong commitment to improving health care management through the application of evidence, (2) a willingness to use and share management data from compatible management information systems to track and monitor strategic interventions and organizational performance, (3) an interest in participating in applied research, and (4) an interest in being involved in demonstration projects to improve health system performance. In return, collaborative partners would receive comparative information on current ways of organizing services; access to the collective experiences of other cooperative members; results from applied research projects; and an array of technical assistance on statistical, management, and marketing issues (Kovner et al., 2000).

A critical partner in these endeavors would be a research center, typically university-based, with an interest and capacity in applied research on health systems and performance, strategic initiatives, and related management and financial issues. The academic partner could provide expertise in data analysis, survey design, program evaluation, and professional education. In addition to serving its collaborative members, the EBMC could assist in disseminating its findings to a broader community of HCOs through peer-reviewed journals, and in training new evidence-based managers and health services researchers (Kovner et al., 2000).

The prototype EBMC is the Center for Health Management Research (CHMR), led by the University of Washington and codirected by the University of California at Berkeley. CHMR was founded in 1992 by a consortium of HCOs and academic centers to provide a forum for managers, clinicians, and researchers to:

- Develop a health care management research agenda in collaboration with corporate members.
- Undertake research, development, and evaluation projects in pursuit of that agenda.
- Disseminate research findings and successful management practices of other HCOs and other industries to its members.

Now involving 17 academic centers with graduate programs in health services administration (personal communication, T. Rundall, University of California, Berkeley, May 2003), CHMR is sponsored by the National Science Foundation (NSF) under its Industry/University Collaborative Research Centers program. It is the only one of the 50 NSF Collaborative Research Centers to receive this designation for the field of health services administration (Center for Health Management Research, 2003). CHMR is also supported by its 10 member health systems, which provide financial resources, collaborate on setting research priorities, and allow researchers to collect data at their various facilities. These members are thereby able to develop and implement a research agenda focused on their defined interests and needs. By serving as the primary sites for CHMR research, member institutions also are able to develop, test, and evaluate management practices, as well as other innovations and new technologies. CHMR practices are disseminated to entities not part of the collaboration through published reports and journal papers. Studies are designed with the transferability of research findings in mind. Other activities include commissioning papers to review and synthesize research findings on selected topics, conducting roundtable discussions on management topics, and holding dissemination conferences where members receive oral and written presentations from researchers (Walshe and Rundall, 2001).

CHMR has undertaken a wide range of research projects to enable evidence-based managerial decision making in its member health systems. By design, its corporate members are integrated delivery systems, and the overarching theme of its research projects has been the strategies, structures, processes, and performance of such systems. One recent research project addressed mechanisms for building more effective relationships between the HCO members and physicians (Walshe and Rundall, 2001). Similar initiatives could address the work environments of nurses and patient safety.

The committee concludes that broader use of such collaboratives could hasten the uptake of the evidence-based management practices described in this chapter, and therefore makes the following recommendation:

Recommendation 4-4. Professional associations, philanthropic organizations, and other organizational leaders within the health care industry should sponsor collaboratives that incorporate multiple academic and other research-based organizations to support HCOs in the identification and adoption of evidence-based management practices.

REFERENCES

Aiken L. 2002. Superior outcomes for magnet hospitals: The evidence base. In: McClure M, Hinshaw A, eds. *Magnet Hospitals Revisited: Attraction and Retention of Professional Nurses*. Washington, DC: American Nurses Publishing. Pp. 61–81.

Aiken L, Smith H, Lake E. 1994. Lower Medicare mortality among a set of hospitals known for good nursing care. *Medical Care* 32(8):771–787.

Aiken L, Sochalski J, Lake E. 1997. Studying outcomes of organizational change in health services. *Medical Care* 35(11 Supplement):NS6–18.

Aiken L, Sloane D, Lake E, Sochalski J, Weber A. 1999. Organization and outcomes of inpatient AIDS care. *Medical Care* 37(8):760–772.

Aiken L, Clarke S, Sloane D. 2000. Hospital restructuring: Does it adversely affect care and outcomes? *Journal of Nursing Administration* 30(10):457–465.

Aiken L, Clarke S, Sloane D, Sochalski J, Busse R, Clarke H, Giovannetti P, Hunt J, Rafferty A, Shamian J. 2001. Nurses' reports on hospital care in five countries. *Health Affairs* 20(3):43–53.

Appleby C. 2002. Industrial strength. *Trustee* 55(1):10–14.

Axelsson R. 1998. Towards an evidence based health care management. *International Journal of Health Planning and Management* 13:307–317.

Baer M, Frese M. 2003. Innovation is not enough: Climates for initiative and psychological safety, process innovations, and firm performance. *Journal of Organizational Behavior* 24:45–68.

Baldridge National Quality Program. 2003. *Criteria for Performance Excellence*. [Online]. Available: http://www.quality.nist.gov/PDF_files/2003_Business_Criteria.pdf [accessed April 24, 2003].

Barry-Walker J. 2000. The impact of system redesign on staff, patient, and financial outcomes. *Journal of Nursing Administration* 30(2):77–89.

Bazzoli G, LoSasso A, Arnould R, Shalowitz M. 2002. Hospital reorganization and restructuring achieved through merger. *Health Care Management Review* 27(1):7–20.

Beaulieu R, Shamian J, Donner G, Pringle D. 1997. Empowerment and commitment of nurses in long-term care. *Nursing Economics* 15(1):32–41.

Bigley G, Roberts K. 2001. Structuring temporary systems for high reliability. *Academy of Management Journal* 44:1281–1300.

Blackler F. 1995. Knowledge, knowledge work and organizations: An overview and interpretation. *Organization Studies* 16(6):1021–1046.

Bryman A, Brensen M, Beadsworth A, Ford J, Keil E. 1987. The concept of the temporary system: The case of the construction project. *Research in the Sociology of Organizations* 5:253–283.

Bunderson J. 2001. How work ideologies shape the psychological contracts of professional employees: Doctors responses to perceived breach. *Journal of Organizational Behavior* 22:717–741.

Burns J. 1978. *Leadership*. New York, NY: Harper and Row.

Carnino A, Director, Division of Nuclear Installation Safety, International Atomic Energy Agency. Undated. *Management of Safety, Safety Culture and Self Assessment: International Atomic Energy Agency*. [Online]. Available: http://www.iaea.org/ns/nusafe/publish/papers/mng_safe.htm [accessed January 15, 2003].

Center for Health Management Research. 2003. *About CHMR: Who We Are*. [Online]. Available: http://dept.washington.edu/chmr/about [accessed May 6, 2003].

Ciborra, C. 1996. The platform organization: Recombining strategies, structures, and surprises. *Organizational Science* 7:103–118.

Clifford J. 1998. *Restructuring: The Impact of Hospital Organization on Nursing Leadership.* Chicago, IL: AHA Press-American Hospital Publishing, Inc. and the American Organization of Nurse Executives.

Coff R, Rousseau D. 2000. Sustainable competitive advantage from relational wealth. In: Leana CR, Rousseau DM, eds. *Relational Wealth: The Advantages of Stability in a Changing Economy.* New York, NY: Oxford University Press. Pp. 27–48.

Conger J, Kanungo R. 1988. The empowerment process: Integrating theory and practice. *Academy of Management Review* 13(3):471–482.

Cooper M. 2000. Towards a model of safety culture. *Safety Science* 36:111–136.

Davenport T, DeLong D, Beers M. 1998. Successful knowledge management projects. *Sloan Management Review* Winter:43–57.

Decker D, Wheeler G, Johnson J, Parsons R. 2001. Effect of organizational change on the individual employee. *The Health Care Manager* 19(4):1–12.

DeLong D, Fahey L. 2000. Diagnosing cultural barriers to knowledge management. *Academy of Management Executive* 14(4):113–127.

Donaldson N, Rutledge D. 1998. Expediting the harvest and transfer of knowledge for practice in nursing: Catalyst for a journal. *The Online Journal of Cinical Innovations* 1(2):1–25.

Edmondson A. 1999. Psychological safety and learning behavior in work teams. *Administrative Sciences Quarterly* 44:350–383.

Feinstein K, Chair, Pittsburgh Regional Healthcare Initiative and President, Jewish Healthcare Foundation of Pittsburgh. 2002. Invited testimony on March 7, 2002 on the subject of medical errors before the House of Representatives Committee on Ways and Means Subcommittee on Health.

Feinstein K, Grunden N, Harrison E. 2002. A region addresses patient safety. *AJIC: American Journal of Infection Control* 30(4):248–251.

Fox R, Fox D, Wells P. 1999. Performance of first-line management functions on productivity of hospital unit personnel. *Journal of Nursing Administration* 29(9):12–18.

Freeman R, Rogers J. 1999. *What Workers Want.* Ithaca, NY: ILR Press.

Frese N, Teng E, Wijnene C. 1999. Helping to improve suggestion systems: Predictors of giving suggestions in companies. *Journal of Organizational Behavior* 20:1139–1155.

Garvin D. 1993. Building a learning organization. *Harvard Business Review* July–August:78–91.

Gelinas L, Manthey M. 1995. Improving patient outcomes through system change: A focus on the changing roles of healthcare organization executives. *Journal of Nursing Administration* 25(5):55–63.

Gelinas L, Manthey M. 1997. The impact of organizational redesign on nurse executive leadership. *Journal of Nursing Administration* 27(10):35–42.

Gifford B, Zammuto R, Goodman E. 2002. The relationship between hospital unit culture and nurses' quality of work life. *Journal of Healthcare Management* 47(1):13–25.

Goodman P. 2001. *Missing Organizational Linkages: Tools for Cross-Level Organizational Research.* Thousand Oaks, CA: Sage Publications.

Goodman P, Garber S. 1988. The effects of absenteeism on accidents in a dangerous environment. *Journal of Applied Psychology* 73:81–86.

Goodman P, Leyden D. 1991. Familiarity and group performance. *Journal of Applied Psychology* 76:578–586.

Goodman P, Darr E. 1996. Exchanging best practices through computer-aided systems. *Academy of Management Executive* 10:7–19.

Graen G, Novak MA, Sommerkamp P. 1982. The effect of leader-member exchange and job design on productivity and satisfaction: Testing a dual attachment model. *Organizational Behavior and Human Performance* 30:109–131.

Hansen M, Nohria N, Tierney T. 1999. What's your strategy for managing knowledge? *Harvard Business Review* March–April:106–117.

Havens D. 2001. Comparing nursing infrastructure and outcomes: AANC magnet and nonmagnet CNEs report. *Nursing Economics* 19(6):258–266.

Heifetz R, Laurie D. 2001. The work of leadership. *Harvard Business Review* 79(11):131–140.

Heller F. 2003. Participation and power: A critical assessment. *Applied Psychology: An International Review* 52:144–163.

Hewison A. 1997. Evidence-based medicine: What about evidence-based management? *Journal of Nursing Management* 5:195–198.

Hinshaw A. 2002. Building magnetism into health organizations. *Magnet Hospitals Revisited: Attraction and Retention of Professional Nurses*. Washington, DC: American Nurses Publishing.

Ho S, Chan L, Kidwell R. 1999. The implementation of business process reengineering in American and Canadian hospitals. *Health Care Management Review* 24:19–31.

Huselid M. 1995. The impact of human resource practices on turnover, productivity, and corporate financial performance. *Academy of Management Journal* 38:635–672.

Ilinitch A, D'Aveni R, Lewin A. 1996. New organizational forms and strategies for managing in hyper competitive environments. *Organization Science* 7:211–220.

Ingersoll G, Fisher M, Ross B, Soja M, Kidd N. 2001. Employee response to major organizational redesign. *Applied Nursing Research* 14(1):18–28.

Institute for Healthcare Improvement. Undated. *Collaboratives*. [Online]. Available: http://www.ihi.org/collaboratives/ [accessed May 7, 2003].

IOM (Institute of Medicine). 2001. *Crossing the Quality Chasm: A New Health System for the 21st Century*. Washington, DC: National Academy Press.

Kimberly J, Quinn R. 1984. *Managing Organizational Transitions*. Homewood, IL: Dow Jones-Irwin.

Knox S, Irving J. 1997. Nurse manager perceptions of healthcare executive behaviors during organizational change. *Journal of Nursing Administration* 27(11):33–39.

Kovner A, Elton J, Billings J. 2000. Evidence-Based Management. *Frontiers of Health Services Management* 16(4):3–24.

Kramer M. 1990a. The magnet hospitals: Excellence revisited. *Journal of Nursing Administration* 20(9):35–44.

Kramer M. 1990b. Trends to watch at the magnet hospital. *Nursing* 2(4):67–74.

Kramer M, Schmalenberg C. 1988a. Magnet hospitals—Part I: Institutions of excellence. *Journal of Nursing Administration* 18(1):13–24.

Kramer M, Schmalenberg C. 1988b. Magnet hospitals—Part II: Institutions of excellence. *Journal of Nursing Administration* 18(2):1–11.

Kramer M, Hafner L. 1989. Shared values: Impact on staff nurse job satisfaction and perceived productivity. *Nursing Research* 38(3):172–177.

Kramer M, Schmalenberg C. 1991. Job satisfaction and retention: Insights for the 90s, Part I. *Nursing* 3(3):50–55.

Kramer M, Schmalenberg C. 1993. Learning from success: Autonomy and empowerment. *Nursing Management* 24(5):58–64.

Kramer M, Schmalenberg C. 2002. Staff nurses identify essentials of magnetism. In: McClure M, Hinshaw A, eds. *Magnet Hospitals Revisited: Attraction and Retention of Professional Nurses*. Washington, DC: American Nurses Publishing. Pp. 25–59.

Kramer M, Schmalenberg C. 2003. Magnet hospital staff nurses describe clinical autonomy. *Nursing Outlook* 51(1):13–19.

Kramer M, Schmalenberg C, Hafner L. 1989. What causes job satisfaction and perceived productivity of quality nursing care? *Managing the Nursing Shortage: A Guide to Recruitment and Retention*. Rockville, MD: Aspen. Pp. 12–32.

Laschinger H, Havens D. 1996. Staff nurse work empowerment and perceived control over nursing practice: Conditions for work effectiveness. *Journal of Nursing Administration* 26(9):27–35.

Laschinger H, Finegan J, Shamian J, Casier S. 2000. Organizational trust and empowerment in restructured healthcare settings: Effects on staff nurse commitment. *Journal of Nursing Administration* 30(9):413–425.

Laschinger H, Finegan J, Shamian J. 2001a. The impact of workplace empowerment, organizational trust on staff nurses' work satisfaction and organizational commitment. *Health Care Management Review* 26(3):7–23.

Laschinger H, Shamian J, Thomson D. 2001b. Impact of magnet hospital characteristics on nurses' perceptions of trust, burnout, quality of care, and work satisfaction. *Nursing Economics* 19(5):209–219.

Leana C, Rousseau D. 2000. *Relational Wealth: The Advantages of Stability in a Changing Economy.* New York, NY: Oxford University Press.

Lowin A, Craig J. 1968. The influence of level of performance on managerial style: An experimental object lesson in the ambiguity of correlational data. *Organizational Behavior and Human Performance* 3:440–458.

Maas M, Specht J. 2001. Shared governance models in nursing: What is shared, who governs, and who benefits. *Current Issues in Nursing* (6th Edition). St. Louis, MO: Mosby, Inc.

MacDuffie J. 1995. Human resource bundles and manufacturing performance: Organizational logic and flexible production systems in the world auto industry. *Industrial and Labor Relations Review* 48:197–221.

MacDuffie J, Pil F. 1996. *"High Involvement" Work Practices and Human Resource Policies: An International Overview.* Kochan T, Lansbury R, Macduffie J, eds. New York, NY: Oxford University Press.

Mayer R, Davis J, Schoorman F. 1995. An integrative model of organizational trust. *The Academy of Management Review* 20(3):709–734.

McClure M, Poulin M, Sovie M. 1983. *Magnet Hospitals: Attraction and Retention of Professional Nurses.* Kansas City, MO: American Academy of Nurses.

McClure M, Poulin M, Sovie M, Wandelt M. 2002. Magnet hospitals: Attraction and retention of professional nurses (The Original Study). In: McClure M, Hinshaw A, eds. *Magnet Hospitals Revisited.* Washington, DC: American Nurses Publishing. Pp. 1–24.

McNeese-Smith D. 1995. Job satisfaction, productivity, and organizational commitment: The result of leadership. *Journal of Nursing Administration* 25(9):17–26.

McNeese-Smith D. 1997. The influence of manager behavior on nurses' job satisfaction, productivity, and commitment. *Journal of Nursing Administration* 27(9):47–55.

Miles R, Snow C. 1984. Designing strategic human resource systems. *Organizational Dynamics* Summer:36–52.

Miles R, Creed W. 1995. Organizational forms and managerial philosophies: A descriptive and analytical review. In: Cummings L, Staw B, eds. *Research in Organizational Behavior.* Vol. 17. Greenwich, CT: JAI Press. Pp. 333–372.

Mintzberg H. 1997. Toward healthier hospitals. *Health Care Management Review* 22(34):9–18.

Mohr J, Abelson H, Barach P. 2002. Creating effective leadership for improving patient safety. *Quality Management in Health Care* 11(1):69–78.

Moorman C, Miner A. 1998. Organizational improvisation and organizational memory. *Academy of Management Review* 23:698–723.

Norrish B, Rundall T. 2001. Hospital restructuring and the work of registered nurses. *Milbank Quarterly* 79(1):55–79.

O'May F, Buchan J. 1999. Shared governance: A literature review. *International Journal of Nursing Studies* 36:281–300.

Parker S. 1998. Enhancing role breadth self-efficacy: The role of job enrichment and other organizational interventions. *Journal of Applied Psychology* 83:835–852.

Pearce J. 2000. Trustworthiness. *Relational Wealth: Advantages of Stability in a Changing Economy.* New York, NY: Oxford University Press.

Petersen D. 1996. *Human Error Reduction and Safety Management.* New York, NY: Van Nostrand Reinhold.

Quinn J. 1992. *Intelligent Enterprise: A Knowledge and Service Based Paradigm for Industry.* New York, NY: The Free Press, a division of Macmillan, Inc.

Reason J. 1990. *Human Error.* Cambridge, UK: Cambridge University Press.

Roberts K. 1990. Managing high reliability organizations. *California Management Review* 32:101–113.

Roberts K, Bea R. 2001a. Must accidents happen? Lessons from high-reliability organizations. *Academy of Management Executive* 15(3):70–78.

Roberts K, Bea R. 2001b. When systems fail. *Organizational Dynamics* 29(3):179–191.

Roberts K, Stout S, Halpern J. 1994. Decision dynamics in two high reliability military organizations. *Management Science* 40:614–24.

Robinet J. 2002, January 4. Regional healthcare initiative moves forward in relative obscurity. *Pittsburgh Business Times Journal.* p. 6.

Rousseau D. 1995. *Psychological Contracts in Organizations: Understanding Written and Unwritten Agreements.* Newbury Park, CA: Sage Publications.

Rousseau D, Tijoriwala S. 1999. What's a good reason to change? Motivated reasoning and social accounts in organizational change. *Journal of Applied Psychology* 84:514–528.

Rousseau D, Sitkin S, Burt R, Camerer C. 1998. Not so different after all: A cross-disciplinary view of trust. *Academy of Management Review* 23:1–12.

Sabiston J, Laschinger H. 1995. Staff nurse work empowerment and perceived autonomy: Testing Kanter's theory of structural power in organizations. *Journal of Nursing Administration* 25(9):42–50.

Sackett D, Rosenberg W, Muir-Gray J, Haynes R, Richardson W. 1996. Evidence-based medicine: What it is and what it isn't. *British Medical Journal* 312(7023):71–72.

Schiff G. 2000. Fatal distraction: Finance vs. vigilance in our nation's hospitals. *JGIM: Journal of General Internal Medicine* 15(4):269.

Scott JG, Sochalski J, Aiken L. 1999. Review of magnet hospital research: Findings and implications for professional nursing practice. *Journal of Nursing Administration* 29(1):9–19.

SEIU Nurse Alliance. 2001. *The Shortage of Care.* Washington, DC: Service Employees International Union, AFL-CIO, CLC.

Sovie M, Jawad A. 2001. Hospital restructuring and its impact on outcomes. *The Journal of Nursing Administration* 31(12):588–600.

Spath P. 2000. Does your facility have a "patient-safe" climate? *Hospital Peer Review* 25:80–82.

Spear S, Bowen H. 1999. Decoding the DNA of the Toyota Production System. *Harvard Business Review* 77(5):97–106.

Stewart T. 1999. Telling tales at BP Amoco. *Fortune* 139(11):220.

Stone R, Reinhard S, Bowers B, Zimmerman D, Phillips C, Hawes C, Fielding J, Jacobson N. 2002. *Evaluation of the Wellspring Model for Improving Nursing Home Quality.* The Commonwealth Fund.

Strebel P. 1996. Why do employees resist change? *Harvard Business Review* May–June:86–92.

The Campbell Collaboration. Undated. *About the Campbell Collaboration.* [Online]. Available: http://www.campbellcollaboration.org/About.html [accessed April 18, 2002].

The Health Technology Center (HealthTech). 2003. *Learn About HealthTech.* [Online]. Available: www.healthtech.org/Common_site/learn_about_healthtech.asp [accessed May 7, 2003].

The Jewish Healthcare Foundation of Pittsburgh. 2002. The Pittsburgh Perfecting Patient Care System: A New Design for Delivering Health. *Branches*, January:1-16. Branches is a publication of the Jewish Healthcare Foundation; Pittsburgh, PA. [Online]. Available: http://jhf.org/reports/branches/pdfs/bran_jan.pdf.

Thomas E, Orav J, Brennan T. 2000. Hospital ownership and preventable adverse events. *Journal of General Internal Medicine* 15:211–219.

Thompson J, Bunderson J. In press. Violations of principle: Ideology currency in the psychological contract. *Academy of Management Review*.

Tucker A, Edmondson A. 2002. Managing routine exceptions: A model of nurse problem solving behavior. *Advances in Health Care Management* 3:87–113.

Tucker A, Edmondson A. 2003. Why hospitals don't learn from failures: Organizational and psychological dynamics that inhibit system change. *California Management Review* 45(2):1–18.

Tucker A, Edmondson A, Spear S. 2002. When problem solving prevents organizational learning. *Journal of Organizational Change Management* 15(2):122–137.

VHA. 2003. *What Is VHA?* [Online]. Available: https://www.vha.com/aboutvha/public/about_whatisvha.asp [accessed May 7, 2003].

Walshe K, Rundall T. 2001. Evidence-based management: From theory to practice in health care. *The Milbank Quarterly* 79(3):429–458.

Walston S, Kimberly J. 1997. Reengineering hospitals: Evidence from the field. *Hospital and Health Services Administration* 42(2):143–163.

Walston S, Burns J, Kimberley J. 2000. Does reengineering really work? An examination of the context and outcomes of hospital reengineering initiatives. *Health Services Research* 34(6):1363–1388.

Ward G, Burns R, Burns K. 1990. *The Civil War.* Warner Home Video, an AOL Time Warner Company. 1990 DVD Video. A production of Florentine Films and WETA-TV.

Weick K, Roberts K. 1993. Collective mind and organizational reliability: The case of flight operations on an aircraft carrier deck. *Administrative Science Quarterly* 38:357–381.

Zucker L. 1986. Production of trust: Institutional sources of economic structure, 1840–1920. In: Staw B, Cummings L, eds. *Research in Organizational Behavior*. Greenwich, CT: JAI Press. Pp. 53–111.

5

Maximizing Workforce Capability

Monitoring patient health status, performing therapeutic treatments, and integrating patient care to avoid gaps in health care are nursing functions that directly affect patient safety. Accomplishing these activities requires an adequate number of nursing staff with the clinical knowledge and skills needed to carry out these interventions, and with the ability to effectively communicate findings and coordinate care with the interventions of other members of the patient's health care team. The committee finds strong evidence that nurse staffing levels, the knowledge and skill levels of nursing staff, and the extent to which workers collaborate in sharing their knowledge and skills affect patient outcomes and safety. The committee also finds that staffing levels in hospitals and long-term care facilities are uneven, posing risks to patient safety. Further, the knowledge base for effective clinical care and new health care technologies are advancing rapidly, making it impossible for nurses (and other clinicians) without organizational support to incorporate this information and these technologies into their clinical decision making and practice. Finally, there is evidence of inconsistent interprofessional collaboration among nursing staff and other health care providers.

Health care organizations (HCOs) need to address all three of these barriers to workforce capability and patient safety by taking action to promote safe staffing levels, support nurses' ongoing knowledge and skill acquisition and clinical decision making at the point of care, and foster interdisciplinary collaboration. The federal government can assist by revising outdated regulations regarding staffing in long-term care facilities and implementing a system for collecting and managing accurate and reliable data on hospital and nursing home staffing.

PROMOTING SAFE STAFFING LEVELS

I knew it was going to be a busy shift. After all, it was Wednesday—that meant elective surgery admissions from PACU [postanesthesia care unit], direct admissions from the clinic, and anything else the emergency room sent us. Each of us already had five patients apiece, some of them needing a lot of nursing care. There was no secretary available to put charts together and the nurse manager had already said that there was "no nurse in the system" to send to help us.

When the ER called to report on my second admission for the shift, I asked if they could please hold the patient until I finished a blood transfusion on one patient and completed the admission on the patient I had gotten from the recovery room. The nurse from the ER told me the patient would be up in five minutes and before I could say another word, she hung up the phone. I called my supervisor and explained that we were overwhelmed with all of the activity on the unit and asked if she could send another nurse to help us get settled or assign the admission to another unit. She told me that she would "look around" but that she had no one she could send right away. I asked her if she could delay the admission for a while until I could stabilize my other patients. She responded that the ER was "backed up" and that I had to take the patient right now or she would have to "write me up."

When the patient came, I had to leave a new mastectomy patient who was crying each time she looked at her surgical dressing and whose PCA [patient-controlled analgesia] pump was alarming. I left her with a promise to get back as soon as I could and went to check the ER admission. The shift ended and I never got back to her except to check her IV fluid totals for the shift.

It was only after I got home that I remembered that I had not put the allergy band for seafood and penicillin on the ER admission. I called back to the unit just as the patient was being sent down to the operating room and asked them to put the allergy band on the patient and note on the front of the chart.

I could not rest. Every time I closed my eyes I thought about the fact that she could have been prepped using an iodine scrub and/or that they might have given her penicillin as a peri-operative antibiotic. A reaction from either of them could have been fatal.

An Adequate Number of Nurses: Essential to Patient Safety

The number of nursing staff available to provide in-patient nursing care is linked to patient safety by a substantial and growing number of research studies. Although there have been no experimental controlled studies of interventions that increased or decreased nurse staffing levels and measured the subsequent effect on patients, substantial evidence on the relationship between nurse staffing levels and patient outcomes has been produced by observational studies. This research has been conducted separately for acute care hospital and nursing home care.

Acute Care Hospitals

Because of the substantial changes that have occurred in the environment of acute care hospitals (see Chapter 1), studies based on older data are
not the most useful for understanding staffing effects. Rather, the strongest
evidence comes from studies published in the last 15 years (Aiken et al.,
1999, 2002; Amaravadi et al., 2000; Blegen and Vaughn, 1998; Blegen et
al., 1998; Bolton et al., 2001; Bond et al., 1999; Dimick et al., 2001; Flood
and Diers, 1988; Hartz et al., 1989; Hunt and Hagen, 1998; Kovner and
Gergen, 1998; Kovner et al., 2002; Lichtig et al., 1999; Needleman et al.,
2002; Pronovost et al., 2001; Shortell et al., 1994). All of these are cross-
sectional studies that explored correlations between measures of nurse staffing levels and rates of adverse occurrences. They examined in-hospital
deaths and nonfatal adverse outcomes, including various types of nosocomial infections, decubitus ulcers, and falls. A variety of acute care hospital
settings were examined, including intensive care units (ICUs), general medical–surgical units, and various specialty units. In some studies, process errors were measured, including medication errors.

The amount of nursing service (staffing level) in a given unit or hospital
typically is expressed administratively as nursing hours per patient per day
(hppd). It is also expressed as a nurse-to-patient ratio, or the average number of patients for each nurse; for example, 1:4 or 1:6 represents one nurse
for every four or six patients, respectively. Higher levels of hppd indicate
higher nurse-to-patient ratios.[1]

An important methodological issue in studies of hospital staffing is the
unit of analysis. Sometimes staffing-level data are obtained for individual
nursing units within hospitals; at other times, staffing data are aggregated
across the entire hospital. Measures of outcomes similarly are aggregated
across individual patients to the unit or hospital level to produce an incidence rate of adverse events. A problem with hospital-level aggregation is
that heterogeneous nursing units, such as pediatric units, labor and delivery
units, adult medical and surgical units, and ICUs, are combined. As a result,
data on hospital-wide staffing levels may not well represent the staffing
levels experienced by patients in a given nursing unit or of interest to poten-

---

[1]Discussions of nurse-to-patient ratios can often be confusing. A nurse-to-patient ratio is
expressed as a numerical relation; e.g., one nurse for each six patients is a nurse-to-patient
ratio of 1:6. Because this figure often resembles a fraction (e.g., 1/6), a "higher" nurse-to-
patient ratio is one in which the ratio of nurses to patients, expressed as a fraction, comes
closest to the whole number 1. That is, a 1:2 ratio (one nurse for every two patients) is a higher
nurse-to-patient ratio than one nurse for every six patients (1:6). In this chapter, we attempt to
avoid this confusion by using the expressions "more nurses" or "fewer nurses" per patient.

tial patients. These data can also sometimes cloud the findings of research (Seago, 2001). This issue is less significant in nursing homes, where heterogeneous nursing units are much less likely to exist, the resident population is more homogeneous, and variation in patients can be addressed for research studies as needed through case-mix adjustment.

A number of studies of the effect of nurse staffing levels on patient outcomes have attempted to use patient mortality as an outcome measure. However, patient mortality is a problematic nurse-staffing outcome for several reasons. First, patient death is not common; its low frequency makes detecting statistically significant differences difficult (Hartz et al., 1989). Second, while some patients die as a result of injuries related to health care, others die as a result of overwhelming disease. While some studies evaluating the quality of hospital care have used methods to assess the reasons for in-hospital deaths (Brennan et al., 1991; Thomas et al., 2000), studies of nurse staffing that have used patient mortality as an outcome measure have lacked methods for attributing the cause of death to preventable or nonpreventable causes. Thus, it is not surprising that these studies do not agree on whether lower nurse-to-patient ratios (i.e., fewer nurses per patient) are associated with higher patient mortality (measured as either in-hospital mortality or death within 30 days of admission). The strongest evidence supporting such a mortality relationship was derived from a study of patients with AIDS (Aiken et al., 1999). This study was conducted in 20 hospitals, aggregated data at the nursing unit level, and had good case-mix controls. Other diagnosis-specific studies have not been able to demonstrate a relationship between nurse staffing levels and patient mortality.

Studies in which patients were not selected by diagnosis also have yielded inconsistent findings about the effect of staffing levels on mortality. Two nationwide studies that aggregated data at the hospital level (Aiken et al., 2002; Bond et al., 1999) found that lower nurse-to-patient ratios were associated with higher patient mortality. This association was not found, however, in other studies examining multiple ICUs (Amaravadi et al., 2000; Shortell et al., 1994) and hospital-level staffing ratios (Hunt and Hagen, 1998; Needleman et al., 2002).

Nonfatal adverse events, such as nosocomial infections and decubitus ulcers, are thought to have a more plausible direct relationship to the availability of hospital nursing staff. A consistent finding across multiple recent studies is that lower nurse-to-patient staffing ratios are associated with higher rates of nonfatal adverse events, including nosocomial infections, pressure ulcers, and cardiac and respiratory failure (Aiken et al., 2002; Cho et al., 2003; Kovner et al., 2002; Needleman et al., 2002). Similarly, a review of evidence pertaining to acute care hospital staffing published in the health professions literature from 1990 to 2001 revealed that of 16 hospital-based studies of the relationship between levels of nursing staff and patient outcomes,[2] 11 found a positive effect on patient outcomes from higher levels of nurse staffing. The 5 studies that did not detect such an association tended to be older, and/or used smaller samples or less sophisticated methods for controlling for confounding variables. This evidence review concludes that "there is strong evidence that leaner nurse staffing is associated with increased length of stay, nosocomial infection (urinary tract infection, postoperative infection, and pneumonia), and pressure ulcers." It concludes further that "these studies had various types and acuities of patients and, taken together, provide substantial evidence that richer nurse staffing is associated with better patient outcomes" (Seago, 2001:430).

Nursing Homes

The relationship between nurse staffing levels and patient outcomes in nursing homes has also been shown in numerous studies (Gustafson et al., 1990; Kayser-Jones et al., 1989; Nyman, 1988). Higher levels of registered nurse (RN) hours per patient have been significantly associated with patient survival, improved functional status, and discharge from the nursing home (Linn et al., 1977). Higher staff levels and lower turnover among RNs also have been found to be related to functional improvement in residents (Spector and Takada, 1991). Increased RN hours have been associated with improved mortality and the probability of discharge (Braun, 1991); with fewer pressure ulcers, catheterized residents, and urinary tract infections; and with lower rates of antibiotic use (Cherry, 1991). Higher staffing also has been related to fewer pressure sores (but more use of physical restraints) (Aaronson et al., 1994).

In addition, higher RN levels, adjusted for case mix, have been shown to be associated with lower mortality rates. An economic analysis using 1987 data from the National Medical Expenditure Survey found that an increase of 0.5 full-time equivalent (FTE) RNs per 100 residents (an approximately 10 percent increase in average RN staffing at that time) would have reduced the probability of dying by about 1 percent. Although this percentage may appear small, the researchers point out that it translates to an estimated 3,000 fewer deaths annually for nursing home residents. Moreover, a higher level of licensed practical nurse/licensed vocational nurse (LPN/LVN) staffing was found to be related to improved functional status as measured by activities of daily living (ADL) dependency (Cohen and Spector, 1996). Inadequate nurse staffing has been shown to be associated

---

[2]The review included observational studies that used controls to protect against threats to validity—e.g., case control, cohort, and pre- and post-design studies and studies using data from large public databases. Observational studies without controls were excluded.

with malnutrition, starvation, and dehydration in nursing home residents (Kayser-Jones, 1996, 1997; Kayser-Jones and Schell, 1997; Kayser-Jones et al., 1999). Licensed nursing hours (but not unlicensed hours) have been found to be significantly related to improved functional ability, increased probability of discharge to home, and reduced mortality in the first year after admission (Bliesmer et al., 1998). And higher total nurse staffing hours, particularly higher RN hours, were shown to be associated with fewer facility deficiencies in a study of all U.S. nursing homes (Harrington et al., 2000b). Other studies have found that gerontological nurse specialists and geriatric nurse practitioners also contribute to improved quality outcomes in nursing homes (Buchanan et al., 1990; Kane et al., 1988; Mezey and Lynaugh, 1989).

These and other studies are reviewed in two Institute of Medicine (IOM) reports (IOM, 1996, 2001b) that confirm the important relationship between staffing and quality. The 1996 IOM report *Nursing Staff in Hospitals and Nursing Homes: Is It Adequate*, found that "the preponderance of evidence from a number of studies using different types of quality measures has shown a positive relationship between nursing staff levels and quality of nursing home care." Based on this evidence, "a relationship between RN-to-resident staffing and quality of care in nursing facilities has been established" (IOM, 1996:153).

Subsequent, additional strong evidence of the effect of nurse staffing on nursing home resident outcomes is provided by a congressionally mandated study on the *Appropriateness of Minimum Nurse Staffing Ratios in Nursing Homes* carried out under the auspices of the U.S. Department of Health and Humans Services' (DHHS) Centers for Medicare and Medicaid Services (CMS) between 1998 and 2002. This study was conducted in two phases, with a Phase I report being provided in July 2000 (CMS, 2000) and a Phase II report in December 2001 (CMS, 2001). The Phase I study involved the development of methodologies and a preliminary assessment of relationships between patient (resident) outcomes and staffing levels using 1996 and 1997 data from three states and over 3,000 facilities. The Phase I report provides a discussion of relevant policy issues, including trends in payment and staffing levels in nursing homes; a discussion of how current federal regulatory staffing requirements are implemented; stakeholder perspectives; a literature review; and an analysis of different staffing data sources. The report also includes two other approaches to determining staffing needs: a time-motion study and use of operations research models.

The Phase II report provides further analysis of staffing–outcome associations using 1999 data from almost 9,000 facilities in 10 states. This report includes a refinement of the previous operations research estimates, studies of nursing staff turnover and retention, case studies of the relationship between care outcomes and nurse staffing issues beyond staffing levels, an assessment of training and education for certified nurse assistants (CNAs), discussion of the adequacy of the nursing workforce to meet higher minimum nurse staffing standards, the development of improved nurse staffing data collection approaches, and an examination of payment options for improving nurse staffing. In combination, these reports provide a comprehensive assessment of staffing-related issues in long-term care and the policy context for addressing these issues. However, the core of this research was empirical work that demonstrated consistent associations between staffing levels and quality of care.

The Phase II empirical study included two separate samples of nursing home residents and facilities (CMS, 2001). The first was a Medicare admission sample designed to evaluate the relationship between staffing and outcomes of postacute nursing home care—care for those residents with acute conditions who are admitted to skilled nursing facilities (SNFs) generally for a relatively short stay. This short-stay sample included all SNF nursing homes from the 10 study states and used claims data linked to data from the federal government's nursing home minimum data set (MDS), which contains information on each resident's diagnoses, physical functioning, and other health conditions, as well as demographic and additional health status information.[3] Outcome measures for this sample related to patient safety were rehospitalizations within 30 days of admission for potentially avoidable causes, including congestive heart failure, electrolyte imbalance, respiratory infection, urinary tract infection (UTI), and sepsis. These resident-level measures were aggregated to the facility level to obtain a nursing home rate[4] for each outcome measure.

The second sample, of long-stay residents, was used to examine the relationship between staffing and care outcomes for nursing home residents. This sample included all residents with two MDS assessments 90 days apart. Outcome measures relevant to patient safety included incidents of pressure ulcers, skin trauma, and weight loss, which were then aggregated to the nursing home level. These outcome measures were selected because they were likely to be affected by nurse staffing, had sufficient incidence for stable estimates, had a measurable set of risk adjustors that could be used to control for differences in risk, and were based on accurate secondary data elements.

A much larger set of measures was evaluated initially. Data sources for hospital-transfer outcome measures were hospital claims, whereas long-stay outcome measures utilized MDS data. Risk factors were obtained from both

---

[3]Further information on the MDS is available at the CMS website: http://cms.hhs.gov/medicaid/mds20/man-form.asp [accessed September 26, 2003].

[4]Facilities with fewer than 25 admissions were excluded.

data sets. Staffing data were obtained from Medicaid cost reports for the 10 states, which were found to have a higher correlation with payroll data than the Medicaid On-line Survey and Certification Report (OSCAR) data that are provided to state survey agencies and the federal government by facilities.

Analysis involved the generation of resident-level risk models for each outcome, which were then used to estimate resident-level risk scores, calculate a facility average risk score, and assess the association between staffing levels and rate of adverse events, adjusting for the facility average risk score. Facilities in the worst 10th percentile were considered to have an inappropriately high level of untoward events, which generally reflected a rate that was three or more times the mean rate for the outcome (e.g. overall UTI hospitalization mean = 0.03; 10th percentile mean = 0.09). Consistently, associations were found between different staffing levels and whether facilities were in the worst 10th percentile. These significant associations persisted until a staffing threshold was reached, above which there was no further detectable benefit from additional staffing. These findings occurred for all three types of nursing staff separately (nursing assistant [NA], licensed [LPN/LVN and RN combined], and RN). The thresholds occurred at staffing levels that exceeded the current levels of 75–90 percent of facilities, depending on the type of staff and the measure. Thus, most facilities fell considerably below the staffing thresholds. These thresholds were between 2.4 and 2.8 hours per resident day for NAs, between 1.1 and 1.3 hours per resident day for licensed staff, and between 0.55 and 0.75 hours per resident day for RNs. However, incremental improvements in quality occurred at all levels until these staffing thresholds were reached.

This study also found (based on an analysis of 631 facilities in California for which information on staff turnover and retention was available) a strong relationship between staff retention and outcomes related to patient safety. For example, improved annual retention of nursing staff up to a threshold of about 51 percent (i.e., half the staff stay for a full year) was associated with a substantially higher likelihood (odds ratio 3.66) that a nursing home would not be in the worst 10 percent of facilities. However, retention of less than 51 percent was associated with a high risk of adverse events, such as hospitalizations for UTIs and pressure ulcers.

Explanations for the Causal Relationship Between Staffing Levels and Patient Outcomes

Several studies have attempted to explain the relationship between higher levels of nurse staffing and improved patient outcomes. The results of these studies support the position that as the numbers of nursing staff increase, the staff are proportionately able to provide increasing amounts of necessary care. Once necessary care is provided, one would expect to see no additional improvement in health outcomes from greater numbers of staff. This point is supported by the above-referenced CMS study of nursing home staffing, which identified a threshold level of nurse staffing above which no further improvements in patient outcomes were detected (CMS, 2001).

An HCO's staffing level is traditionally considered a structural measure of quality that can affect the processes and outcomes of care (Donabedian, 1980; IOM, 1996). In nursing homes, the processes of care include a range of nursing activities, such as assistance with ADLs and monitoring of health status; therapeutic services, such as dressing changes and administration of medications; and other nursing activities, such as the management of incontinence. The outcomes of care can be measured as weight loss, pressure ulcers, incontinence, or other markers of physical decline (Zimmerman et al., 1995).

In long-term care, higher staff levels and lower RN turnover have been shown to be related to better care processes, such as lower urinary catheter use, better skin care, and better resident participation rates (Spector and Takada, 1991). Inadequate nurse staffing is correlated with inadequate feeding assistance and poor oral health (Kayser-Jones, 1996, 1997; Kayser-Jones and Schell, 1997; Kayser-Jones et al., 1999). NAs with inadequate time to provide care have been documented to cut corners in order to manage their workloads (Bowers and Becker, 1992).

Schnelle et al. (2002) conducted a blinded study to determine whether there were differences in the quality of care processes among 34 randomly selected California long-term care facilities with different staffing levels. Three groups of homes were identified in the sample. Group 1 (nine homes at the 0 to 25th percentile of staffing levels) reported 2.7 mean total (RNs, LVNs, and NAs) direct-care hours per resident/day (hprd). Group 2 (six homes in the 75th to 90th percentile) reported 3.4 hprd; and Group 3 (six homes in the 91st to 100th percentile) reported 4.9 hprd. During a 3-day on-site visit, research staff used standardized protocols for direct observation, resident assessment, resident interview, and medical record review to assess 16 care processes delivered by NAs and 11 care processes delivered by licensed nurses. NAs in Group 3 homes reported significantly lower resident care loads across the day and evening shifts in 2001–2002 (7.6 residents per NA) compared with NAs in all of the remaining homes. Group 3 homes also performed significantly better on 12 of 16 care processes implemented by NAs compared with all other remaining homes combined. Residents in the Group 3, or highest-staffed, homes were significantly more likely to be out of bed and engaged in activities during the day and to receive more feeding assistance and incontinence care. The researchers concluded that there is a relationship between nursing home reports of total staffing, NA reports of resident care load, and the quality of implementation of care processes. Comparing these findings with those of studies of eight separate quality indicators (weight loss, bedfast, physical restraints, pressure ulcers, incontinence, loss of physical activity, pain, and depression), the researchers concluded that staffing levels are a better predictor of high-quality care processes than the eight quality indicators (Schnelle et al., 2002).

For acute hospital care, the relationship between licensed nurse staffing levels and patient outcomes also has been attributed in part to the surveillance function of nursing described in Chapters 1 and 3. As the staffing level rises, so does the availability of nurses to spend more time in surveillance (monitoring) of patients for changes in their condition, which in turn enables quicker detection of changes in health status and more prompt rescue activities by the health care team. When this does not happen, "failure to rescue" is said to occur. The concept of failure to rescue has been tested and validated as an indicator of the quality of acute hospital care for surgical patients (Silber et al., 1992). When higher levels of nurse staffing are present in hospitals, failure to rescue is reduced (Aiken et al., 2002; Needleman et al., 2002).

Other attempts to understand how overall staffing affects patient safety in acute care hospitals have examined ratios of RNs to nonlicensed nursing personnel. Two studies found that higher ratios of RNs to unlicensed nurses are associated with lower rates of both medication errors and decubiti (Blegen et al., 1998) and with lower mortality rates (Hartz et al., 1989). However, one study that did not include case-mix adjustment found no association between the ratio of RNs to unlicensed nurses and nonfatal complications (Bolton et al., 2001).

Variation in Hospital and Nursing Home Staffing Levels

Acute Care Hospital Staffing

There is no national database on hospital nurse staffing levels that (1) reports staffing levels by type of patient care unit; (2) distinguishes direct-care nursing staff from nursing staff in administrative, managerial, educational, or other non–direct patient care positions; or (3) distinguishes inpatient nurses from those delivering outpatient care in hospitals. However, a few studies and state hospital data sets show that staffing levels vary considerably from hospital to hospital and across inpatient units within hospitals.

Variation in hospital staffing is illustrated by 1998–2000 data from the California Nursing Outcomes Coalition (CalNOC), which maintains a statewide database of nurse staffing levels submitted directly by California hospitals (see also Chapter 3). Although these data constitute a convenience sample of 52 California hospitals voluntarily contributing staffing data to the initiative, the data are useful because they are collected at the level of the nursing unit (as opposed to the aggregate hospital level), use common data definitions and reporting, and have ongoing verification to ensure accuracy. Data reported on the 330 critical care, medical–surgical, and step-down units across nine calendar quarters in these hospitals revealed averages and ranges of RN-to-patient staffing ratios across these facilities:

- ICUs—a range of one RN for every 0.5–5.3 patients (average = one RN for every 1.6 patients)
- Step-down units—a range of one RN for every 1.5–11.6 patients (average = one RN for every 4.2 patients)
- Medical–surgical units—a range of one RN for every 2.7–13.8 patients (average = one RN for every 5.9 patients)

These findings did not vary over the nine quarters or by the size of the hospital (Donaldson et al., 2001).

As discussed in Chapter 3, data from a fiscal year 2002 national convenience sample survey of hospitals on staffing, scheduling, and workforce management of nursing department employees show similar variation. The 135 hospitals responding varied in nurse staffing levels even with the shift and type of patient care unit being held constant. Although the average RN-to-patient ratio in medical–surgical units on the day shift was 1:6, the range was from 1:3 to 1:12. Twenty-three percent of hospitals reported that nurses in their medical–surgical units on the day shift were each responsible for caring for between 7 and 12 patients. On the night shift, 7 patients on average were assigned to each nurse, but 34 percent of hospitals reported between 8 and 12 patients assigned to each nurse. For critical care units, the average number of patients assigned to each nurse was 2 for both the day and the night shifts, but 7.4 percent of hospitals reported having nurses care for 3 or 4 ICU patients during the day shift, and 11 percent reported nurses caring for 3 or 4 ICU patients during the night shift (Cavouras and Suby, 2003).

A 1999 survey (Aiken et al., 2002) of a 50 percent random sample of Pennsylvania hospital RNs working in all hospital units who held staff positions involving direct patient care similarly reported variable nurse-to-patient ratios (see Table 5-1).

Unfortunately, studies that distinguish type of nursing unit or separate direct-care nurses from nurses in administrative positions are rare. Most studies measuring nurse staffing levels collect staffing data aggregated across all hospital units, such as ICUs, general medical–surgical units, emergency rooms, and labor and delivery units (Aiken et al., 1999, 2002; Bolton et al., 2001; Bond et al., 1999; Cho et al., 2003; Flood and Diers, 1988; Kovner

TABLE 5-1   Variations in Nurse-to-Patient Ratios in Pennsylvania Hospitals, 1999

Patients per Nurse	Percent of Respondents Reporting
≤ 4	7.1
5	47.3
6	20.8
7	10.9
≥ 8	4.0

SOURCE: Aiken et al. (2002).

and Gergen, 1998; Kovner et al., 2002; Lichtig et al., 1999; Needleman et al., 2002; Sochalski, 2001). Some studies specific to ICU staffing have been conducted; information on staffing levels in other hospital units, including medical–surgical units, is sparse.

Overall hospital staffing As stated above, a problem with hospital-level aggregation is that when heterogeneous nursing units, such as pediatric units, labor and delivery units, adult medical–surgical units, and ICUs, are combined, hospital-wide staffing levels may not well represent the levels experienced by patients in a given nursing unit, and the findings of research can be clouded. Table 3-3 in Chapter 3 (replicated here as Table 5-2) indi-

TABLE 5-2   Types of Work Units in Which Hospital-Employed RNs Spend More Than Half of Their Direct Patient Care Time

Type of Work Unit	Percent of RNs Employed
General/specialty bed unit	30.9
Intensive care unit	16.9
Operating room	9.0
Labor/delivery	8.2
Emergency department	7.9
Step-down/transition from ICU	5.9
Outpatient department	5.8
Postanesthesia recovery room	3.1
Other area	2.5
No specific area	1.8
Not known	8.0
TOTAL	100

SOURCE: Spratley et al. (2000).

cates that general medical–surgical nurses would likely contribute much of the data on hospital-wide nurse staffing; together, however, ICU, operating room (OR), and labor and delivery nurses could also reasonably be expected to exert significant influence on reported aggregate, hospital-wide nurse staffing levels.

This is an important point because the only source of staffing data on all types of inpatient hospital units (i.e., the California Office of Statewide Health Planning and Development [OSHPD])[5] shows that ICU, labor and delivery (apart from other obstetrics), and step-down/transition units have considerably higher average nurse staffing levels than medical–surgical and other hospital nursing units (Spetz et al., 2000). These data are presented later in this chapter.

When staffing levels are based on hppd estimates[6] from staffing studies that combine nurses in direct patient care positions with those in administrative or other non–direct care positions and are aggregated across multiple hospital units, nurse staffing levels such as those in Table 5-3 are produced.

The high nurse staffing levels suggested by these estimates are in contrast to the unit-specific data and direct patient care nurse-specific data produced by the Donaldson, Cavouras, and Aiken studies cited above. The higher nurse staffing levels in Table 5-3 also reflect the limitations of the available data sources on nurse staffing. The American Hospital Association (AHA) data used in several of the studies included in Table 5-3 aggregate all nursing staff (direct-care nurses and nurses in administrative positions) across all inpatient and outpatient care units, thereby producing higher levels of nurse staffing. State data sets often can distinguish nursing staff by cost center (and thereby by nursing unit), but may suffer from incomplete data. For example, in the Lichtig et al. (1999) study cited above, seven California hospitals did not submit cost reports, 26 submitted reports but did not include data on nursing hours, and 8 reported unrealistic nursing hours. Better understanding of actual nurse staffing levels is provided by studies that have examined staffing levels within specific types of patient care units.

---

[5]OSHPD's survey of hospitals is considered to be the most comprehensive in the United States and is held up as a model for other states. In spite of some limitations, it captures data from nearly every hospital in the state, and data are provided by cost center, allowing examination of care delivered by distinct care units as opposed to all hospital patient care units in the aggregate (Spetz et al., 2000).

[6]Staffing estimates are sometimes calculated by dividing 24 hours by the number of hppd for a facility; e.g., 24 hours divided by 6.2 hppd = 3.9 patients per nurse. Other studies estimate hospital-wide nurse staffing levels using other measures, including the ratio of FTE hospital RNs to total hospital-adjusted days (Kovner and Gergen, 1998) and RN staffing per 100 occupied beds (Bond et al., 1999).

TABLE 5-3 Nurse Staffing Estimates Derived from Staffing Studies[a]

Estimated RN:Patient Ratio	Source of Estimates	Source
1.0:4.0–4.5	Estimates derived from authors' report of average hppd for all nursing staff and % RN nursing staff. Data from 1994 New York and California state databases. Authors note poor quality of these data.	Lichtig et al. (1999)
1.0:3.9	Authors estimated 6.2 RN hppd (adjusted)[b] from national 1996 American Hospital Association (AHA) data.	Kovner et al. (2000)
1.0:3.7	Authors estimated 6.56 RN hppd (adjusted) from 1996 AHA data for hospitals in 13 states.	Kovner et al. (2002)
1.0:3.1	Authors estimated average RN (administrative and direct-care) hppd of 7.8 from 11 states that collected 1997 nurse staffing data from state hospital data sets across all hospital inpatient units.	Needleman et al. (2002)
1.0:3.8	Authors estimated 6.3 RN hppd across medical–surgical, ICU, and coronary care units in 232 California hospitals.	Cho et al. (2003)

[a]Estimates calculated by dividing 24 hours by the number of hppd.

[b]AHA data were adjusted to account for differences between hospital inpatient and outpatient services.

Intensive care units A 1988–1990 study of 42 hospital ICUs, including a combination of volunteer hospitals and a geographically stratified random sample of nonfederal U.S. hospitals with at least 200 beds (the vast majority of all hospitals with ICUs), obtained nurse staffing data on each shift from a questionnaire completed by the director of the nursing unit. In that study, the mean number of patients cared for by an ICU nurse was 1.5 (range of 0.7 to 3.3). Hospitals falling one standard deviation below the mean had staffing ratios of one nurse for every 2.1 patients (Shortell et al., 1994). This average of 1.5 patients per nurse is identical to average ICU staffing levels calculated from hours of ICU nursing care (18 hppd) and the proportion of that care delivered by RNs (90 percent) reported in a 2.5-year study (1993–1995) of nurse staffing and adverse events in eight ICUs in 11 hospitals[7] (Blegen and Vaughn, 1998), and is similar to that observed more recently in California. OSHPD data for 1998–1999 show average nurse-to-patient ICU staffing levels of 1.0:1.5 (medical–surgical), 1.0:1.8 (coronary), 1.0:1.2 (pediatric), and 1.0:2.1 (neonatal) (Spetz et al., 2000).

---

[7]Ninety percent of 18 hppd = 16.2 RN hppd; 24 hours/day/patient divided by 16.2 RN hppd = 1.48 patients per RN.

A series of studies of ICU outcomes conducted between 1994 and 1996 in all nonfederal, short-stay hospitals in Maryland found that 82 percent of these hospitals had day-shift ICU nurse staffing levels of one nurse for every one to two patients. Lower staffing levels—i.e., nurses caring for three or more ICU patients—were reported for 18 percent of hospitals. After adjusting for patient characteristics and for hospital and surgeon volume, patients who had abdominal aortic surgery in hospitals with fewer ICU nurses (i.e., each nurse caring for three or more patients) on the day shift were more likely to have postoperative complications, particularly pulmonary insufficiency and reintubation (Pronovost et al., 2001).

A second analysis of these data examined ICU direct-care nurse staffing on day and night shifts. Nurse staffing was coded as either low intensity (1:3 or greater nurse-to-patient ratio on the day and night shifts); medium intensity (1:3 or greater on either the day or night shifts, but not both), or high intensity (1:2 or lower on both day and night shifts). The majority of hospitals (63 percent) were staffed at a high-intensity level; 21 percent were staffed at a mixed-intensity level; and 16 percent had low-intensity staffing. After controlling for patient and organizational variables, the analysis showed that patients cared for on units with medium-intensity staffing were more likely to have cardiac and other complications than were patients cared for on high-intensity units. Patients cared for on units with low-intensity nurse staffing were more than twice as likely to have respiratory complications as patients on units with high-intensity staffing. Patients were more than five times as likely to develop pulmonary insufficiency and were more than twice as likely to be mechanically ventilated after 96 hours and reintubated when cared for on units with low-intensity staffing as compared with units with high-intensity staffing (Dang et al., 2002).

These sources and others (Amaravadi et al., 2000; Fridkin et al., 1996) indicate that nurse staffing levels of 1:2 or better not only are commonly used by large numbers of ICUs, but also have a protective effect on patients.

Medical–surgical units   Information on medical–surgical staffing levels is available from two states and one multihospital, multistate data set. In California, CalNOC data show an average of 5.9 patients assigned to individual medical–surgical nurses across all shifts (Donaldson et al., 2001). California OSHPD data show similar average nurse-to-patient ratios of 1.0:5.2, with a median of 1.0:5.8 (Spetz et al., 2000). An examination of nurse staffing ratios within individual shifts from a convenience sample of representative medical–surgical units from 28 percent of California hospitals showed variation in staffing across shifts and by rural/urban status. This study estimated staffing levels using two methods: (1) computing a nurse staffing ratio based on the hospital-reported number of hours in a shift and the RN hours per patient for the shift, and (2) using staffing ratios reported directly by the hospital. In general, the hospital-reported ratios were leaner (fewer nurses for the patients) than those computed. These two methods yielded the average nurse-to-patient ratios and ranges of staffing levels by shift and rural/urban hospital status shown in Tables 5-4 and 5-5, respectively. The range of nurse staffing levels is shown by the reported number of patients per RN displayed in quartiles in Table 5-5.

A survey of Pennsylvania RNs working in hospitals in 1999 identified medical–surgical nurses and asked them to provide (for the most recent shift they had worked) information on the type of shift they had worked (i.e., day, evening, or night), the number of patients in their unit during that shift, the number of patients assigned to them, and the number of RNs who had worked in their unit during that shift. The average number of patients assigned to these medical–surgical nurses ranged from six to eight, with

TABLE 5-4   Average Number of Patients per RN, by Shift and Rural/Nonrural Location, in California

Shift	Rural with 12-Hour Shifts	Nonrural with 12-Hour Shifts	Rural with 8-Hour Shifts	Nonrural with 8-Hour Shifts
Computed number of patients per RN				
Day shift	4	4.4	6.2	4.2
Evening shift	NA	NA	3.0	4.7
Night shift	4.4	5.2	3.0	5.7
Reported number of patients per RN				
Day shift	6.7	5.9	6.8	6.1
Evening shift	NA	NA	6.7	6.9
Night shift	7.4	6.9	7.3	8.2

NOTE: NA = not applicable.
SOURCE: Spetz et al. (2000).

TABLE 5-5   Quartiles of Staffing Data in Medical–Surgical Units, in California

Shift	Reported Number of Patients per RN, by Shift			
	25%	50%	75%	100%
Day shift	5	6	7	12
Evening shift	5.1	7	8	12
Night shift	6	8	9	26

SOURCE: Spetz et al. (2000).

progressively higher ratios found on the evening and night shifts compared with the day shift. The number of patients reported by individual nurses as being assigned to them was identical to the average number of patients assigned to nurses as calculated by dividing the total number of patients on the unit by the total number of RNs on the unit (Sochalski, 2001). The higher patient loads reported by the Pennsylvania nurses may be due in part to higher nurse staffing levels in California. AHA data show that California has higher average and median RN hours per adjusted patient day than the nation as a whole. California is ranked 19th among states in median RN and LPN/LVN hppd (Spetz et al., 2000).

Other hospital units   Publicly reported data on nurse staffing in other hospital units are scarce. Information on staffing levels in transition (step-down) units is available from the CalNOC data presented above. Additional information on step-down unit and other inpatient unit staffing comes from California OSHPD data. OSHPD data for 1998–1999 indicate the nurse-to-patient ratios shown in Table 5-6, derived from hospital reports of RN hppd across all shifts and based on the assumption that an average patient day is 24 hours in length. OSHPD data also revealed that rural hospitals had higher staffing levels than urban hospitals (Spetz et al., 2000).

Nursing Home Staffing

Nurse staffing levels in nursing homes also are typically reported in terms of hprd. They are calculated by dividing the total nursing hours worked in the facility by the total resident days of care per year. Although staffing levels vary widely across facilities, since 1997 the average nursing

TABLE 5-6   California Hospital Nurse-to-Patient Ratios: Means, Medians, and Quartiles (1998–1999)

Type of Unit	Mean	Median	25th Percentile	75th Percentile
Pediatric acute	1:3.2	1:3.4	1:4.9	1:2.5
Obstetrics	1:4.0	1:4.8	1:6.5	1:3.4
Newborn nursery	1:5.7	1:6.9	1:10.1	1:4.3
Subacute care	1:11	1:14.7	1:18.5	1:8.7
Definitive observation[a]	1:3.1	1:4.6	1:5.6	1:3.7
Rehabilitation care	1:6.3	1:6.7	1:8.9	1:5.0
Labor and delivery[b]	1:1.3	1:1.4	1:1.8	1:1.1

[a]A level of care between intensive and medical–surgical care. This would equate to step-down and transitional units in the CalNOC data.
[b]Staffing level per delivery.

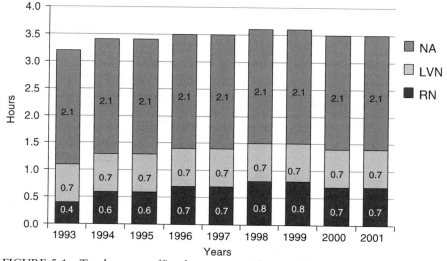

FIGURE 5-1   Total nurse staffing hours per resident in all U.S. nursing facilities, 1993–2001.
SOURCE: Harrington et al. (2002).

home in the United States has provided a combined total of 3.5 to 3.6 hprd of RN, LVN/LPN, NA, and director of nursing time (see Figure 5-1). Most of this time (58 percent or 2.1 hours) is provided by NAs, who on average care for 11 residents. Each RN and LPN/LVN (at 0.7–0.8 hprd) typically oversees care for 32 to 34 residents, although these ratios may vary across shifts and on weekends and holidays (Harrington et al., 2002).

Staffing levels vary widely by facility characteristics. SNFs that admit only Medicare residents have almost double the staffing levels of nonskilled (Medicaid-only) nursing facilities (Harrington et al., 2002). For-profit facilities generally have lower staffing levels than nonprofits, even though there can be high variability in this regard (Aaronson et al., 1994; Harrington et al., 2001). There are also wide variations in staffing levels across states (Harrington et al., 2002).

Federal nursing home regulations require that each facility receiving Medicare or Medicaid payments (the majority of nursing homes) have "sufficient nursing staff to provide nursing and related services to attain or maintain the highest practicable physical, mental, and psychosocial well-being of each resident, as determined by resident assessments and individual plans of care."[8] These regulations also require all Medicare- or Medicaid-certified nursing homes to have an RN who is the director of nursing; at

---

[8] 42 Code of Federal Regulations (CFR) 483.30, revised as of October 1, 2002.

least one RN on duty for 8 hours a day, 7 days a week; and at least one licensed nurse (RN or LVP/LPN) on duty on the other shifts. The director of nursing may also serve as the RN on duty in facilities with 60 or fewer residents. These standards apply regardless of the number of patients in the nursing home; e.g., they apply equally to a facility with 60 patients and a facility with 300 patients. As of April 2001, 25 states had established higher minimum staffing requirements for licensed nurses than those of the federal government, and 15 states had higher RN staffing requirements (Harrington, 2001).

Responding to the Evidence on Staffing and Patient Safety

Given the above evidence, the committee sought to determine what course(s) of action with respect to nurse staffing would be most likely to ensure patient safety. Strategies proposed by consumer, professional, industry, and labor associations and by policy analysts generally include regulatory approaches, adoption of more-effective internal staffing practices by HCOs, and marketplace/consumer-driven approaches. The committee considered the individual merits of these approaches and found that each has both benefits and limitations. We took particular note of the unavailability, incompleteness, and unreliability of nurse staffing data in the United States and the weaknesses of tools for measuring nursing workload and predicting hospital staffing needs. The committee believes the appropriate and coordinated use of all three approaches would have a synergistic effect and be most conducive to achieving safe staffing levels.

Regulatory Approaches

A number of labor, nursing, and consumer advocacy organizations recommend that quantitative ratios of the numbers of nursing staff or nursing hours per patient be mandated, in some form, for nursing homes and/or hospitals to promote safer patient care (Massachusetts Nurses Association, 2003; National Citizens Coalition for Nursing Home Reform, 1998; SEIU, 2001). They point out that minimum personnel standards, expressed as ratios, are used in many other service industries, such as child day care, education, and fire services. In the airline industry, for example, standards require a certain number of personnel on each flight based on the aircraft and number of passengers, and also limit the number of hours personnel can fly without a break. Thus, where safety is a concern, regulatory standards have been deemed appropriate to reduce error. Beyond these minimum standards, organizations compete to provide higher levels of service by using more or better-trained personnel and by exceeding other minimum standards.

The committee believes that, based on currently available evidence, the use of minimum personnel standards is presently and generally more appropriate for nursing homes than for hospitals, for two reasons. First, we find that in general, the evidence for specific numerical staffing standards is stronger for nursing homes (although evidence of the effect of specific ICU staffing levels on patient safety is also strong). The CMS (2001) study on the appropriateness of minimum nurse staffing ratios in nursing homes greatly advanced the knowledge base on the effect of different nursing staff-to-patient ratios on patient outcomes. It identified staffing levels (2.4–2.8 hprd for NAs, 1.1–1.3 hprd for licensed nursing staff, and 0.55–0.75 hprd for RNs) above which no further improvements in patient outcomes were observed, and below which improvements in quality occurred with each incremental increase in staffing.

The purpose of minimum standards for staffing in nursing homes would be to ensure that at least the minimum resources are in place to preserve the safety of nursing home residents. Current requirements for 8 hours of RN and 24 hours of licensed nurse coverage per day are, in fact, minimum standards. Although these minimum standards ensure that long-term care facilities can administer medications 24 hours a day and have an RN available to supervise NAs and respond to issues during 8 hours per day, this minimum is not based on the premise of patient safety. Patient safety requires staff resources that are sufficient to prevent an inappropriately high rate of untoward events that could be avoided with adequate staffing levels. For such a standard to be reasonable, it must at least be based on the number of residents in the nursing home and address NAs, who provide most of the care to nursing home residents. Such minimum staffing standards are not a precise statement of how many staff are required to fully meet the needs of each specific group of residents on each unit, nor are they a quality improvement tool to optimize quality in each nursing home. Rather, a minimum staffing level is one that avoids placing individual residents unnecessarily at risk because of insufficient numbers of staff to provide even the most basic care.

In contrast, with the exception of studies of ICU staffing, the committee identified only one hospital staffing study that measured the effects of different staffing levels within a specific type of hospital patient care unit (i.e., medical–surgical unit [Sochalski, 2001]). In this study, the frequency of adverse events was subjectively reported by nursing staff using a Likert scale, rather than being counted using clinical data sets. The need for hospital unit–specific information is important because, as pointed out previously, the hospital patient population and the nursing units in which they receive care are more heterogeneous than is the case in nursing homes, making hospital-level data more difficult to interpret.

A number of researchers studying hospital staffing levels and patient outcomes have found that evidence does not yet exist to indicate the necessary (minimum) or ideal (optimal) staffing across the various types of hospital inpatient care units (Bolton et al., 2001; Kovner et al., 2002; Spetz et al., 2000). The Agency for Healthcare Research and Quality (AHRQ) evidence report *Making Health Care Safer: A Critical Analysis of Patient Safety Practices* also finds that, for acute hospital care, ". . . there is no definitive evidence as to specific thresholds for RN or total nursing staff hours per patient day, or nursing skill mix for various patient populations or nursing unit types" (Seago, 2001:429). The committee agrees that generalizing the results of studies of the effects of hospital-wide staffing on patient safety to specific types of hospital units is inappropriate. We believe nurse staffing regulations should be based on evidence that demonstrates the effect of specific staffing levels (including skill mix) on patient safety within specific patient care units.

Second, federal and state governments already regulate nursing home staffing levels, as described previously. Although a few states regulate hospital nurse staffing levels for specific types of patient care units (e.g., ICUs and labor and delivery units), none currently regulate all the different types of patient care units found in hospitals. California has proposed regulating hospital staffing for all patient care units; the nurse staffing ratios that California hospitals will be required to meet are scheduled to take effect in January 2004. These standards call for certain *licensed nurse* staffing levels in all hospital patient care units (the state already has hospital staffing requirements for some patient care units, such as ICUs, ORs, and nursery units). However, the regulations do not require the nurses to be RNs as opposed to LPNs/LVNs. California's regulations allow "sufficient flexibility in the type of nurse to be used . . . determined by nursing scope of practice and patient acuity" (Office of the Governor, 2002).

Based on the above considerations, the committee makes the following recommendation:

Recommendation 5-1. The U.S. Department of Health and Human Services (DHHS) should update existing regulations established in 1990 that specify minimum standards for registered and licensed nurse staffing in nursing homes. Updated minimum standards should:

- **Require the presence of at least one RN within the facility at all times.**
- **Specify staffing levels that increase as the number of patients increase, and that are based on the findings and recommendations of the DHHS report to Congress, *Appropriateness of Mini-***

mum Nurse Staffing Ratios in Nursing Homes—Phase II Final Report.
• Address staffing levels for nurse assistants, who provide the majority of patient care.

With respect to requiring the presence of at least one RN in each nursing home at all times, two previous IOM studies made this same recommendation to achieve better patient outcomes (IOM, 1996, 2001b). This committee additionally calls attention to this minimal staffing requirement as essential to patient safety.

With respect to the recommendation that DHHS specify staffing standards in regulations that would increase with the number of patients and be based on the findings and recommendations of the Phase II DHHS report to Congress on the appropriateness of minimum staffing ratios in nursing homes (CMS, 2001), the committee notes that the thresholds identified in that study above which no further benefit from staffing ratios could be identified are above the staffing levels of 75–90 percent of facilities, depending on the type of staff. However, a minimum standard set by DHHS need not approach the threshold level above which there is no further benefit. In fact, such a standard would go beyond the expectation for a *minimum*, which is intended to identify situations in which facilities unequivocally place residents at an unacceptable level of risk. The challenge is that there is no absolute minimum level of risk for untoward events that is considered acceptable.

If every single resident in a nursing home experienced an avoidable untoward event, that would clearly be considered unacceptable. But there is no absolute rate of pressure ulcers, weight loss, or hospitalization for infection that is considered unacceptable. Even if one were assured that every event counted was due to a care error (i.e., avoidable), one would still tolerate some errors and would have to choose an acceptable rate. Thus, it is most defensible to set an unacceptable rate based on relative standards using the distribution of rates across facilities and identifying outliers. In the Phase II CMS study, the worst 10 percent of facilities is used as the relative standard, recognizing that an argument could be made for other standards. Facilities in the worst decile, however, were generally three or more times more likely than those at the mean to have untoward events. The study does not propose a specific minimum standard for RNs, licensed nurses, and NAs because agreement must first be reached about what is an unacceptable level of risk. However, data exist from this national study with which to determine the staffing levels for each type of staff that are associated with any level of risk for untoward events.

The committee believes it is feasible to establish a minimum staffing level for each type of staff based on the consensus of experts about unacceptable levels of risks for untoward events. These standards could be phased in over time such that a greater level of risk would be tolerated in the first year, requiring somewhat lower minimum standards, with decreasing tolerance for errors and hence increasing minimum staffing levels in subsequent years. Any such strategy should be accompanied by an evaluation of the number of facilities affected, the staffing changes that occur in these facilities, and the changes in the rates of untoward events.

At the same time, a number of nursing organizations, policy experts, and HCOs point out the limitations of staffing ratios. While they may help ensure a baseline level of staffing in HCOs that may be outliers, they are poor instruments for achieving optimal staffing. Depending on the skill mix and expertise of nursing staff and patient acuity (defined below), minimum ratios may still not provide the needed levels of safety. Moreover, counts of patients needed to calculate nurse staffing levels consistent with a ratio must be taken at a point or points in time. Yet patient admissions, transfers, and discharges are frequent; therefore, an adequate nurse-to-patient ratio at 7 A.M. may be inadequate at 10 A.M., and an organization that has satisfied a nurse-to-staffing ratio at one point in time may still have inadequate staffing at another point. Thus, while staffing ratios can help protect against the most egregious staffing deficiencies, HCOs will need to employ more sensitive approaches internally to fine-tune staffing levels.

More-Effective Internal Staffing Practices by HCOs

Problems in the application of widely used tools to predict hospital staffing Many hospitals determine the amount of nursing staff they need to provide care on individual patient care units and shifts through the use of staffing tools collectively referred to as patient classification systems (PCSs). PCSs are quantitative formulas that measure patient acuity, translate this measure into projections of actions that need to be performed and the time it will take to perform them (nurse workload), and use those projections to estimate nurse staffing needs. *Acuity* in PCSs refers to the amount of nursing time required to care for an individual patient given that patient's care needs (which may or may not correspond to the severity of the person's medical illness) (Norrish and Rundall, 2001).

In PCSs, the nursing care requirements of individual patients are summed to estimate the total patient care needs for a particular nursing unit. Staffing projections are then based on predetermined time standards for each type of patient or patient-care task. These time standards are intended to be either derived empirically and uniquely for each institution based on work sampling measures, or adopted from standards inherent in a particular PCS.

During the 1980s, the emphasis on PCSs increased as a result of Joint

Commission on Accreditation of Healthcare Organizations (JCAHO) accreditation standards that required nursing departments to have a system for determining nursing care requirements based on patient needs (Norrish and Rundall, 2001). Today, PCSs are widely used by hospitals (but not nursing homes) despite their frequently noted shortcomings. These shortcomings pertain not as much to how patient acuity is measured as to how corresponding work is measured, the extent to which the PCS methodology accommodates variations in staff expertise and work environment, and how HCOs implement the PCS.

PCSs lack desired sensitivity to variations in patient acuity levels. PCS models identify discrete levels of patient acuity and translate them into estimates of the amount of care individuals at that level typically require. However, patient acuity varies *within* classification levels. When HCOs fail to appreciate this fact, they can become locked into average PCS predictions and fail to acknowledge the need for flexibility that is an intrinsic characteristic of PCSs (DeGroot, 1994).

Workload estimates for various patient classification levels may be inaccurate and unreliable. Measurements of workload are the product of three factors: (1) product and service (i.e., patient care) classifications (described above), (2) forecasts of volume demand for each classification, and (3) the standard times for each service (Bayiz, 2003). To translate patient acuity into workload estimates, the work performed by nurses when caring for such patients needs to be sampled (DeGroot, 1994). Work sampling involves identifying the activities that are performed and the average time required for each.

HCOs' use of PCSs has been criticized in several areas pertaining to work sampling. First, work sampling and time estimates are often not derived from the institution using the PCS. Instead, HCOs often use work sampling estimates produced by external PCS vendors or other facilities. To the extent that these external work estimates were derived from work samplings for patient care units that differ from those of the institution using the PCS—in terms of the experience level or skill mix of nursing staff, the availability of support staff, the way patient care is organized and delivered across units, and/or the physical layout of the nursing units and hospital—or are rationally derived using educated "best estimates," they will likely be inaccurate and unreliable estimates of how long it takes nursing staff *within that particular institution* to perform certain activities or care for a given level of patients. There is no "one size fits all" set of standard times that can be used across hospitals (Bayiz, 2003; DeGroot, 1994). Accordingly, some have pointed to PCSs as contributing to the perception that "a nurse is a nurse is a nurse," that all nurses are equal and interchangeable. This perception is inconsistent with the evidence presented in Chapter 3 that nurses vary in their level of knowledge and expertise. It has also been identified as contributing to decreased confidence in the validity and reliability of PCSs and the staff allocations that result from their use (Malloch and Conovaloff, 1999).

Workload estimates used in PCSs also are criticized as not taking into account other factors, such as the frequent interruptions encountered by nurses in performing certain tasks (Malloch and Conovaloff, 1999) or the need for multitasking by nurses—often in the performance of the invisible, cognitive work of nurses described in Chapter 3. For example, while a nurse may be changing intravenous tubing, he or she may also be observing the patient's physical status and pain level and providing patient education (Malloch and Conovaloff, 1999). Workload estimates also are criticized for being derived from measurements of care that is *delivered*, which is often constrained by staffing limits and therefore is not an accurate predictor of the care that is actually *needed* (Jennings et al., 1989).

One study compared PCS predictions with the care actually delivered, as measured by the same classification tool administered retrospectively by nurses who had received intensive training on the use of the PCS tool and had scored high on interrater reliability. This study found significant differences in the average prospective and retrospective classification scores in two of the three nursing units in which the study was conducted. For all three units, the retrospective PSC scores were higher than the prospective scores. The times associated with these differences would result in staffing deficits of 0.24 FTEs, 0.72 FTEs, and 2.99 FTEs in the three units (Hlusko and Nichols, 1996). An earlier study comparing the application of four different PCSs for the same patient population found large statistically and clinically significant differences in hours of care needed by the patients according to those four tools (O'Brien-Pallas et al., 1992).

Such concerns point to the need to validate and evaluate PCSs during their actual implementation (DeGroot, 1994). However, although there are reports in the literature regarding the validity and reliability of a system during its initial implementation (efficacy), there is "a paucity of published research related to patient classification system validation after implementation" (effectiveness) (Hlusko and Nichols, 1996:40). Moreover, continual changes in personnel, work environments, tools and equipment, and technology in most workplaces result in corresponding changes in the time required to perform the work, necessitating revision of the standard times. As a rule of thumb, experts recommend that work measurement reviews and reevaluations be conducted annually and additionally on an ad hoc basis whenever major work redesigns are undertaken (Bayiz, 2003).

Multiple purposes create incentives for gaming. Although PCSs are used to predict staffing needs, they have other uses as well, such as to estimate long-term staffing requirements for budgeting purposes (Seago, 2002). These multiple purposes of PCSs provide incentives for "gaming" or manipulation. While nursing staff can consciously or subconsciously manipulate patient classification levels (and thereby project needs for greater staffing—a phenomenon referred to as "acuity creep"), managers can also influence staffing need projections through their selection of the staffing allowances for the various acuity levels (Norrish and Rundall, 2001).

PCSs are time-consuming. Most PCSs require nurses to check off activities, treatments, and procedures according to their frequency of occurrence for each patient several times a day. A survey of California hospitals, for example, revealed that three-fourths of hospitals must complete 36 items for their PCS, while half must complete 20 items; one PCS was found to contain 200 items (Seago, 2002).

As a result of the above concerns, researchers studying patient staffing and PCSs note "widespread distrust" of virtually all these tools (Spetz et al., 2000), and the AHRQ evidence report *Making Health Care Safer: A Critical Analysis of Patient Safety Practices* (Seago, 2001:427) concludes that "although PCSs are used for multiple purposes, they are an inadequate tool for determining unit staffing on a daily or shift basis. In addition, there are numerous patient classification systems and most are specific to one hospital or one nursing unit. The validity and reliability of PCSs are inconsistent and the systems cannot be compared with one another." Nonetheless, a number of states mandate the use of PCSs. Five states (Texas, Oregon, Kentucky, Nevada, and Virginia) require hospitals to develop and implement nurse staffing plans, methodologies, or systems (ANA, 2002). The California nurse staffing legislation described above requires hospitals to adhere to both nurse staffing ratios and the results of a hospital-selected PCS, whichever is higher. Some speculate that hospitals will have incentives to readjust their PCS staffing factors to predict staffing levels no higher than the ratios mandated by law (Seago, 2002).

For this reason, many researchers, hospital executives, and policy analysts call for more reliable and valid measures of patient acuity (Reed et al., 1998) or the use of approaches other than PCSs to determine nurse staffing in relation to current patient needs (Kovner et al., 2000). Some urge the development of a formula approach to determining nurse staffing levels that would take into account multiple variables in addition to patient acuity, including RN staff expertise; work intensity; unit physical layout; and availability of NAs, other support staff, and physicians (Seago, 2002).

Failure of methods for predicting patient volume to keep pace with changes in hospital admission practices Compounding the above problems with predicting workload on the basis of patient acuity are problems in predicting daily and hourly patient volume. As discussed above, PCSs document the acuity level of patients at a point in time. If patient volume and acuity are assumed to be stable, acuity, workload, and theoretically staffing are predictable for the next shift. However, as the environment becomes less stable as a result of patient turnover (patient discharges and new admissions) and changes in patient status, projections become less accurate. To the extent that input (patient admissions) to a unit is not predictable, PCS predictions will be less accurate (Seago, 2002).

Historically, hospitals have predicted patient volume—and thereby staffing levels—based on a daily census, typically taken at midnight. A midnight census, however, underestimates care requirements. The actual number of patients cared for by nurses during a 24-hour period is actually the total of four patient types—those on the unit for the full 24-hour period, patient admissions, patient discharges, and patients admitted and discharged on the same day (often referred to as "observation-only" patients). The midnight census fails to capture two of these four—discharges prior to midnight and observation-only patients (Lawrenz, 1992). The latter patients often are in need of care because of an outpatient surgical or radiological procedure and frequently require the same level of care as other inpatients. Moreover, admissions and discharges are well known to be high-activity, time-demanding processes. Thus when hospitals base predictions on projected patient volume as indicated by the midnight census alone, they fail to accurately measure the true level of patient volume—and nurses' workload (Budreau et al., 1999; Jacobson et al., 1999).

A 1997 study was conducted at a large midwestern medical center to determine the difference between the midnight census and the actual number of patients receiving nursing care in one unit for a 24-hour period. The midnight census counted 23 patients on the unit, while the unit had actually cared for 35 patients during the day. This study also examined periods of peak activity and found that, contrary to historical patterns of peak activity, the evening shift in today's environment is just as busy as the day shift in terms of total hours of care required. This situation is attributed to several changes brought about by today's health care environment, such as the fact that a late discharge maximizes the number of hours a patient is in the hospital while avoiding incurring an additional "day" charged at midnight. Late discharges also occur because family members often prefer to pick up the patient after their workday, when they will be home to monitor the patient more closely. Because discharges are late, admissions are also late, awaiting the availability of a bed (Jacobson et al., 1999).

Staffing principles that can help compensate for these problems As of 2002, five states had laws requiring hospitals to develop and follow internal nurse staffing plans (as opposed to adhering to nurse staffing ratios) (ANA, 2002). A number of nursing organizations have put forth guidance for HCOs to follow when developing such staffing plans. This guidance often speaks to issues broader than patient safety, including nurses' "degree of involvement in quality initiatives" and their "immersion . . . in activities such as nursing research that add to the body of nursing knowledge" (ANA, 1999:7), as well as their professionalism, satisfaction, and personal values and ethics (American Association of Critical Care Nurses, 1999). From work in the behavioral, organizational, engineering, and health sciences, the committee has identified the following staffing practices that can improve patient safety.

Incorporate admissions, discharges, and "less than 24-hour"patients into estimates of daily patient volume. Evidence presented at the beginning of this chapter makes clear that staffing for patient safety requires, in part, staffing proportionate to patient volume. To this end, HCOs must obtain estimates of patient volume for the upcoming shift, day, weeks, and months that are as accurate as possible. These estimates should be developed not solely by measuring patient volume at one point in time (e.g., the midnight census), but also by including admissions, discharges, and observation-only patients in patient volume measurements for each unit.

Involve direct-care nursing staff in selecting, modifying, and evaluating staffing methods. Despite the limitations of PCSs described above, they provide a degree of objectivity in the allocation of staffing resources (American Association of Critical Care Nurses, 1999). Until more-effective methods are developed for predicting staffing needs, estimates of patients' clinical care needs (patient care workload) and nurse staffing levels are likely to continue to be made using some variant of PCSs. Estimates thus derived ideally should rely on work sampling studies conducted on the unit to which they will be applied, thereby better reflecting variations in the expertise and skill mix of nursing staff, the availability of support staff, the way patient care is organized and delivered across units, and the physical layout of the nursing unit and hospital (Bayiz, 2003; Malloch and Conovaloff, 1999).

Such work sampling can be expensive, however, especially if done individually for multiple nursing units, as well as labor-intensive. HCOs may instead choose to use one of the numerous PCSs that are available commercially or use their own historical nurse staffing models. Further, variables such as the experience and expertise of nursing staff and the availability of support staff frequently change on a shift-to-shift basis. For these reasons, it is important to increase the accuracy of the workload estimates produced by involving direct-care nursing staff in selecting the PCS or other approach (e.g., the HCO's own historical nurse staffing models) used to estimate staffing. Staff should also be involved in evaluating the assumptions and methods used in the selected PCS (i.e., validating the patient classification methods and identifying threats to the generalizeability of the results derived from the PCS to individual patient care units), in developing and applying remedies to make the projections more accurate, and in monitoring the outcomes of the application of the PCS (Malloch and Conovaloff, 1999).

Furthermore, the workload estimates produced with traditional PCSs should be recognized as just one dimension rather than the sole determinant of staffing. In addition to being involved in evaluating the general approach used to estimate nurse staffing levels, nursing staff need to be directly involved in developing approaches to compensate for the inevitable imprecision of volume and workload estimates. This principle of high involvement of nursing staff in selecting, modifying, and evaluating approaches to estimating nurse staffing is based on evidence presented in Chapter 4 describing the benefits of involving workers in work design and work flow decision making.

Provide for "on-time" staffing or demand elasticity to accommodate unpredicted variations in patient volume and/or acuity and resulting workload. The best PCSs and other workload measurement/staffing methodologies available use measures of past populations to project future workload. Like all predictions, these projections are imperfect, and there is always a variance between the anticipated and actual workload (Bayiz, 2003). It has long been established that when using nurse staffing methodologies based on patient classification and workload estimates, corrective allocations or smoothing techniques are needed to respond to variations in patient volume or acuity not predicted by past events (Bayiz, 2003; Hershey et al., 1980). Meeting these unplanned-for needs for additional staffing can be accomplished either by providing for an increase in nurses or by controlling the demand for nursing services.

Providing for "on-time" increases in nurses can be accomplished in several ways: staffing above predicted estimates, developing pools of cross-trained nurses who are floated among units to smooth demand fluctuations, temporarily reallocating a nurse to a unit other than the one he/she normally works (often called "pulling" a nurse (Hershey et al., 1980), and using nurses obtained from external sources (e.g., temporary employment agencies). While staffing above predicted levels may be costly and difficult because of the existing nursing shortage, this approach offers higher patient safety benefit than floating, pulling, or using nurses from external agencies. Nursing staff are immediately available to accommodate quick changes in patient status or volume—not available in the situation described below:

> I was the nurse-in-charge of a 19-bed labor, deliver and recovery unit. Every bed was full and one patient was being cared for in a "room" in the hallway. Normally charge duties would consist of supervising and providing back-up for nursing staff and handling all logistical issues for the unit. On this day, every nurse was caring for as much or more than she could handle. I took on patient triage (determining if pregnant women were ready to be admitted for delivery or sent home) and caring for a patient recovering from a postpartum hemorrhage of about 2000 ccs (blood pressure 54/32 and pulse = 200 at her worst point).

After triaging the first patient, I left her to check again on my patient with the post-partum hemorrhage, leaving the first and a new triage patient under the watchful eye of a wonderful, but not fully trained "scrub tech," telling the tech to call me if the patient needed anything. No sooner had I got to the post-partum hemorrhage patient, than I had to leave her. I was the only nurse available to assist with a patient in active labor (she delivered in less than 20 minutes) while still (in theory) monitoring the post-partum hemorrhage patient (fortunately her husband was an emergency medical technician and I pressed him into monitoring her condition) and two triage patients.

On another shift, only luck and great teamwork kept a disaster from happening when we admitted an emergency C-section for abruption with hemorrhaging. I and several other nurses (all also responsible for two patients apiece) went to assist. Once the case was underway, the other nurses returned to care for their patients. I reminded my charge nurse that one of my patients was on Pitocin (a drug that causes contractions) and had earlier had fetal distress. She gave a worried laugh and said that there as no one else to watch them but that she would try. When I came out of the OR to get drugs for anesthesia, I glanced at the fetal monitor and saw my patient back in fetal distress. I dropped off the drugs, ran out of the OR leaving the other nurse on her own with the C-section, turned off the Pitocin, and went to notify my patient's doctor. If anesthesia has not needed the drugs, the distress would have continued because every other nurse was going as fast as they could caring for other patients.

Staffing above predicted levels follows the principle of redundancy that is employed by high-reliability organizations (Roberts, 1990). Such redundancy is not wasteful. Determining optimal workforce size by considering the trade-offs between the costs of excess demand and excess capacity is a well-studied area of operations research. Statistical modeling incorporating the costs of both undersupply and oversupply of personnel is often employed to calculate a critical ratio that is used to determine how many extra employees should be maintained (Bayiz, 2003). Moreover, this redundancy or "slack" is necessary for learning and training to occur. Studies of effective learning environments (see Chapter 4) have revealed that staff must have sufficient time for reflection and analysis to assess current work systems and devise new work processes. Learning is difficult when employees are harried or rushed; it tends to be driven out by the pressures of the moment. Only if management allows employees time for the purpose does learning occur with any frequency (Garvin, 1993). High-reliability organizations also illustrate this principle by regularly freeing up workers' time for ongoing training.

However, staffing above projected need *for each nursing unit* will result in additional supply and higher labor costs. When staffing above predicted levels for each unit is not possible, additional staff will need to be obtained in other ways. Use of internal HCO employees is preferred to use of temporary employees from outside sources. As described in Chapter 3, the latter employees are less familiar with an organization's information systems, patient care technology, facility layout, critical pathways, work components' interdependency, ways of coordinating and managing work, and other work processes. Consequently, the use of temporary nursing staff from external sources can pose a threat to patient safety. Use of external temporary employees also decreases continuity of care.

Moreover, work systems with high worker involvement as described in Chapter 4 are more difficult to implement where there is extensive use of such labor because of the lesser quality of communication between management and temporary workers and lower trust levels. Firms that rely on temporary staff (e.g., registry or travel nurses) are less likely to have high-involvement work practices because of lower levels of shared information and common experience (Rousseau and Libuser, 1997; Wells et al., 1991).

A pool of internal HCO "float nurses," having received the training necessary to provide care to patients with diverse clinical needs in different patient care units, can meet the need for additional staff (Barry-Walker et al., 1994). Use of cross-trained float nurses is safer than pulling nurses from the units in which they work because the cross-trained float pool will have the knowledge and expertise to function in a variety of nursing units. Use of a float pool reduces the number of extra staff in a facility, in contrast to staffing each unit above projections. It is cost-efficient because variation in staffing needs is often more dramatic on a unit-by-unit basis than for the institution as a whole. However, it does have some limitations. Float nurses need to be cross-trained, requiring investments in their education on the part of the HCO. Second, unless these positions are well designed and supported, they can be a source of job dissatisfaction. Having no single work group with which to identify can be isolating, and performance evaluation is made difficult by the frequent changes in job assignment and different clinical supervisors on each unit. Frequent changes in assignment may also affect quality of care (Bayiz, 2003).

An alternative to decreasing workload by increasing the supply side of personnel is to moderate the demand side. Advocates of work sampling tools to reengineer nurses' work assert that achieving optimum nursing work distribution requires empowered nursing staff who are allowed to use their creativity and search for more efficient ways to delivery quality patient care (Upenieks, 1998). Allowing staff to regulate work flow will reduce the need for a float pool (Bayiz, 2003). This point is illustrated by the approach used by Luther Midelfort hospital in Wisconsin, which regulates patient flow through a unit assessment tool administered by nursing staff. Nursing staff have the authority to limit new admissions, even when there are empty beds, when in their judgment the number of available staff (number and experience level of RNs and other factors, such as support staff) is insufficient for the workload, and patient safety is endangered (Rozich and Resar, 2002). A similar approach has been used elsewhere (Knaus et al., 1986).

Minimize staff turnover and use of nursing staff from external agencies. As discussed in Chapter 3, high turnover of nursing staff and the use of temporary staff from external agencies threaten patient safety by decreasing the continuity of patient care and introducing personnel with less knowledge of nursing unit policies and practices. All of the above observations regarding the use of temporary external staff apply as well to situations of high staff turnover. Both reducing staff turnover and limiting use of registry personnel are priority strategies for achieving adequate staffing.

Continually assess staffing methodologies and their relationship to patient safety. HCOs should not assume that their staffing work is done once they have complied with state and federal staffing regulations, purchased a proprietary PCS, or successfully negotiated staffing standards with their labor partners. Ongoing research is producing better information about the relationship between staffing and patient outcomes, and the science of measuring workload and estimating staffing is still evolving. Moreover, the costs of implementing sophisticated staffing technologies for application across every nursing unit may be prohibitive for many HCOs, and the nurse workforce (as discussed in Chapter 3) is characterized by high rates of turnover. For these reasons, HCOs need to continually assess the effectiveness of their approach to staffing and its effect on patient safety. This precept is similar to that contained in JCAHO's accreditation standards, which require hospitals to use data on clinical services in combination with personnel resource data to assess their own staffing effectiveness and identify and implement strategies for improvement (JCAHO, 2003). The JCAHO standards became effective for hospitals in July 2002 and are currently being tested in nonhospital programs (e.g., nursing facilities).

The committee believes that, in addition to evaluating the effect of staffing on certain clinical and human resource *outcomes*, HCOs need to frequently evaluate the overall *process* used for determining staffing levels. Doing so is important because studies of health care quality have well documented that the outcomes measured by a subset of clinical quality indicators cannot be generalized to health care quality overall (Brook et al., 1996). It is possible for an HCO to score highly on its chosen clinical indicators and still have staffing that contributes to poor outcomes as measured by other indicators.

In sum, the committee strongly believes that safe patient care requires frequent and ongoing review of staffing methods and patient care outcomes and efficient use of staff. Regardless of the approach used by hospitals (and nursing homes, for which there is no comparable literature describing the methods used to predict staffing needs), the committee recommends that all hospitals and nursing homes take the following actions to increase the safety of their staffing levels:

> Recommendation 5-2. Hospitals and nursing homes should employ nurse staffing practices that identify needed nurse staffing for each patient care unit per shift. These practices should:
>
> - Incorporate estimates of patient volume that count admissions, discharges, and "less than full-day" patients in addition to a census of patients at a point in time.
> - Involve direct-care nursing staff in determining and evaluating the approaches used to determine appropriate unit staffing levels for each shift.
> - Provide for staffing "elasticity" or "slack" within each shift's scheduling to accommodate unpredicted variations in patient volume and acuity and resulting workload. Methods used to provide slack should give preference to scheduling excess staff and creating cross-trained float pools within the HCO. Use of nurses from external agencies should be avoided.
> - Empower nursing unit staff to regulate unit work flow and set criteria for unit closures to new admissions and transfers as nursing workload and staffing necessitate.
> - Involve direct-care nursing staff in identifying the causes of nursing staff turnover and in developing methods to improve nursing staff retention.
>
> Recommendation 5-3. Hospitals and nursing homes should perform ongoing evaluation of the effectiveness of their nurse staffing practices with respect to patient safety, and increase internal oversight of their staffing methods, levels, and effects on patient safety whenever staffing falls below the following levels for a 24-hour day:
>
> - In hospital ICUs—one licensed nurse for every 2 patients (12 hours of licensed nursing staff per patient day).
> - In nursing homes, for long-stay residents—one RN for every 32 patients (0.75 hours per resident day), one licensed nurse for every 18 patients (1.3 hours per resident day), and one nurse assistant for every 8.5 patients (2.8 hours per resident day).

The staffing thresholds identified in recommendation 5.3 for nursing homes are those identified in the CMS (2001) study of the appropriateness of minimum nurse staffing ratios in nursing homes discussed at the beginning of this chapter. The ICU thresholds were taken from published studies cited previously that found that ICUs in which individual nurses are responsible for more than two patients are associated with specific types of patient complications, including respiratory problems, cardiac arrest, and infections.

The committee was disappointed that, although higher levels of nurse staffing are clearly strongly related to better patient outcomes and reduced adverse events, the research that has produced this evidence has not yet included sufficient studies of staffing levels within specific types of patient care units (e.g., medical–surgical units and labor and deliver units). As a result, with the exception of studies of ICU care, the committee was not able to identify quantitative staffing levels that could be used by hospitals in evaluating the appropriateness of their staffing levels for medical–surgical units, labor and delivery units, or other types of hospital patient care units.

The committee strongly recommends that researchers studying the effects of staffing on patient safety take the next step of conducting research for specific types of patient care units. We note that such research will be challenging because the smaller numbers of patients found in individual patient care units will make statistical analysis more difficult. Moreover, the lack of a standardized approach to classifying patients by their level of nursing care acuity will confound interpretation of the findings of such research. The different acuity levels of patients found in, for example, medical–surgical units or step-down/transition units heightens the importance of being able to adjust for the acuity level of patients. Thus a strong, standardized approach for classifying patient care acuity in terms of nursing care is needed. The committee calls this need to the attention of researchers and those who fund health services research.

With respect to the recommendation that hospitals and nursing homes perform ongoing evaluation of the effectiveness of their nurse staffing practices with respect to patient safety and increase their internal oversight of their staffing methods, levels, and effects on patient safety whenever staffing levels fall below the identified levels, we wish to offer the following clarification: these staffing levels are not intended to be rules that should never be violated, but to serve as yardsticks against which each hospital and nursing home can compare the results of the methods it uses to predict its staffing needs on a daily basis, across all shifts in the aggregate. Because of the very strong evidence linking staffing levels to patient safety, we believe that all hospitals and nursing homes should examine trends in their staffing levels and the daily patterns that emerge when their staffing levels are compared against these standards. For example, if a facility found that it routinely met the standards but infrequently did not, it would want to examine what happened on those days when staffing diverged from the norm. Was it because of staff absences, higher-than-predicted patient volume, or some other reason? How had the HCO planned to deal with such variations, and were those plans effective? This is the rationale behind the committee's recommendation that all HCOs provide for staffing elasticity or slack within each shift's scheduling to accommodate unpredicted variations in patient volume and acuity and resulting workload.

Alternatively, if an HCO's staffing were consistently below these levels, it might want to pay particular attention to the recommendation to involve direct-care nursing staff in determining and evaluating approaches used to calculate appropriate unit staffing levels for each shift. If nursing staff believe the HCO's methodology is producing safe staffing levels, the HCO can be assured that it is using its nursing staff safely as well as efficiently (i.e., not valuing efficiency and productivity over safety, as discussed in Chapter 4). If nursing staff express that the methodology is not routinely providing safe staffing levels, the HCO should reexamine its staffing methodology, assumptions, and underlying data.

Marketplace/Consumer-Driven Approaches

Hospital and nursing home report cards Providing consumers with information about health care quality is widely identified as a means of enabling them to make better health care choices and leverage the power of the marketplace to encourage all HCOs to take the sometimes difficult actions needed to improve health care quality (Hibbard et al., 2002). Report cards on performance have been used primarily for hospitals, health plans, and physician groups (Corrigan, 1995; Luft et al., 1990; Mukamel and Mushlin, 1998; Simon and Monroe, 2001). Many researchers have examined whether these efforts are effective and how to make report cards more useful to consumers (Goldstein and Fyock, 2001; Hibbard et al., 2000, 2002). Because staffing levels in hospitals and long-term care facilities are important components of patient safety (a dimension of quality), information about staffing levels could be made available to the public. Several organizations are providing such information with respect to nursing homes, but such has not been the case for acute care hospitals.

Nursing home report cards CMS began publishing information on nurse staffing on its website in 1999.[9] This website provides comparative data for all nursing homes in the United States that are certified to provide services to Medicare and Medicaid beneficiaries. The data are collected at the time of the annual nursing home survey conducted by states and reflect

---

[9]This website also includes other basic information about nursing homes, such as location, bed size, occupancy, complaints and deficiencies, and quality indicators. See www.Medicare.gov/NHCompare/home.asp [accessed September 26, 2003].

a 2-week period. Nurse staffing levels are typically reported in terms of average hprd of care for each type of nursing staff (RN, LPN/LVN, NA) and the director of nursing (CMS, 2003a).

Nursing home report cards are also produced by state governments. As of 2002, 24 states and the District of Columbia had created websites making a variety of information from these report cards available to users. A review of these sites found that they varied in scope and detail, and four contained very limited information. While most offered information on facility characteristics, only seven provided data on nurse staffing, and none had data on staff turnover rates (Harrington et al., 2003). California Nursing Home Search (Calnhs) is a comprehensive consumer nursing home website launched by the California HealthCare Foundation in October 2002.[10] Calnhs indicators include staffing data, as well as facility characteristics and ownership; resident characteristics and case mix; measures of quality performance; data on deficiencies, complaints, and enforcement actions; and financial indicators. The website interprets the data and offers nursing home ratings and guidance to assist consumers in comparing and selecting facilities.

Calnhs staffing indicators provide information on hprd for total nursing staff and by type of staff. Each nursing home is then rated based on its staffing levels. Total nurse staffing levels are compared against the California minimum staffing requirement (set at 3.2 hprd in 1999, excluding directors of nursing). Nursing homes that do not meet the minimum standard are given a one-star rating, while facilities that meet the standard are given two stars. To receive a three-star rating (the highest level), a nursing home is required to meet a staffing goal of 4.1 hprd, which is based on the CMS (2001) study on the appropriateness of minimum nurse staffing ratios in nursing homes. Calnhs uses resident assessment data to categorize facilities based on resident case mix. Facilities receive a three-star rating if those with low resident needs have 4.1 hprd, if those with average resident needs have 4.3 hprd, and if those with high resident needs have 4.5 hprd. Calnhs also presents information on the type of staff in each nursing home (RNs, LPNs, and NAs) and compares the facility's hprd with that in the CMS study (0.75 RN hprd, 0.55 LVN/LPN hprd, and 2.8–3.2 NA hprd). Also presented on the website are detailed guides to understanding staffing levels for consumers, as well as information on staff turnover rates and wages paid to NAs. As discussed in Chapter 3, both high turnover rates and very low wages pose threats to patient safety.

Hospital report cards   The federal government has announced plans to publish a hospital report card on its website. The report card will include

---

[10]See www.calnhs.org [accessed September 26, 2003].

10 measures of basic procedures used to treat patients with heart attacks, congestive heart failure, or pneumonia. Nurse staffing levels are not one of the 10 measures. The website will also show how patients responded to an experience-with-care survey they will be asked to fill out when they are discharged (Brown, 2002). A draft of this Hospital Patient Perspectives on Care instrument is currently being tested by CMS in a voluntary pilot project. Although the draft does not ask about nurse staffing levels, it does contain questions about patients' care from nurses that could be indicative of staffing adequacy (e.g., "How often did nurses spend enough time with you?"). However, the survey instrument does not define "nurse," and is not expected, at present, to generate nursing unit–level data (CMS, 2003b). These omissions will limit the interpretability of the data by consumers.

Most states also publish hospital report cards; 37 states are required to provide some data on the quality of their hospitals. However, state hospital report cards typically do not include data on nurse staffing levels, in spite of this being identified by consumers as one of the three most important features of high-quality hospital care (in addition to good systems for coordinating care and experience in treating specific medical conditions) (Consumers Union, 2003a,b). A number of private-sector consumer organizations and purchasing coalitions also sponsor consumer report cards on HCOs—most often hospitals and health plans.

Establishing quantitative measures of nurse staffing levels for hospitals will be more difficult than for nursing homes. As discussed at the beginning of this chapter, hospitals have a large number of heterogeneous nursing units (e.g., labor and delivery, oncology, ICU, pediatrics). Nursing homes typically have a comparatively small number of heterogeneous units; many have none. For this reason, as discussed previously, a *hospital-wide* numerical measure of nurse staffing will not well represent the nurse staffing on a particular unit. For example, tertiary hospitals with multiple ICUs (which tend to have greater staffing relative to other units) may appear to have higher staffing levels than a community hospital without ICUs, even though the community hospital may have higher staffing on a general medical floor. Developing staffing measures for hospital report cards will likely be complex. Patients' reports of their perceptions of the sufficiency of nursing services on an experience-of-care survey may be a useful measure.

Need for more accurate and reliable staffing data to inform these efforts and research on staffing At present, staffing data from both hospitals and long-term care facilities are widely noted as unreliable.

Nursing home staffing data Staffing data for nursing homes collected by the Medicare and Medicaid programs are widely acknowledged to be limited and unreliable. For this reason, the CMS (2000) study on the appropriateness of minimum nurse staffing ratios in nursing homes had to use payroll records and invoices for contract nurses to measure staffing accurately. The only electronic sources of nursing home staffing data currently and routinely available are Medicaid Cost Reports and CMS' OSCAR.

Medicaid Cost Reports are financial reports of all nursing home facility costs, including those for staffing, submitted annually by all nursing facilities to their state Medicaid agencies for reimbursement and accounting purposes. Cost Report data are not available for all states or for facilities that are not Medicaid certified (CMS, 2001). The OSCAR database contains staffing and other information on every nursing home in the United States certified by Medicare and/or Medicaid. The data are collected as part of the process for certifying each nursing home initially and annually for Medicare and/or Medicaid reimbursement, but represent only facility-reported staff positions for the 2-week period immediately prior to annual certification. While some edit checks of these data are performed by CMS, the staffing data are currently not audited, and concerns have been expressed about their accuracy and validity.

The Phase I report of the CMS (2000) study on the appropriateness of minimum nurse staffing ratios in nursing homes states that a new staffing reporting and auditing system is needed for nursing facilities. During this phase of the study, payroll data were collected from nursing facilities in one state to assess the validity and reliability of staffing data from the Medicaid Cost Reports and OSCAR. The analysis found that both were limited in their ability to provide an accurate depiction of staffing levels over multiple, distinct time periods. The Medicaid Cost Reports contained more-accurate staffing data than did OSCAR, but did not include staffing definitions or report consistent staffing measures across states. In addition, there is a considerable time lag from the reporting period to data availability (CMS, 2000). CMS currently is funding a project to develop and test a more accurate reporting form for nursing homes and a mechanism for auditing what is reported, as well as to determine the most efficient method of transmitting staffing data for public reporting (CMS, 2001).

To improve the staffing data in OSCAR, CMS could develop a methodology for conducting payroll audits at the time of the annual survey or develop a new staffing reporting system, or both (CMS, 2000, 2001). Advocates suggest that a new staffing report should be developed so facilities would submit a uniform, standardized, and computerized data report on all nursing staff (by numbers and types of staff and residents) for each day on a quarterly basis—at the same time they submit their resident assessment data from the MDS each quarter. Use of such a standardized quarterly report would provide staffing data that would be more accurate and current, which could then be audited on a regular basis by state surveyors.

Legislation is being considered that would require more-detailed reporting on staffing.

Hospital staffing data   A lack of uniform, reliable, and readily available data on hospital staffing similarly is widely cited as preventing better understanding of nurse staffing (Kovner et al., 2000; Needleman et al., 2001; Sochalski, 2001; Unruh, 2002). Researchers who want to examine national patterns of staffing frequently use data collected by AHA's Annual Survey of Hospitals. However, this survey does not ask for staffing data by hospital unit; it collects aggregate staffing data at the level of the hospital, combining all different types of inpatient units (e.g., ICUs, labor and delivery, pediatrics), outpatient units, and any hospital-based long-term care units (Kovner et al., 2000; Spetz et al., 2000). It further collects data on all nurses and does not distinguish nurses providing direct patient care from those in purely administrative or managerial positions (Kovner et al., 2002). Moreover, while the survey asks hospitals to report full-time and part-time licensed nurses, it does not define "full-time" RNs and assumes that part-time licensed nurses work 20 hours per week on average. This assumption is inconsistent with data from the National Sample Survey of RNs, which indicate that part-time nurses work closer to 30 hours per week. The AHA staffing numbers are thereby likely to underestimate the hours worked by nursing personnel (Spetz et al., 2000). Furthermore, when hospitals do not respond to the survey, the AHA "imputes" a response. Therefore, some of the data are estimates rather than true self-reports, which may substantially reduce their accuracy (Spetz et al., 2000). Because of these limitations, some researchers use staffing data obtained from states (Lichtig et al., 1999; Needleman et al., 2002). However, not all states collect these data, and those that do often receive data that are incomplete and unreliable (Lichtig et al., 1999).

Specific ways of improving data on hospital nurse staffing include (1) counting all nursing staff (RNs, LVNs/LPNs, and NAs) in nurse staffing reports, (2) developing universal definitions of nurse categories and procedures for calculating full-time and part-time nursing staff, and (3) separately reporting staffing for inpatient and outpatient care and for specific nursing units (Needleman et al., 2001; Sovie and Jawad, 2001). Based on the importance of nurse staffing levels to patient safety, the role of the health care marketplace in promoting patient safety, and the current poor quality of nurse staffing data, the committee makes the following recommendation:

Recommendation 5-4. DHHS should implement a nationwide, publicly accessible system for collecting and managing valid and reli-

able staffing and turnover data from hospitals and nursing homes. Information on individual hospital and nursing home staffing at the level of individual nursing units and the facility in the aggregate should be disclosed routinely to the public.

- Federal and state nursing home report cards should include standardized, case-mix–adjusted information on the average hours per patient day of RN, licensed, and nurse assistant care provided to residents and a comparison with federal and state standards.
- During the next 3 years, public and private sponsors of the new hospital report card to be located on the federal government website should undertake an initiative—in collaboration with experts in acute hospital care, nurse staffing, and consumer information—to develop, test, and implement measures of hospital nurse staffing levels for the public.

The creation of such a system for collecting staffing data from hospitals and nursing homes should remedy the lack of a national database on hospital nurse staffing levels that, as previously cited, (1) reports staffing levels by type of patient care unit; (2) distinguishes direct-care nursing staff from nursing staff in administrative, managerial, educational, or other non–direct patient care positions; and (3) distinguishes inpatient nurses from those delivering outpatient care in hospitals. These problems have thwarted researchers' and managers' attempts to better understand the role of nurse staffing in patient care and the more efficient and effective deployment of nursing staff.

SUPPORTING KNOWLEDGE AND SKILL ACQUISITION AND CLINICAL DECISION MAKING[11]

The IOM (2001a) report *Crossing the Quality Chasm* cites the growing complexity of science and technology as one of the four main attributes of the U.S. health system affecting health care quality. This tremendous expansion of clinical knowledge, drugs, medical devices, and technologies continues unabated, and likely provides ongoing benefits to patients. In a study of hospital organizational and structural features associated with patient

---

[11]This report addresses *postemployment* knowledge and skill acquisition. Issues pertaining to prelicensure nursing education were outside of the scope of this study. However, recommendations addressing the education of all health professions with respect to improving health care quality are contained in a recent IOM report *Health Professions Education: A Bridge to Quality* (IOM, 2003).

mortality, the presence of high technology or its proxies was consistently found to be associated with lower mortality (Mitchell and Shortell, 1997).

Crossing the Quality Chasm also calls attention to the threats to patient safety posed by this expansion in knowledge, noting, "Today, no one clinician can retain all the information necessary for sound, evidence-based practice. No *unaided* human being can read, recall and act effectively on the volume of clinically relevant scientific literature" (IOM, 2001a:25). This observation has implications for the work environment of nurses and patient safety. As advances in science and technology emerge, nurses—like all health care providers—will need to adopt and implement those that have proven beneficial to patients. Doing so will require that nurses continually acquire new knowledge and skills and apply them in the clinical decisions they make at the point of care.

If, however, human beings cannot without assistance identify, incorporate into their personal knowledge base, and recall when needed all clinical information pertinent to the care of a patient at a given point in time, where are they to obtain such assistance? Evidence presented in Chapter 4 indicates that the ongoing acquisition and management of knowledge is an essential responsibility of high-performing organizations in today's society. The discussion in that chapter highlights the important role that employer organizations play in actively managing the learning process of their organization and transferring knowledge quickly and efficiently throughout the organization. This role of HCOs is critical to supporting nurses' knowledge and skills. While many nurses pursue continuing education activities as a matter of professional commitment and/or at the behest of state licensing boards, studies of research-based innovation in nursing indicate that practicing nurses are often not aware of new knowledge that is applicable to their practice; if they are aware, they can be hampered in integrating that knowledge into their practice because targeted adoption of certain practice innovations may involve multiple disciplines, departments, and processes within the HCO (Donaldson and Rutledge, 1998). Moreover, because many NAs live at or below the poverty level (see Chapter 3), they frequently lack the resources to pursue continuing education on their own. Thus while the individual nurse is responsible for her or his own continuing education and training, all HCOs need to provide actively for their nursing staff's ongoing acquisition of new knowledge and skills, and to support the application of this knowledge and offer other decision support at the point of care delivery.

Need to Strengthen Ongoing Assistance in Knowledge and Skill Acquisition

Knowledge and skills are the fundamental building blocks of worker capability (Rousseau and Libuser, 1997). However, it is not reasonable to expect that all nurses (especially those newly licensed) will come to a place of employment possessing the knowledge and skills needed to practice at a high level of expertise. Dreyfus and Dreyfus' (1986) careful studies of the skill acquisition process across a wide range of learners and workers (e.g., airline pilots, chess players, auto drivers, and adult learners of a second language) show that individuals usually pass through at least five stages of qualitatively different perceptions of work tasks and decision making as skill improves through the cumulative effects of substantial experience. Learners progress along a pathway from novice to advanced beginner, competence, proficiency, and finally expert (Benner, 1984; Dreyfus and Dreyfus, 1986).

Prelicensure or pre-employment education cannot provide sufficient frequency and diversity of experiences (and sometimes offer no experience) in the performance of every clinical nursing intervention needed for every clinical condition found in patients, especially as the breadth of knowledge and technology expands. Nurses, therefore, like physicians, come to their initial place of employment as novices without certain skills and knowledge—their limited skill and expertise reflecting the limitations of time and experience in their academic education.

Furthermore, after licensure, nurses may practice clinically in a certain area, such as general medical–surgical nursing, for a number of years and gain high levels of expertise. They may then desire to practice in a more clinically specialized area, such as oncology or ICU, in which they have less expertise, necessitating the acquisition of new knowledge and skills. Finally, it will always be impossible for prelicensure education of nurses and pre-employment education of NAs to teach students about diagnostic and therapeutic advances that have not yet been invented. Both the medical and nursing professions are grappling with the need to ensure the continuing competency of licensed health professions in the face of the growing base of new knowledge and technology.

In 1996, the National Advisory Council on Nurse Education and Practice (NACNEP) noted that advances in medical therapeutics and technology had led to increasing complexity for nurses caring for individuals with a variety of health conditions and that a large portion of existing RNs had not been adequately prepared to meet the health care needs of their patients in the face of the rapidly expanding base of knowledge. NACNEP (1996) determined that actions were needed to upgrade the knowledge, skills, and abilities of the existing RN workforce. This position is echoed by organizations employing nurses, organizations concerned with patient safety and quality of care, and nurses themselves.

Likewise, in a statement before the Senate Committee on Health, Education, Labor and Pensions, JCAHO (2001) called attention to nurses' lack of appropriate education, orientation, and training to manage increasingly sophisticated care. And in a national, stratified, representative sample survey of nursing administrators from acute care hospitals and long-term care facilities conducted in 2001 by the National Council of State Boards of Nursing, fewer than half of nursing administrators evaluated newly licensed nurses as possessing the overall educational preparation to provide safe, effective care. RNs were viewed as particularly lacking skills in recognizing abnormal physical and diagnostic findings and responding to emergencies (Smith and Crawford, 2002a). These findings were quite similar to the responses of a nationally representative survey of newly graduated nurses conducted by the same organization in 2001. These nurses also reported needing better educational preparation or work orientation in recognizing abnormal laboratory findings and responding to emergency situations (Smith and Crawford, 2002b).

This lack of knowledge is not just a result of the inability of prelicensure programs to provide education on all therapies needed for all clinical conditions. At present, a number of state boards of nursing have no mechanisms in place to promote ongoing acquisition of knowledge and skills to maintain clinical competency. As of March 2001, 24 of the 56 U.S. states and jurisdictions required RNs to engage in continuing education, and 4 required competency examinations (National Council of State Boards of Nursing, 2001). Moreover, both AHA and JCAHO have stated that many hospitals have scaled back their orientation programs for newly hired nurses and ongoing in-service training and continuing education programs for nurses as a result of financial pressures (Berens, 2000; JCAHO, 2002). Inadequate training of hospital nurses has been cited as a key contributor to medical errors (Berens, 2000). Table 5-7 shows the types of orientation programs

TABLE 5-7 Types and Average Length of Orientation Programs for Newly Licensed RNs

Type of Program	Percent	Average Length (in weeks)
No formal orientation	5.5	—
Classroom instruction/skills lab only	0.7	3.7
Classroom instruction and/or skills lab plus supervised work with patients	13.1	7.1
Work with an assigned preceptor with or without additional classroom instruction or skills lab work	72.1	8.0
Formal internship with or without additional classroom instruction or skills lab work	6.1	12.3
Other	2.5	7.5

SOURCE: Smith and Crawford (2003).

provided to newly licensed RNs and the average duration of each according to a 2002 national, stratified random sample survey of 4,000 newly licensed RNs practicing in all settings of care (84 percent in hospitals).

The need for ongoing training of NAs in hospitals (Hurley, 2000) and nursing homes has also been documented. The CMS (2001) Phase II final report on the appropriateness of minimum nurse staffing ratios in nursing homes includes a review of the training and education of NAs in nursing homes. NAs working in Medicare- or Medicaid-certified nursing homes (the majority of facilities) are required to have a minimum of 75 hours of initial training (including at least 16 hours of supervised practical training in performing hands-on care of individuals) and/or to pass a certification and skills test prior to employment, and must receive 12 hours per year of in-service education. The report notes that while the acuity level of nursing home residents has increased over the 13 years since these training regulations were established, the requirements for training have not. Further, NAs themselves identify the training they receive as inadequate. Continuing education is in the form of in-service education—taking place in the nursing home while the NAs are on the job, sometimes being interrupted for patient care. Education usually is presented in 1-hour segments, allowing little time for reflection. Educational material is typically presented in lecture or videotape form (CMS, 2001).

The report notes further that most NAs and NA educators agree that current initial certification education is insufficient, and that in-service education should be enhanced and tailored to the needs of staff members, with more advanced topics being covered for more experienced workers (CMS, 2001). A study of training methods in health care settings identifies the following key components of successful NA in-service programs: (1) didactic instruction presented in writing and verbally, followed by modeling by the trainer, demonstration by the trainee, and immediate feedback by the trainer; (2) further assessment of skill performance in a prototype situation, allowing for additional feedback on performance; and (3) assessment of trainees' performance on the job (Burgio and Burgio, 1990).

Ongoing training is an especially important issue in nursing homes because of the extremely high turnover rates cited in Chapter 3. HCOs with high turnover rates must provide more training than those with low turnover rates because they have higher levels of new employees.

Training also is especially important when work is being reengineered or redesigned. In a study of 14 hospitals reengineering their work processes, it was found that many hospitals underestimated the amount of initial training and retraining needed by NAs to perform such tasks as electrocardiograms and phlebotomies. In interviews, researchers were told that new workers were often assigned patient responsibilities after initial, short training periods (some as brief as 3 days) only to function very inadequately, so that much of the rework fell back on nursing staff. The researchers note that training costs are high when addressed comprehensively. One 500-bed hospital spent $700,000 on its training in the first 2 years of its reengineering initiative. This hospital also performed a gap analysis to identify those roles not being performed adequately and to evaluate what additional training was needed. The reviewers conclude that such continual evaluation of training needs is important to implementing new roles and responsibilities effectively (Walston and Kimberly, 1997). As noted in Chapter 3, unlike NAs working in nursing homes, there are no federal requirements for the amount of training NAs working in hospitals must receive.

Benchmark Training Practices in Other Industries and Health Care

Worker training is not an issue unique to the health care industry. Many technology-dependent industries, safety-conscious industries, and industries that simply find themselves in a competitive marketplace understand ongoing worker training to be an essential part of doing business. Developing and managing human skills and intellect—more than managing physical and capital assets—is increasingly recognized as a dominant concern of managers in successful companies (Quinn, 1992).

High-reliability organizations spend more money than other organizations on training workers to recognize and respond to problems. Operators at Diablo Canyon Nuclear Power Plant, for example, work their regular shifts 3 weeks of every month. During the fourth week, they train for a wide range of unusual and potentially dangerous situations. This training keeps them alert to all the things that can go wrong. It also reinforces the idea that the organization is taking seriously the likelihood of errors, and the need for ongoing vigilance and action on the part of employees to detect errors before they result in adverse events (Roberts and Bea, 2001). Likewise, the International Atomic Energy Agency cites employee training as key to an organization's safety culture (Carnino, undated). And findings from the aviation industry indicate that training needs to be ongoing and tailored to conditions and the experience within organizations. In the absence of recurrent training, attitudes and practices decay (Helmreich, 2000).

The American Society for Training and Development (ASTD) provides a voluntary benchmarking service for organizations across all industries to report their training practices and commitment of resources. In 2001, 270 public and private employers submitted data to the service showing an average training budget of 1.9 percent of payroll ("payroll" is defined as including wages and salaries but not benefits). The average for HCOs using the service was 1.4 percent. The range across all industries from 1996 to 2001 was 1.5 to 2.0. Organizations considered "leaders in training investment" dedicated an average of 3.2–3.6 percent of payroll to training between 1998 and 2001 (Thompson et al., 2002).

In health care, studies of magnet hospitals have found them to be characterized by high levels of training and education among nursing staff, beginning with orientation and lasting several weeks to months. Nursing staff in these hospitals also were frequently assigned preceptors who served as role models and mentors. Once orientation had been completed, continuing education was viewed as essential and supplied in sufficient quantity and quality. Magnet hospitals also typically provided further support for formal education through tuition reimbursement, flexible scheduling, and leaves of absence (McClure and Hinshaw, 2002).

Strategies to Support Nursing Staff in Ongoing Acquisition of Knowledge and Skills

Continuing and in-service education using formal and informal classroom-style group lectures traditionally has been used to provide ongoing knowledge and skill acquisition in health care. However, traditional methods of continuing education, such as conferences and dissemination of written materials, have been shown to have little effect in changing clinical practice (IOM, 2001a). Additional strategies that can be employed to help nursing staff acquire new knowledge and skills are described below.

Preceptorships and Residencies for New Nurses

Nurse residencies or internships are used by some hospitals to transition new nurse graduates into clinical practice. Residencies are usually described in formal contracts between the employer and the new graduate that specify the clinical activities to be performed by the nurse in exchange for further education and experience to advance the individual's professional development. A survey of chief nursing officers of the University HealthSystem Consortium revealed that 85 percent reported having an extended program of orientation for new graduates (AACN, 2002). This finding is consistent with practices observed in other industries. A large proportion of employers (81 percent) reporting to the ASTD education and training benchmarking service cited the use of mentoring/coaching programs (Thompson et al., 2002).

The University HealthSystem Consortium and the American Association of Colleges of Nursing recently undertook a joint initiative to develop a standardized postbaccalaureate residency program to support new baccalaureate-prepared nursing graduates as they transition into their first professional position in direct-care nursing. Designed for academic acute care hospitals, the 1-year residency program consists of a series of learning and work experiences addressing resource management, communication, patient safety, pain management, evidence-based care, emergency responses, end-of-life care, and critical thinking, among other knowledge and skill competencies. The residency program was implemented at six medical centers in 2002, with 259 nursing residents being enrolled under the guidance of assigned, individual preceptors and resident facilitators within each institution.[12]

Individualized Training

Research shows that not everyone learns the same way. While many individuals learn well through reading, some learn better through auditory mechanisms, such as lectures. Others learn better through approaches that allow them to use their motor skills. Teaching adult learners therefore requires different styles of education and training or supplements to lecture-style continuing education (Lazear, 1991), and nursing staff can benefit from being helped to learn individually, rather than as group learners, at a pace suited to their particular learning styles. CD-ROM-based and individualized text-based programs can be used to provide this individualized learning (Rauen, 2001). Peer support groups also are helpful to NAs in nursing homes in internalizing new knowledge (CMS, 2000).

Simulation

Simulation is the use of an artificially created, "practice" event or situation constructed to resemble an actual event or situation that an individual is likely to encounter and that requires critical decision making and/or physical skills. Simulation exercises often emphasize the application and integration of knowledge, skills, and critical thinking (Rauen, 2001). Simulation training allows workers to practice dealing with error-inducing situations without jeopardy to themselves or patients and to receive feedback on both individual and team performance (Helmreich, 2000). Use of simulation training has been cited by 23 percent of employers reporting to the ASTD education and training benchmarking service (Thompson et al., 2002).

In nursing, simulations of clinical practice using varying degrees of technological sophistication can be used to teach clinical assessment skills, nursing procedures, and use of technology. Body-part simulators allow the practice of such skills as inserting catheters and tracheostomy care and suctioning. Computers have greatly aided the use of simulation as an education

---

[12]Personal communication, A. Rhome, American Association of Colleges of Nursing, June 11, 2003.

tool. They can be used, for example, to simulate electrocardiograms and hemodynamic body functions. Full-body, computer-integrated, physiologically accurate simulators, originally created for anesthesia training, can be used for critical care nursing education, although they require additional expenditures, space, computer literacy, and technical support (Rauen, 2001).

Decision Support at the Point of Care Delivery

Nurses also need mechanisms to help identify new sources of knowledge and integrate them into their ongoing practice at the point of care delivery. At a June 2002 invitational conference on Using Innovative Technology to Enhance Patient Care Delivery, sponsored by the American Academy of Nursing, attendees representing national health care associations, health care provider organizations, clinicians, and health care technology vendors identified minimal decision support for nurses within HCOs as a deficiency in their work environments (Bolton, 2002).

Such supports can be both low-tech and high-tech. Health care literature on decision support has addressed primarily high-tech, computer-assisted support for physicians in making diagnostic and treatment decisions (Brailer et al., 1996). Deploying informatics to develop and maintain databases and providing health care practitioners with such information as clinical practice guidelines when they need it at the point of care are recommended ways of assisting practitioners in acquiring new knowledge (Eisenberg, 2000).

Crossing the Quality Chasm (IOM, 2001a) also highlights the importance of using information technology to improve access to information and support clinical decision making. It calls attention to software that integrates information on individual patients with a computerized knowledge base to generate patient-specific assessments or recommendations, thereby helping clinicians or patients make clinical decisions. Decision supports for nurses are described less frequently; publications most often address the use of clinical pathways and automated support for medication administration. Other low-tech decision supports include using memory/cognition aids, such as protocols and checklists, and providing access to clinical information at the point of care delivery. The use of clinical pathways can also provide support to nurses in integrating evidence-based knowledge.

Clinical pathways Clinical pathways are disease- or procedure-specific blueprints for clinical care specifying actions that need to be performed by nurses and other members of a patient's health care team, and in what sequence. They frequently map the expected course of an illness or procedure and provide prompts to clinicians that identify appropriate clinical interventions in response to individualized patient characteristics or clinical developments. Clinical pathways are often evidence-based and are typically multidisciplinary—specifying the responsibilities of nurses, physicians, and other members of the health care team. They sometimes are a component of or replace documentation in the chart and may be paper-based or automated. Most clinical pathways are locally developed—frequently within a hospital—serving both cost-containment and quality assurance purposes (Trowbridge and Weingarten, 2001a). There is evidence that they are increasingly being used to manage and standardize both nursing care processes and interdisciplinary care in hospitals (Anonymous, 2001; Bridgeman et al., 1997; Helfrich Jones et al., 1999; Schriefer and Botter, 2001).

The AHRQ evidence-based report *Making Health Care Safer: A Critical Analysis of Patient Safety Practices* cites conflicting evidence on the efficacy of clinical pathways in influencing provider behavior and patient safety (Trowbridge and Weingarten, 2001a). However, experts on mechanisms for promoting interdisciplinary collaboration point out that such care delivery protocols and care maps equate to the use of standard operating procedures that are useful in other high-risk environments. These prewritten documents assist team members in providing consistent quality care while ensuring that other team members know what is occurring with the patient. They also facilitate the assumption of care by team members if the lead person is unable to carry out his or her responsibilities (Ingersoll and Schmitt, 2003).

Computer-supported clinical decision support systems Clinical decision support systems (CDSSs) assist clinicians in applying new information to patient care through the analysis of patient-specific clinical variables. They vary in complexity, function, and application. Some but not all are computer-based. *Crossing the Quality Chasm* (IOM, 2001a) highlights the potential of automated CDSSs—software that integrates information on the characteristics of individual patients with a computerized knowledge base for the purpose of generating patient-specific assessments or recommendations designed to aid clinicians or patients in making clinical decisions. The AHRQ evidence-based report *Making Health Care Safer: A Critical Analysis of Patient Safety Practices* notes that the preponderance of evidence suggests that CDSSs are at least somewhat effective, especially with respect to the prevention of medical errors (Trowbridge and Weingarten, 2001b). CDSSs are widely implemented and evaluated with respect to physician practice, but less so in nursing.

Point-of-care decision support devices can be mobile, stationary, or hand-held. They allow nurses to gather patient information (e.g., on allergies, intake restrictions) automatically from patient records or from data repositories that can be Internet-based or accessed from another source. Point-of-care decision support systems for medication administration are an example. These systems can support nurses in medication administration by providing information on drug actions, dosages, interactions, and side effects at the point of medication administration. When integrated with an automated medication administration record, they allow nurses to verify the five "rights" of medication administration—the right patient, medication, dose, route, and time (Ball et al., 2003).

An automated integrated clinical information system used by Our Lady of the Lake (OLOL) Regional Medical Center in Louisiana illustrates the potential of such advanced systems to provide decision support to nurses. This system provides online access to patient charts and the ability to capture vital signs at the point of care, as well as intake and output, weights, and alerts of medical orders. Rules for care are embedded in system components that capture nursing documentation, results of laboratory tests, and medication orders. The system is accessed through wireless laptop devices used by nurses for input of care documentation; it includes a clinical repository for access to the patient's electronic medical record, and a pharmacy system with a reference database that enables checking for drug–drug interactions and adverse drug event rules. Additional rules built into the system identify patients at risk for falls, pressure ulcers, and other medical errors. When one of these rules is triggered, the system sends an alert from the clinical documentation that produces care protocols with simultaneous orders to all the departments involved in the response (e.g., nursing, physicians, dietary, supplies). During a 12-month study of the use of the system, falls decreased from 4.45. to 3.70 per 1000 inpatient days, and the risk of pressure sore development decreased from 9 to 1 percent. Two years after implementation, the medical center took advantage of planned system down time to measure the differences in documentation time with and without the system. This evaluation revealed time savings gained through use of the system; moreover, nurses complained about the loss of reminders for work organization when the system was available (Ball et al., 2003).

Given the career-long need for nursing staff to maintain competency through the acquisition of new knowledge and skills, and the essential role of HCOs in helping to meet this need, the committee makes the following recommendation:

Recommendation 5-5. HCOs should dedicate budgetary resources equal to a defined percentage of nursing payroll to support nursing staff in their ongoing acquisition and maintenance of knowledge and skills. These resources should be sufficient for and used to implement policies and practices that:

- Assign experienced nursing staff to precept nurses newly practicing in a clinical area to address knowledge and skill gaps.
- Annually ensure that each licensed nurse and nurse assistant has
  an individualized plan and resources for educational development within health care.
- Provide education and training of staff as new technology or
  changes in the workplace are introduced.
- Provide decision support technology identified with the active
  involvement of direct-care nursing staff to enable point-of-care
  learning.
- Disseminate to individual staff organizational learning as captured in clinical tools, algorithms, and pathways.

Although the committee does not specify in recommendation 5.5 a particular percentage of nursing payroll that HCOs should dedicate to ongoing
knowledge and skill acquisition by nursing staff, we call attention to ASTD
data showing average training budgets across all industries of 1.9 percent of
payroll and an average for HCOs of 1.4 percent. These numbers can serve
as initial benchmarks for HCOs in assessing their own level of commitment
to employee education and training. As HCOs begin to prospectively set
aside a certain percentage of payroll for staff education and training, they
are encouraged to report this information to organizations providing
benchmarking services.

FOSTERING INTERDISCIPLINARY COLLABORATION

Because of the increasing acuity of their health care needs, individual
patients are often attended to by an array of different health care providers
with whom nursing staff must interact, including physicians, pharmacists,
allied health providers, social workers, and unlicensed health care technicians. Sometime nurses interact with these providers as members of a formal interdisciplinary team of health care providers, such as in the OR or
emergency department. In such cases, promoting more effective team functioning is a key strategy that HCOs should undertake to improve patient
safety (IOM, 2000).

However, not all nurses function as part of a single team with fixed
membership and defined roles. More often, nurses interact with an array of
providers that changes from day to day and often is different for each patient in their care as shift and patient assignments change; attending physicians, resident physicians, and NAs change or rotate; and float nurses and
temporary workers are brought in as short-term fixes for nursing shortages.
Thus a nurse caring for four patients on a single shift is likely to be involved
with four different groups of health care providers as residents, attending

physicians, specialty physicians, social workers, family members, and community agencies vary for each patient. And a float nurse may find himself or herself interacting with different configurations of providers on a daily basis. Hence, the paradigm of highly functioning teams may not be the best model for all nurse–provider interactions (Ingersoll and Schmitt, 2003; Thomas and Helmeich, 2002). Rather, interdisciplinary collaboration may be a more widely applicable model for effective nurse–provider interactions and strategies for achieving safe and effective health care.

As part of this study, the committee commissioned a review of published research on the effectiveness of team functioning and interdisciplinary collaboration in achieving patient safety and related outcomes. The evidence analyzed in this review (see Appendix B) generally supports the effectiveness of both teams and interdisciplinary collaboration in improving patient outcomes. Although findings concerning the relationship between the existence and performance of health care teams and patient outcomes are mixed, evidence suggests that the relationship is positive when measured carefully and with clear indication of team processes and interactions. Moreover, the concept of collaboration within and apart from prescribed teams appears to be an important dimension of what makes teams (and individuals, dyads, or small groups) successful.

Hallmarks of Effective Interdisciplinary Collaboration

Health services researchers note that interdisciplinary collaboration, like team care, has not yet been well conceptualized. Further, "Team care is not a single homogeneous treatment variable. Teams, as work groups, vary in the quality of their functioning . . . collaboration is not a dichotomous variable, simply present or absent, but present to varying degrees" (Schmitt, 2001:51). There is, however, agreement among health services researchers, as well as researchers in organizational and psychological sciences, that collaboration is multidimensional and typically characterized by necessary precursors and distinct behaviors.

Necessary Precursors to Collaboration

Individual clinical competence   Clinical competence was first identified as an essential precursor for collaborative practice between nurses and physicians by a National Joint Practice Commission convened in 1981 (Baggs and Schmitt, 1988). Clinical competence as a component of effective interaction and coordination of medical and nursing staff has been associated with lower risk-adjusted length of stay (Shortell et al., 1994), lower nurse turnover, higher professionally evaluated technical quality of care (Mitchell et al., 1996; Shortell et al., 1994), and greater professionally evaluated ability to meet family member needs (Shortell et al., 1994). Findings from a study of nurse–physician collaboration in a medical ICU reinforce that nurses and physicians are more likely to collaborate with each other when they perceive the other as having the knowledge necessary for good clinical care (Baggs and Schmitt, 1997). The theme of respect for one another's capabilities is present throughout almost all of the writings on interdisciplinary collaboration (Rice, 2000).

Mutual trust and respect   Respect has been described as being manifested by politeness, manners, and being diplomatic and pleasant (Baggs and Schmitt, 1988, 1997; Rice, 2000). At the same time, personal respect and trust are intertwined with respect for and trust in clinical competence.

Characteristics of Collaboration

Collaboration is frequently described as the aggregation of several behaviors, including those described below.

Shared understanding of goals and roles   Collaboration is enhanced by shared understanding of an agreed-upon collective goal (Gittell et al., 2000). Role confusion and role conflict are a frequent barrier to interdisciplinary collaboration (Rice, 2000).

Effective communication   Multiple studies identify effective communication as a key feature of collaboration (Baggs and Schmitt, 1988; Knaus et al., 1986; Schmitt, 2001; Shortell et al., 1994). "Effective" communication is described variously as frequent, timely, understandable, accurate, and satisfying (Gittell et al., 2000; Shortell et al., 1994). It is characterized by discussion with contributions by all parties, active listening, openness, a willingness to consider other ideas and ask for opinions, questioning (Baggs and Schmitt, 1997; Shortell et al., 1994), and the free flow of information among participants who feel they are able to speak out. It is also characterized as nonhierarchical.

Shared decision making   In shared decision making, problems and strategies are discussed openly (Baggs and Schmitt, 1997; Baggs et al., 1999; Rice, 2000; Schmitt, 2001). Moreover, consensus is often used to arrive at a decision.

Conflict management   Disagreements over treatment approaches and philosophies, roles and responsibilities, and ethical questions are commonplace in health care settings. Positive ways of addressing these inevitable differences are identified as a key component of effective caregiver interactions (Shortell et al., 1994).

Inconsistent Collaboration Between Nursing Staff and Other Health Care Providers

While the literature on interdisciplinary teams has focused on a broad array of disciplines involved in health care delivery, the literature concerning collaboration has focused primarily on nurse–physician interactions (Ingersoll and Schmitt, 2003). The limited existing evidence indicates that most nurses experience positive relationships with their physician colleagues. However, the extent to which a "positive relationship" is indicative of collaboration is unknown. There are also indications that positive relationships with physicians are not experienced by all nurses.

There are numerous anecdotal and historical reports of poor nurse–physician relationships, including reports of generally poor communication (Greenfield, 1999; Schmitt, 2001), hierarchical communication patterns (Disch et al., 2001), unilateral decision making by physicians (Schmitt, 2001), and verbal abuse of nurses by physicians (Manderino and Berkey, 1997; Rosenstein, 2002). These problems are sometimes attributed to differences in power, sex, class, economics, and education (McMahan and Hoffman, 1994). However, interpretation of these reports is impeded by the absence of any representative survey of practicing nurses across health care delivery settings regarding the levels of collaboration they experience with physicians and other health care providers. Studies that have attempted to measure nurse–physician interactions are often convenience samples without controls for sampling bias. Further, surveys that have attempted to measure the incidence of verbal abuse of nurses have not used physicians as the unit of analysis, so it is not known whether abusive behavior characterizes a small minority of physicians or is more widely practiced.

In two representative samples of nurses, large majorities reported "good" working relationships with physicians. In 2002–2003, a random sample survey of nurses licensed to work in Illinois and North Carolina[13] was conducted as part of a longitudinal study of nurses' worklife and health funded by the National Institute for Occupational Safety and Health (NIOSH) of the U.S. Centers for Disease Control and Prevention (CDC). Of the 674 RN respondents to this survey who were currently employed as full-time hospital or nursing home general-duty staff, 82.4 percent agreed or agreed strongly with the statement, "In my job, doctors and nurses have

---

[13]These states were selected because they have large ethnic diversity in their RN populations and because they renew RN licenses annually, providing up-to-date mailing lists.

good working relationships."[14] Likewise, in a survey of 50 percent of RNs living in Pennsylvania, 83.4 percent of nurses working in hospitals reported that "physicians and nurses have good working relationships" (Aiken et al., 2001). Positive and collaborative relationships between nurses and physicians are also characteristically found in magnet hospitals (Kramer and Schmalenberg, 2002).

The use of agency staff, high turnover rates among nursing staff (Disch et al., 2001), and short rotation periods for medical residents (Baggs and Schmitt, 1997) also threaten collaborative relationships. Building collaborative relationships takes time, and these phenomena have been cited as making it difficult to form the sustained relationships that are essential for the development of trust and a precursor to collaboration.

Heavy workloads are also cited as interfering with the formation of collaborative relationships. When staff are overwhelmed with caregiving responsibilities, they may not take the time to collaborate. Yet while unilateral decision making is easier in the short run, collaborative relationships are viewed as saving time in the long run (Baggs and Schmitt, 1997; Disch et al., 2001).

Building and Nurturing Collaboration

There is some evidence that collaboration can be facilitated by supportive organizational structures and processes including the following:

- *Leadership modeling of collaborative behaviors*—This approach can help other medical staff improve their relationships with nursing staff (Disch et al., 2001).
- *Commitment of resources to build nurse expertise*—The strong evidence cited above that individual clinical competency is an essential precursor to collaborative practice is further reinforcement for recommendation 5.5 regarding the actions HCOs should take to support nursing staff in their ongoing acquisition and maintenance of knowledge and skills.
- *Design of work and workspace to facilitate collaboration*—Collaboration is facilitated by providing workspaces that encourage physical proximity among those performing the work and by ensuring that staff have the time to participate in collaborative activities, such as conducting interdisciplinary patient rounds (Baggs and Schmitt, 1997). Hospital unit design and staffing approaches should reflect attention to whether they will promote or discourage interdisciplinary collaboration. This observation further sup-

---

[14]Unpublished data from Alison Trinkoff, Ph.D., University of Maryland at Baltimore, NIOSH grant R01OH3702 (personal communication, April 9, 2003).

ports the staffing recommendations made earlier in this chapter. A discussion of workspace design is presented in Chapter 6.

• *Interdisciplinary practice mechanisms*—There is some evidence that using structured interdisciplinary forums, such as interdisciplinary rounds, can be effective in improving patient care (Curley et al., 1998). Regularly scheduled interdisciplinary meetings also can be held at the patient care unit level. During these meetings, nursing, medical, pharmacy, and other clinical providers can work together to address issues pertaining to the running of the unit and patient care. Small work groups can be formed to address specific concerns and report back to the larger group (Disch et al., 2001). Interdisciplinary practice can also be facilitated by patient record and documentation practices that promote interdisciplinary information sharing, such as the use of interdisciplinary clinical pathways (Lange et al., 1998).

• *Training*—Training and development may be needed in collaborative practice behaviors, such as effective communication and conflict resolution (Disch et al., 2001).

• *Human resource policies*—Human resource policies that identify verbal abuse and other hostile behaviors as unacceptable, along with procedures for addressing such behaviors, may be helpful (Manderino and Berkey, 1997). Some have suggested identifying interpersonal components of organizational practice expectations for clinicians. Such components might include, for example, expectations that all health care providers involved in clinical services within the organization cooperate and communicate with other providers while displaying regard for their dignity; refrain from foul language, shouting, and rudeness; and use conflict management skills in handling disagreements (Pfifferling, 1999). Performance evaluation also can include measures of the extent to which health care providers are viewed as collaborators by those in other disciplines.

HCOs can act on this information to build and nurture collaboration across health care providers. Many strategies to this end have already been addressed in the committee's recommendations pertaining to evidence-based management, staffing, and the acquisition of new knowledge and skills by nursing staff. In addition, the committee makes the following recommendation:

Recommendation 5-6. HCOs should take action to support interdisciplinary collaboration by adopting such interdisciplinary practice mechanisms as interdisciplinary rounds, and by providing ongoing formal education and training in interdisciplinary collaboration for all health care providers on a regularly scheduled, continuous basis (e.g., monthly, quarterly, or semiannually).

REFERENCES

AACN (American Association of Colleges of Nursing). 2002. *Hallmarks of the Professional Nursing Practice Environment.* Washington, DC: AACN.

Aaronson W, Zinn J, Rosko M. 1994. Do for-profit and not-for-profit nursing homes behave differently? *Gerontologist* 34(6):775–786.

Aiken L, Sloane D, Lake E, Sochalski J, Weber A. 1999. Organization and outcomes of inpatient AIDS care. *Medical Care* 37(8):760–772.

Aiken L, Clarke S, Sloane D, Sochalski J, Busse R, Clarke H, Giovannetti P, Hunt J, Rafferty A, Shamian J. 2001. Nurses' reports on hospital care in five countries. *Health Affairs* 20(3):43–53.

Aiken L, Clarke S, Sloane D, Sochalski J, Silber J. 2002. Hospital nurse staffing and patient mortality, nurse burnout, and job dissatisfaction. *Journal of the American Medical Association* 288:1987–1993.

Amaravadi R, Dimick J, Pronovost P, Lipsett P. 2000. ICU nurse-to-patient ratio is associated with complications and resource use after esophagectomy. *Intensive Care Medicine* 26:1857–1862.

American Association of Critical Care Nurses. 1999. Medina J, ed. *Staffing Blueprint: Constructing Your Staffing Solutions.* AlisoViejo, CA: AACCN.

ANA (American Nurses Association). 1999. *Principles for Nurse Staffing.* Washington, DC: American Nurses Publishing.

ANA. 2000. *Nurse Staffing and Patient Outcomes in the Inpatient Hospital Setting.* Washington, DC: American Nurses Publishing.

ANA. 2002. *State Legislative Trends and Analysis.* Washington, DC: ANA.

Anonymous. 2001. Clinical pathways: A special report. *Hospital Case Management* 9(4):49–63.

Baggs J, Schmitt M. 1988. Collaboration between nurses and physicians. *IMAGE: Journal of Nursing Scholarship* 20(3):145–149.

Baggs J, Schmitt M. 1997. Nurses' and resident physicians' perceptions of the process of collaboration in an MICU. *Research in Nursing & Health* 20(1):71–80.

Baggs J, Schmitt M, Mushlin A, Mitchell P, Eldredge D, Oakes D, Hutson A. 1999. Association between nurse–physician collaboration and patient outcomes in three intensive care units. *Critical Care Medicine* 27(9):1991–1998.

Ball M, Weaver C, Abbott P. 2003. Enabling technologies promise to revitalize the role of nursing in an era of patient safety. *International Journal of Medical Informatics* 69:29–38.

Barry-Walker J, Bulechek G, McCloskey J. 1994. A description of medical–surgical nursing. *MEDSURG Nursing* 3(4):261–268.

Bayiz M. 2003. The Anderson School of Management, UCLA. *Work and Workload Measurement in Nurse Staffing.* Paper commissioned by the Institute of Medicine Committee on the Work Environment for Nurses and Patient Safety.

Benner P. 1984. *From Novice to Expert: Excellence and Power in Clinical Nursing Practice.* Menlo Park, CA: Addison-Wesley Publishing Company.

Berens M. 2000 (September 11). Training often takes a back seat; budget pressures, lack of state laws aggravate trend. *Chicago Tribune.* News. p. 7.

Blegen M, Vaughn T. 1998. A multisite study of nurse staffing and patient occurrences. *Nursing Economics* 16(4):196–203.

Blegen M, Goode C, Reed L. 1998. Nurse staffing and patient outcomes. *Nursing Research* 47(1):43–50.

Bliesmer M, Smayling M, Kane R, Shannon I. 1998. The relationship between nursing staffing levels and nursing home outcomes. *Journal of Aging and Health* 10(3):351–371.

Bolton L, American Academy of Nursing. 2002. *Statement to the Committee on the Work Environment for Nurses and Patient Safety.* Testimony presented on September 24, 2002, at IOM committee meeting in Washington, DC.

Bolton L, Jones D, Aydin C, Donaldson N, Brown D, Lowe M, McFarland P, Harms D. 2001. A response to California's mandated nursing ratios. *Journal of Nursing Scholarship* 33:179–184.

Bond C, Raehl C, Pitterle M, Franke T. 1999. Health care professional staffing, hospital characteristics, and hospital mortality rates. *Pharmacotherapy* 19:130–138.

Bowers B, Becker M. 1992. Nurse's aides in nursing homes: The relationship between organization and quality. *The Gerontologist* 32(3):360–366.

Brailer D, Goldfarb S, Horgan M, Katz F, Paulus R, Zakrewski K. 1996. Improving performance with clinical decision support. *Joint Commission Journal on Quality Improvement* 22(7):443–456.

Braun B. 1991. The effect of nursing home quality on patient outcome. *Journal of the American Geriatrics Society* 39(4):329–338.

Brennan T, Leape L, Laird NHL, Loaclio R, Lawthers A, Newhouse J, Weiler P, Hiatt H. 1991. Incidence of adverse events and negligence in hospitalized patients: Results of the Harvard Medical Practice Study. *The New England Journal of Medicine* 324:370–376.

Bridgeman T, Flores M, Rosenbluth J, Pierog J. 1997. One emergency department's experience: Clinical algorithms and documentation. *Journal of Emergency Nursing* 23(4):316–325.

Brook R, McGlynn E, Cleary P. 1996. Quality of health care part 2: Measuring quality of care. *The New England Journal of Medicine* 335(13):966–970.

Brown D. 2002 (December 13). Hospitals Will Be Rated on Their Performance. *The Washington Post.* p. A1, A32–A33.

Buchanan J, Bell R, Arnold S, Witsberger C, Kane R, Garrard J. 1990. Assessing cost effects of nursing-home-based geriatric nurse practitioners. *Health Care Financing Review* 11(3):67–78.

Budreau G, Balakrishnan R, Titler M, Hafner M. 1999. Caregiver–patient ratio: Capturing census and staffing variability. *Nursing Economics* 17(6):317–324.

Burgio L, Burgio K. 1990. Institutional staff training and management: A review of the literature and a model for geriatric, long-term-care facilities. *International Journal of Aging and Human Development* 30(4):287–302.

Carnino A, Director, Division of Nuclear Installation Safety, International Atomic Energy Agency. Undated. *Management of Safety, Safety Culture and Self Assessment.* [Online]. Available: http://www.iaea.org/ns/nusafe/publish/papers/mng_safe.htm [accessed January 15, 2003].

Cavouras C, Suby C. 2003. *2003 Survey of Hours Report: Direct and Total Hours per Patient Day (HPPD) by Patient Care Units.* Phoenix, AZ: Labor Management Institute.

Cherry R. 1991. Agents of nursing home quality of care: Ombudsmen and staff ratios revisited. *The Gerontologist* 21(2):302–308.

Cho S, Ketefian S, Barkauskas V, Smith D. 2003. The effects of nurse staffing on adverse events, morbidity, mortality, and medical costs. *Nursing Research* 52(2):71–79.

CMS (Centers for Medicare and Medicaid Services). 2000. *Report to Congress: Appropriateness of Minimum Nurse Staffing Ratios in Nursing Homes—Phase I Report.* [Online]. Available: www.cms.gov/medicaid [accessed April 22, 2002].

CMS. 2001. *Report to Congress: Appropriateness of Minimum Nurse Staffing Ratios in Nursing Homes—Phase II Final Report.* [Online]. Available: www.cms.gov/medicaid/reports/rp1201home.asp [accessed June 25, 2002]. Site stated, "last modified on Wednesday June 12, 2002."

CMS. 2003a. *Nursing Home Compare*. [Online]. Available: http://www.medicare.gov/NH Compare/Home.asp [accessed on June 7, 2003].

CMS. 2003b. *Hospital CAHPS: CMS Pilot Test Questionnaire*. January 15, 2003, draft.

Cohen J, Spector W. 1996. The effect of Medicaid reimbursement on quality of care in nursing homes. *Journal of Health Economics* 15:23–28.

Consumers Union. 2003a. Hospitals: Your right to know. *Consumer Reports* 68(1):6.

Consumers Union. 2003b. How safe is your hospital? *Consumer Reports* 68(1):12–18.

Corrigan J. 1995. How do purchasers develop and use performance measures? *Medical Care* 33:JS18–JS24.

Curley C, McEachern JE, Speroff T. 1998. A firm trial of interdisciplinary rounds on the inpatient medical wards: An intervention designed using continuous quality improvement. *Medical Care* 36(8 Supplement):AS4–AS12.

Dang D, Johantgen M, Pronovost P, Jenckes M, Bass E. 2002. Postoperative complications: Does intensive care unit staff nursing make a difference? *Heart & Lung: Journal of Acute & Critical Care* 31(3):219–228.

DeGroot H. 1994. Patient Classification Systems: Part 1, Problems and Promise. *Journal of Nursing Administration* 24(9):43–51.

Dimick J, Swoboda S, Pronovost P, Lipsett P. 2001. Effect of nurse-to-patient ratio in the intensive care unit on pulmonary complications and resource use after hepatectomy. *American Journal of Critical Care* 10:376–382.

Disch J, Beilmann G, Ingbar D. 2001. Medical directors as partners in creating healthy work environments. *AACN Clinical Issues* 12(3):366–377.

Donabedian A. 1980. *The Definitions of Quality and Approaches to Its Assessment*. Volume 1: Explorations in Quality Assessment and Monitoring. Ann Arbor, MI: Health Administration Press.

Donaldson N, Rutledge D. 1998. Expediting the harvest and transfer of knowledge for practice in nursing: Catalyst for a journal. *The Online Journal of Clinical Innovations* 1(2):1–25.

Donaldson N, Brown D, Aydin C, Bolton L. 2001. Nurse staffing in California hospitals 1998–2000: Findings from the California Nursing Outcomes Coalition Database Project. *Policy, Politics, & Nursing Practice* 2(1):19–28.

Dreyfus H, Dreyfus S. 1986. *Mind Over Machine*. New York, NY: The Free Press, a Division of Macmillan, Inc.

Eisenberg J. 2000. Continuing education meets the learning organization: The challenge of a systems approach to patient safety. *The Journal of Continuing Education in the Health Professions* 20:197–207.

Flood S, Diers D. 1988. Nurse staffing, patient outcome and cost. *Nursing Management* 19:34–35, 38–39, 42–43.

Fridkin S, Pear S, Williamson T, Galgiani J, Jarvis W. 1996. The role of understaffing in central venous catheter–associated bloodstream infections. *Infection Control Hospital Epidemiology* 17:150–158.

Garvin D. 1993. Building a learning organization. *Harvard Business Review* July–August:78–91.

Gittell J, Fairfield K, Bierbaum B, Head W, Jackson R, Kelly M, Laskin R, Lipson S, Siliski J, Thornhill T, Zuckerman J. 2000. Impact of relational coordination on quality of care, postoperative pain and functioning, and length of stay. *Medical Care* 38(8):807–819.

Goldstein E, Fyock J. 2001. Reporting of CAHPS® Quality Information to Medicare Beneficiaries. *Health Services Research* 36(3):478–488.

Greenfield L. 1999. Doctors and nurses: A troubled partnership. *Annals of Surgery* 230(3):279–288.

Gustafson D, Sainfort F, Van Konigsveld R, Zimmerman D. 1990. The Quality Assessment Index (QAI) for Measuring Nursing Home Quality. *Health Services Research* 25(1):97–127.

Harrington C. 2001. *Nursing Home Staffing Standards in State Statutes and Regulations.* Washington, DC: National Citizens Coalition for Nursing Home Reform.

Harrington C, Zimmerman D, Karon SL, Robinson J, Beutel P. 2000. Nursing home staffing and its relationship to deficiencies. *Journal of Gerontology: Social Sciences* 55B (5):S278–S287.

Harrington C, Woolhandler S, Mullan J, Carrillo H, Himmelstein D. 2001. Does investor-ownership of nursing homes compromise the quality of care. *American Journal of Public Health* 91(9):1452–1455.

Harrington C, Carrillo H, Wellin V, Shemirani B. 2002. *Nursing Facilities, Staffing, Residents, and Facility Deficiencies, 1995-2001.* San Francisco, CA: University of California. [Online]. Available: http://www.nccnhr.org/public/50_155_3801.cfm [accessed June 1, 2003].

Harrington C, Collier E, O'Meara J, Kitchener M, Simon L, Schnelle J. 2003. Federal and state nursing facility websites: Just what the consumer needs? *American Journal of Medical Quality* 18(1):21–37.

Hartz A, Kranauer H, Kuhn E, Young H, Jacobsen S, Gay G, Muenz L, Katzoff M, Bailey R, Rimm A. 1989. Hospital characteristics and mortality rates. *The New England Journal of Medicine* 321(25):1720–1725.

Helfrich Jones M, Day S, Creeley J, Woodland M, Gerdes J. 1999. Implementation of a clinical pathway system in maternal newborn care. *Journal of Perinatal and Neonatal Nursing* 13(3):1–20.

Helmreich R. 2000. On error management: Lessons from aviation. *British Medical Journal* 320:781–785.

Hershey J, Pierskalla W, Wandel S. 1980. Nurse staffing management. In: Boldy D, ed. *Operational Research Applied to Health Services.* London: Ctroom-Helm Ltd. Pp. 189–220.

Hibbard J, Harris-Kojetin L, Mullin P, Lubalin J, Garfinkel S. 2000. Increasing the impact of health plan report cards by addressing consumers' concerns. *Health Affairs* 19(5):138–143.

Hibbard J, Slovic P, Peters E, Finucane M. 2002. Strategies for reporting health plan performance information to consumers: Evidence from controlled studies. *Health Services Research* 37(2):291–313.

Hlusko D, Nichols B. 1996. Can you depend on your patient classification system? *Journal of Nursing Administration* 26(4):39–44.

Hunt J, Hagen S. 1998. Nurse to patient ratios and patient outcomes. *Nursing Times* 94:63–66.

Hurley M. 2000. Workload, UAPs, and you. *RN* 63(12):47–49.

Ingersoll G, Schmitt M, University of Rochester Medical Center. 2003. *Work Groups and Patient Safety.* Paper commissioned by the Institute of Medicine Committee on the Work Environment for Nurses and Patient Safety.

IOM (Institute of Medicine). 1996. Wunderlich G, Sloan F, Davis C, eds. *Nursing Staff in Hospitals and Nursing Homes: Is It Adequate?* Washington, DC: National Academy Press.

IOM. 2000. *To Err Is Human: Building a Safer Health System.* Washington, DC: National Academy Press.

IOM. 2001a. *Crossing the Quality Chasm: A New Health System for the 21st Century.* Washington, DC: National Academy Press.

IOM. 2001b. *Improving the Quality of Long-Term Care.* Wunderlich G, Kohler P, eds. Washington, DC: National Academy Press.

IOM. 2003. Greiner A, Knebel E, eds. *Health Professions Education: A Bridge to Quality.* Washington, DC: The National Academies Press.

Jacobson A, Seltzer J, Dam E. 1999. New methodology for analyzing fluctuating unit activity. *Nursing Economics* 17(1):55–59.

JCAHO (Joint Commission on Accreditation of Healthcare Organizations). 2001. *Statement on Direct Care Staffing Shortages.* Statement before the Senate Committee on Health, Education, Labor and Pensions on May 17, 2001, at a hearing on Addressing Direct Care Staffing Shortages.

JCAHO. 2002. *Health Care at the Crossroads: Strategies for Addressing the Evolving Nursing Crisis.* JCAHO.

JCAHO. 2003. *2003 Hospital Accreditation Standards.* Oakbrook Terrace, IL: Joint Commission Resources.

Jennings B, Rea R, Antopol B, Carty J. 1989. Selecting, implementing, and evaluating patient classification systems: A measure of productivity. *Nursing Administration Quarterly* 14(1):24–35.

Kane R, Kane R, Arnold S, Garrard J, McDermott S, Kepferle L. 1988. Geriatric nurse practitioners as nursing home employees: Implementing the role. *The Gerontologist* 28(4):469–477.

Kayser-Jones J. 1996. Mealtime in nursing homes: The importance of individualized care. *Journal of Gerontological Nursing* 22(3):26–31.

Kayser-Jones J. 1997. Inadequate staffing at mealtime: Implications for nursing and health policy. *Journal of Gerontological Nursing* 23(8):14–21.

Kayser-Jones J, Schell E. 1997. The effect of staffing on the quality of care at mealtime. *Nursing Outlook* 45(2):64–72.

Kayser-Jones J, Wiener C, Barbaccia J. 1989. Factors contributing to the hospitalization of nursing home residents. *The Gerontologist* 290:1502–1510.

Kayser-Jones J, Schell E, Porter C, Barbaccia J, Shaw H. 1999. Factors contributing to dehydration in nursing homes: Inadequate staffing and lack of professional supervision. *Journal of the American Geriatrics Society* 47(10):1187–1194.

Knaus W, Draper E, Wagner D, Zimmerman J. 1986. An evaluation of outcome from intensive care in major medical centers. *Annals of Internal Medicine* 104(3):410–418.

Kovner C, Gergen P. 1998. Nurse staffing levels and adverse events following surgery in U.S. hospitals. *Image: The Journal of Nursing Scholarship* 30(4):315–321.

Kovner C, Jones C, Gergen P. 2000. Nurse staffing in acute care hospitals, 1990–1996. *Policy, Politics, & Nursing Practice* 1(3):194–204.

Kovner C, Jones C, Zhan C, Gergen P, Basu J. 2002. Nurse staffing and postsurgical adverse events: An analysis of administrative data from a sample of U.S. hospitals, 1990–1996. *Health Services Research* 37(3):611–629.

Kramer M, Schmalenberg C. 2002. Staff nurses identify essentials of magnetism. In: McClure M, Hinshaw A, eds. *Magnet Hospitals Revisited: Attraction and Retention of Professional Nurses.* Washington, DC: American Nurses Publishing. Pp. 25–59.

Lange L, Mengwasser M, Kretzinger C, Michaelis L. 1998. Preparing for automation: Integrating standards of care and documentation in surgical services. *Surgical Services Management* 4(11):36–38, 40–41.

Lawrenz E. 1992. Are patient classification systems still the best way to measure workload? *Perspectives on Staffing and Scheduling* XI(5):1–4.

Lazear D. 1991. *Seven Ways of Knowing: Teaching to Multiple Intelligences.* Palatine, IL: Skylight Publishing.

Lichtig L, Knauf R, Milholland D. 1999. Some impacts of nursing on acute care hospital outcomes. *Journal of Nursing Administration* 29:25–33.

Linn M, Gurel L, Linn B. 1977. Patient outcome as a measure of quality of nursing home care. *American Journal of Public Health* 67:337–344.

Luft H, Garnick D, Mark D, Peltzman D, Phibbs C, Lichtenberg E, McPhee S. 1990. Does quality influence choice of hospital? *Journal of the American Medical Association* 263(21):2899–2906.

Malloch K, Conovaloff A. 1999. Patient classification systems, Part 1. The third generation. *Journal of Nursing Administration* 29(7-8):49–56.

Manderino M, Berkey N. 1997. Verbal abuse of staff nurses by physicians. *Journal of Professional Nursing* 13(1):48–55.

Massachusetts Nurses Association. 2003. *MNA Files Quality Patient Care/Safe RN Staffing Bill to Regulate RN-Patient Ratios in Massachusetts Hospitals.* [Online]. Available: http://www.massnurses.org/news/safestaff/200212BillFiled.htm [accessed June 2, 2003].

McClure M, Hinshaw A, eds. 2002. *Magnet Hospitals Revisited: Attraction and Retention of Professional Nurses.* Washington, DC: American Nurses Publishing.

McMahan E, Hoffman K. 1994. Physician–nurse relationships in clinical settings: A review and critique of the literature, 1966–1992. *Medical Care Review* 51(1):83–112.

Mezey M, Lynaugh J. 1989. The teaching nursing home program: Outcomes of care. *Nursing Clinics of North America* 24(3):769–780.

Mitchell P, Shortell S. 1997. Adverse outcomes and variations in organization of care delivery. *Medical Care* 35(Supplement 11):NS19–NS32.

Mitchell P, Shannon S, Cain K, Hegyvary S. 1996. Critical care outcomes: Linking structures, processes, and organizational and clinical outcomes. *American Journal of Critical Care* 5(5):353–363.

Mukamel D, Mushlin A. 1998. Quality of care information makes a difference: An analysis of market share and price changes after publication of the New York State Cardiac Surgery Mortality Reports. *Medical Care* 36:945–954.

NACNEP (National Advisory Council on Nurse Education and Practice). Report to the Secretary of the U.S. Department of Health and Human Services. 1996. *Report on the Basic Registered Nurse Workforce.* Washington, DC: U.S. Government Printing Office.

National Citizens Coalition for Nursing Home Reform. 1998. *NCCNHR Minimum Staffing Standards.* [Online]. Available: www.nchnccnhr.org/govpolicy/51_162_472.cfm [accessed January 25, 2003].

National Council of State Boards of Nursing. 2001. *Profiles of Member Boards—2000.* Chicago, IL: National Council of State Boards of Nursing, Inc.

Needleman J, Buerhaus P, Mattke S, Stewart M, Zelevinsky K. 2001. Nurse Staffing and Patient Outcomes in Hospitals. *Final Report for Health Resources Services Administration* 1–457.

Needleman J, Buerhaus P, Mattke S, Stewart M, Zelevinsky K. 2002. Nurse-staffing levels and the quality of care in hospitals. *The New England Journal of Medicine* 346(22):1715–1722.

Norrish B, Rundall T. 2001. Hospital restructuring and the work of registered nurses. *Milbank Quarterly* 79(1):55.

Nyman J. 1988. Improving the quality of nursing home outcomes: Are adequacy- or incentive-oriented policies more effective. *Medical Care* 12:1158–1171.

O'Brien-Pallas L, Cockerill R, Leatt P. 1992. Different systems, different costs? An examination of the comparability of workload measurement systems. *Journal of Nursing Administration* 22(12):17–22.

Office of the Governor. 2002. *Governor Davis Moves to Improve Nursing Care:* California Department of Health Services. Press release dated September 29, 2002. [Online]. Available: http://www.governor.ca.gov/state/govsite/gov [accessed August 27, 2003].

Pfifferling J. 1999. The disruptive physician: A quality of professional life factor. *The Physician Executive* 25(2):56–61.

Pronovost P, Dang D, Dorman T, Lipsett P, Garrett E, Jenckes M, Bass E. 2001. Intensive care unit nurse staffing and the risk for complications after abdominal aortic surgery. *Effective Clinical Practice* 4(5):199–206.

Quinn J. 1992. *Intelligent Enterprise: A Knowledge and Service Based Paradigm for Industry.* New York, NY: The Free Press, a division of Macmillan, Inc.

Rauen C. 2001. Using simulation to teach critical thinking skills: You can't just throw the book at them. *Critical Care Nursing Clinics of North America* 13(1):93–103.

Reed L, Blegen M, Goode C. 1998. Adverse patient occurrences as a measure of nursing care quality. *Journal of Nursing Administration* 28(5):62–69.

Rice A. 2000. Interdisciplinary collaboration in health care: Education, practice, and research. *National Academies of Practice Forum: Issues in Interdisciplinary Care* 2(1):59–73.

Roberts K. 1990. Managing high reliability organizations. *California Managment Review* 32:101–113.

Roberts K, Bea R. 2001. Must accidents happen? Lessons from high-reliability organizations. *Academy of Management Executive* 15(3):70–78.

Rosenstein A. 2002. Nurse–physician relationships: Impact on nurse satisfaction and retention. *American Journal of Nursing* 102(6):26–34.

Rousseau D, Libuser C. 1997. Contingent workers in high risk organizations. *California Management Review* 39(2):103–123.

Rozich J, Resar R. 2002. Using a unit assessment tool to optimize patient flow and staffing in a community hospital. *Journal on Quality Improvement* 28(1):31–41.

Schmitt M. 2001. Collaboration improves the quality of care: Methodological challenges and evidence from U.S. health care research. *Journal of Interprofessional Care* 15(1):47–66.

Schnelle J, Simmons S, Harrington C, Cadogan M, Garcia E, Bates-Jensen B. 2002. University of California Los Angeles Borun Center for Gerontological Research and the Los Angeles Jewish Home for the Aging. *Nursing Home Staffing Information: Does It Reflect Differences in Quality of Care?* Los Angeles, CA: California HealthCare Foundation.

Schriefer J, Botter M. 2001. Tools and systems for improved outcomes. *Outcomes Management for Nursing Practice* 5(3).

Seago J. 2001. Nurse staffing, models of care delivery, and interventions. In: Shojania K, Duncan B, McDonald K, Wachter R, eds. *Making Health Care Safer: A Critical Analysis of Patient Safety Practices. Evidence Report/Technology Assessment No. 43.* Rockville, MD: AHRQ.

Seago J. 2002. The California experiment: Alternatives for minimum nurse-to-patient ratios. *Journal of Nursing Administration* 32(1):48–58.

Seago J, Spetz J, Coffman J, Rosenoff E, O'Neil E. 2003. Minimum staffing ratios: The California Workforce Initiative Survey. *Nursing Economics* 21(2):65–70.

SEIU (Service Employees International Union). 2001. *The Shortage of Care: A Study by the SEIU Nurse Alliance.* Washington, DC: SEIO, AFL-CIO, CLC.

Shortell S, Zimmerman J, Rousseau D, Gillies R, Wagner D, Draper E, Knaus W, Duffy J. 1994. The performance of intensive care units: Does good management make a difference? *Medical Care* 32(5):508–525.

Silber J, Williams S, Krakauer H, Schwartz S. 1992. Hospital and patient characteristics associated with death after surgery: A study of adverse occurrence and failure to rescue. *Medical Care* 30(7):615–627.

Simon L, Monroe A. 2001. California provider group report cards: What do they tell us? *American Journal of Medical Quality* 16(2):61–70.

Smith J, Crawford L. 2002a. *Report of Findings from the 2001 Employers Survey.* NCSBN Research Brief. 3. Chicago, IL: National Council of State Boards of Nursing, Inc.

Smith J, Crawford L. 2002b. *Report of Findings from the Practice and Professional Issues Survey—Spring 2001.* NCSBN Research Brief. 2. Chicago, IL: National Council of State Boards of Nursing, Inc.

Smith J, Crawford L. 2003. *Report of Findings from the 2002 RN Practice Analysis.* NCSBN Research Brief. 9. Chicago, IL: National Council of State Boards of Nursing, Inc.

Sochalski J. 2001. Quality of care, nurse staffing, and patient outcomes. *Policy, Politics, & Nursing Practice* 2(1):9–18.

Sovie M, Jawad A. 2001. Hospital restructuring and its impact on outcomes. *Journal of Nursing Administration* 31(12):588–600.

Spector W, Takada H. 1991. Characteristics of nursing facilities that affect resident outcomes. *Journal of Aging and Health* 3(4):427–454.

Spetz J, Seago J, Coffman J, Rosenoff E, O-Neil E, California Workforce Initiative. 2000. *Minimum Nurse Staffing Ratios in California Acute Care Hospitals.* Oakland, CA: California HealthCare Foundation.

Spratley E, Johnson A, Sochalski J, Fritz M, Spencer W. 2000. *The Registered Nurse Population: Findings from the National Sample Survey of Registered Nurses.* DHHS, HRSA. [Online]. Available: http://bhpr.hrsa.gov/healthworkforce/reports/rnsurvey/rnss1.htmm [accessed October 4, 2003].

Thomas E, Studdert D, Burstin H, Orav E, Zeena T, Willimas E, Howard K, Weiler P, Brennan T. 2000. Incidence and types of adverse events and negligent care in Utah and Colorado. *Medical Care* 38:261–271.

Thomas E, Helmeich R. 2002. Will airline safety models work in medicine? In: Rosenthal M, Sutcliffe K, eds. *Medical Error: What Do We Know? What Do We Do?* San Francisco, CA: Jossey-Bass.

Thompson C, Koon E, Woodwell W, Beauvais J. 2002. *Training for the Next Economy: An ASTD State of the Industry Report on Trends in Employer-Provided Training in the United States.* Alexandria, VA: American Society of Training and Development.

Trowbridge R, Weingarten S. 2001a. Clinical pathways. In: Shojania K, Duncan B, McDonald K, Wachter R, eds. *Making Health Care Safer: A Critical Analysis of Patient Safety Practices.* Evidence Report/Technology Assessment Number 43. AHRQ Publication No. 01-E058. Rockville, MD: AHRQ.

Trowbridge R, Weingarten S. 2001b. Clinical decision support systems. In: Shojania K, Duncan B, McDonald K, Wachter R, eds. *Making Health Care Safer: A Critical Analysis of Patient Safety Practices.* Evidence Report/Technology Assessment Number 43. AHRQ Publication No. 01-E058. Rockville, MD: AHRQ.

Unruh L. 2002. Nursing staff reductions in Pennsylvania hospitals: Exploring the discrepancy between perceptions and data. *Medical Care Research and Review* 59(2):197–214.

Upenieks V. 1998. Work sampling: Assessing nursing efficiency. *Nursing Management* 29(4): 27–29.

Walston S, Kimberly J. 1997. Reengineering hospitals: Evidence from the field. *Hospital and Health Services Administration* 42(2):143-163.

Wells J, Kochan T, Smith M. 1991. *Managing Workforce Safety and Health: The Case of Contract Labor in the U.S. Petrochemical Industry.* Beaumont, TX: John Gray Institute.

Zimmerman D, Karon S, Arling G. 1995. Development and testing of nursing home quality indicators. *Health Care Financing Review* 16(4):107–127.

6

Work and Workspace Design to Prevent and Mitigate Errors

The largest, best-trained, and most dedicated workforce will still make errors; its fallibility is an immutable part of human nature. However, this innate fallibility can be compounded when the practices, procedures, tools, techniques, and devices used by workers are unreliable, complex, and themselves unsafe—having been designed, selected, and maintained by other fallible humans.

The two Institute of Medicine (IOM) reports discussed earlier in this report—*To Err Is Human* (IOM, 2000) and *Crossing the Quality Chasm* (IOM, 2001)—call for better design of work processes to improve patient care and safety. *To Err Is Human* recommends that health care organizations (HCOs) incorporate safety principles in work design. *Crossing the Quality Chasm* underscores this recommendation by observing that "health care has safety and quality problems because it relies on outmoded systems of work. Poor designs set up the workforce to fail, regardless of how hard they try (IOM, 2001: 4)." The report reiterates that safer health care requires redesigned health care processes.

Some nursing processes, such as medication administration, are well documented to have multiple features conducive to the commission of health care errors. The long work hours of some nurses also cause fatigue and contribute to their making errors. Inefficient care processes and workspace design, while not intrinsically dangerous to patients, decrease patient safety to the extent that they reduce the time nurses have for monitoring patients and providing therapeutic care. Documentation and paperwork requirements are well known to involve such inefficiencies.

226

The committee agrees that nurses' work processes and workspace need to be designed to make them more efficient, less conducive to the commission of errors, and more amenable to detecting and remedying errors when they occur. In addition, limiting the number of hours worked per day and consecutive days of work by nursing staff, as is done in other safety-sensitive industries, is a fundamental patient safety precaution. It is also essential to foster collaboration of nursing staff with other health care personnel in identifying high-risk and inefficient work processes and workspaces and (re)designing them for patient safety and efficiency. Redesign of patient care documentation practices, however, cannot be accomplished solely by nursing staff and internal HCO efforts. Because many documentation practices are driven by external parties, such as regulators and oversight organizations, these organizations will need to assist in the redesign of those practices.

This chapter reviews the evidence on the design of nurses' work hours, work processes, and workspaces, primarily as they relate to patient safety, but also with respect to efficiency (which, as noted above, is a contributory factor in safety). We present findings and recommendations derived from this evidence on designing these elements of the nursing environment so as to enhance safety.

DESIGN OF WORK HOURS

This section reviews the evidence related to the design of nurses' work hours: the effect of fatigue from shift work and extended work hours on work performance, the relationship between nurse work hours and the commission of errors, and data on hours worked by both hospital and nursing home nursing personnel. The committee's responses to this evidence in the form of conclusions and a recommendation are then presented.

Effect of Fatigue from Shift Work and Extended Work Hours on Work Performance[1]

Fatigue results from continuous physical or mental activity, inadequate rest, sleep loss, or nonstandard work schedules (e.g., working at night). Whatever the origin of physical or mental fatigue, it is accompanied by a subjective feeling of tiredness and a diminished capacity to do work. The effects of fatigue include slowed reaction time, diminished attention to detail, errors of omission, compromised problem solving (Van-Griever and

---

[1]This section incorporates content from a paper on "Work Hour Regulation in Safety-Sensitive Industries" commissioned by the committee and included in this report as Appendix C.

Meijman, 1987), reduced motivation, and decreased vigor for successful completion of required tasks (Gravenstein et al., 1990). Thus, fatigue also causes decreased productivity. Tired workers accomplish less, especially if their tasks demand accuracy (Krueger, 1994; Rosa and Colligan, 1988). In nurses' work environments, fatigue is produced by shift work and extended work hours.

Shift Work

Since almost all physiological and behavioral functions are affected by circadian rhythms, the time of day when work must be completed is important. The human circadian rhythm strongly favors sleeping during night-time hours. Overall capacity for physical work is reduced at night (Cabri et al., 1988; Cohen and Muehl, 1977; Rosa, 2001; Wojtczak-Jaroszowa and Banaszkiewicz, 1974). Reaction times, visual search, perceptual–motor tracking, and short-term memory are worse at night than during the day (Folkard, 1996; Monk, 1990). On-the-job performance also deteriorates. At night, railroad signal and meter reading errors increase, minor errors occur more frequently in hospitals, and switchboard operators take longer to respond to phone calls (Monk et al., 1996).

Night shift workers also have difficulty staying awake. In a survey of nurses working in seven West Coast hospitals, 19.3 percent of those working night and rotating shifts reported struggling to stay awake at least once during the previous month while taking care of patients, compared with 3.8 percent of day and evening shift nurses (Lee, 1992). In a 1986 study of nurses in one hospital, 35.3 percent of those who routinely rotated to the night shift, 32.4 percent of those who always worked nights, and 20.7 percent of day/evening shift nurses who worked occasional nights reported falling asleep during the night shift at least once a week. Nurses working night shifts or rotating shifts also made more on-the-job procedural and medication errors due to sleepiness than did nurses working other shifts. Sleepiness appeared to be confined to the night shift, as none of the shift rotators or day/evening nurses who worked occasional nights reported significant difficulties remaining alert on other shifts (Gold et al., 1992). Likewise, objective findings of sleeping on duty were reported in a study of 15 French nurses working at night. Only 4 of the 15 were able to remain awake all night while at work as measured by activity (wrist actigraphy) and sleep (polysomnographic) recordings; the remaining nurses averaged 86.5 (standard deviation ± 77.6) minutes of sleep while on duty (Delafosse et al., 2000). Difficulties in maintaining alertness at night are not confined to nurses. Self-reported and objective measures of sleep were recorded in U.S. Air Force traffic controllers on duty at night (Luna et al., 1997). And the most consistent factor influencing truck driver fatigue and alertness over a

16-week study of 80 commercial truck drivers was time of day. Episodes of drowsiness at the wheel were observed in the majority of drivers. Drowsiness was markedly greater during nighttime than daytime driving (Wylie et al., 1996).

Coping with nonstandard work hours (nights or rotating shifts) is easier for someone fully rested. A person who is not sleep deprived performs tasks more efficiently after prolonged wakefulness (Dinges et al., 1996). However, individuals working nights and rotating shifts rarely obtain optimal amounts of quality sleep. Their sleep is shorter, lighter, more fragmented, and less restorative than sleep at night (Knauth et al., 1980; Lavie et al., 1989; Walsh et al., 1981).

A number of interventions have been proposed to mitigate the effect of shift work. Clockwise shift rotations—day shift, progressing to evening, then night shifts—appear to be tolerated more easily than the reverse. Scheduled, on-the-job naps and use of bright lighting also have been found to combat fatigue to some extent. However, the way in which they are best implemented has not been established. The speed of shift rotation, how to counteract the sleep inertia that commonly accompanies the taking of naps, and how to provide bright lighting for nurses while maintaining optimal darkness for patients are some of the issues not yet resolved. Consequently, experts on fatigue have recommended modifying work tasks and processes to reduce the risk for error and creating mechanisms to detect errors at the time they are committed to reduce their adverse effects (Office of Technology Assessment, 1991; Jha et al., 2001).

Extended Work Hours

Shifts of 12 or more hours with limited opportunity for rest and no opportunity for sleep are referred to as "sustained operations" (Kruger, 1989). Workers engaged in sustained operations in a variety of occupations report greater fatigue at the end of their shifts than do those who work 8-hour shifts (Mills et al., 1983; Rosa, 1995; Ugrovics and Wright, 1990).[2]

Studies in a variety of industries also show that accident rates increase during overtime hours (Kogi, 1991; Schuster, 1985); rates rise after 9 consecutive hours, double after 12 hours (Hanecke et al., 1998), and triple after 16 hours (Akerstedt, 1994). Data from aircraft accident investigations

---

[2]In two studies, however, mine workers reported no differences in fatigue after 8- and 12-hour shifts despite high physical workloads (Duchon et al., 1994), and computer operators reported reduced tiredness throughout the shift after switching from 8-hour to 12-hour shifts (Williamson et al., 1994). Neither study reports the timing and duration of meal and "coffee" breaks. In the case of unionized mine workers, it is likely they were provided brief rest periods during their work shifts.

conducted by the National Transportation Safety Board also show higher rates of error after 12 hours (National Transportation Safety Board, 1994). Finally, night shifts longer than 12 hours and day shifts longer than 16 hours have consistently been found to be associated with reduced productivity and more accidents (Rosa, 1995).

Laboratory studies have shown that moderate levels of prolonged wakefulness can produce performance impairments equal to or greater than those due to levels of intoxication deemed unacceptable for driving, working, and/or operating dangerous equipment. Prolonged periods of wakefulness (e.g., 17 hours without sleep) can produce performance decrements equivalent to a blood alcohol concentration (BAC) of 0.05 percent, the level defined as alcohol intoxication in many western industrialized countries.[3] After 24 hours of sustained wakefulness, cognitive psychomotor performance decreases to a level equivalent to a BAC of 0.10 percent (Dawson and Reid, 1997; Lamond and Dawson, 1998). Performance on neurobehavioral tests decreases linearly after 17 hours of wakefulness, with the poorest performance occurring after 25–27 hours. Performance on the most complex task—grammatical reasoning—was found to be impaired several hours earlier than performance on vigilance accuracy and response latency (20.3 hours versus 22.3 and 24.9 hours, respectively) (Lamond and Dawson, 1998). Prolonged wakefulness also significantly impairs speed and accuracy, hand–eye coordination, decision making, and memory (Babkoff et al., 1988; Florica et al., 1968; Gillberg et al., 1994; Linde and Bergstrom, 1992; Mullaney et al., 1983). A nurse who worked on average one mandatory double shift (16 hours) every 2 weeks for a 2-month period reported, "By 4 a.m., I was so exhausted that I would stop between going from one baby to the next and completely forget why I was going to the other bedside. Another time, again about 4 a.m., I would sometimes stop in the middle of the floor and forget what I was doing" (California Nurses Association, 2003).

Fatigue is also exacerbated by working increased numbers of shifts without a day off (Dirks, 1993; Knauth, 1993) and by having only short durations between work shifts. Working more than four consecutive 12-hour shifts is associated with excessive fatigue and longer recovery times (Wallace and Greenwood, 1995). Very short off-duty periods—8 hours or less—do not provide enough time for commuting, recovery sleep, or time to take care of domestic responsibilities (Dinges et al., 1996; Rosa, 1995, 2001). Most adults require at least 6–8 hours of sleep to function adequately at work (Krueger, 1994). The loss of even 2 hours of sleep affects waking

---

[3]In the United States, BAC-level definitions of intoxication are set by the states. Limits of 0.08 and 0.10 are typical for adult drivers; the majority of states set lower levels for drivers under 21 years of age, such as 0.00–0.07 (Wagenaar et al., 2001).

performance and alertness the next day (Dinges et al., 1996). After 5 to 10 days of shortened sleep periods, the sleep debt (sleep loss) is significant enough to impair decision making, initiative, information integration, planning, and plan execution (Krueger, 1994). The effects of sleep loss are insidious and usually not recognized by the sleep-deprived individual until they have become severe (Dinges et al., 1996; Rosenkind et al., 1999). Schedules that require workers to return to work after an 8-hour rest period or to transition from night to day or evening shifts without at least 24 hours off are considered particularly dangerous (Olson and Ambrogetti, 1998; Rosa and Colligan, 1988).

Recovery from extended work periods requires more than 1 day. Off-duty intervals ranging from 10 to 16 hours are either suggested or already mandated for many transportation workers (Dinges et al., 1996; Gander et al., 1991; Mitler et al., 1997). Two consecutive nights of recovery sleep can return performance and alertness to normal levels, even following two or three 12-hour shifts (Dinges et al., 1996; Tucker et al., 1996); longer intervals between works days are even more beneficial. Workers obtain more sleep and start their next shift with less fatigue. The first or second night on a new series of night shifts, however, may be the most fatiguing because of circadian desynchrony (Rosa, 2001).

The combination of sustained wakefulness and working at night is particularly hazardous (Gold et al., 1992; Smith et al., 1994). When the *Exxon Valdez* ran aground around midnight on March 23, 1989, the third mate had been awake 18 hours and anticipated working several more hours (Alaska Oil Spill Commission, 1990). Although the explosion of the Challenger space shuttle occurred during the daytime, the decisions made the night before the launch by mission control staff have been cited as a major factor contributing to the explosion (Mitler et al., 1988). In a small study of the use of extended (16-hour) night shifts in seven wards of a Japanese university hospital, several compensatory measures were employed to protect against the dual effects of sustained operations and night shift work. These measures included increases in the numbers of night staff to allow all nursing staff to take a 2-hour nap in a dedicated resting room. Staff was also allowed to take at least one recovery day off after a 16-hour shift. The increase in staff, 2-hour nap, and day off were believed to contribute to the extended shift nurses' less frequent complaints of fatigue and general decreased physical activity as compared with nurses working 8-hour shifts (Fukuda et al., 1999). The study also found that sleep inertia (characterized by sleepiness, fatigue, and dullness) increased immediately after the nap, but then decreased to the same levels as existed before the nap. The researchers concluded that nap length would need to be carefully regulated to avoid persistent sleep inertia and its attendant risks (Takahashi et al., 1999).

A review of evidence on the effects of worker fatigue on patient safety is included in the Agency for Healthcare Research and Quality's (AHRQ) report *Making Health Care Safer: A Critical Analysis of Patient Safety Practice* (Jha et al. 2001). Consistent with the above evidence, the report notes that sleep deprivation leads to decreased alertness and poor performance on standardized testing, and that shift workers in particular experience disturbances in their circadian rhythms and tend to perform less well on reasoning and nonstimulating tasks.

Evidence on Nurse Work Hours and the Commission of Errors

Researchers conducting the evidence review presented in the AHRQ report cited above (Jha et al., 2001) were unable to locate research that could help identify the specific numbers of hours worked by health care personnel, including nurses, beyond which patient safety is threatened. These researchers noted inconsistent research findings with respect to ideal shift length for enhanced worker performance. The report suggests that while multiple studies have sought to document the impact of fatigue on the performance of medical personnel, these studies have been limited by poor design or outcomes that did not correlate well with medical error.

This situation has been improved by a 2002 study funded as part of AHRQ's initiative to examine the effects of working conditions on patient safety. This study documented the work patterns of a sample of hospital staff nurses randomly selected from the membership of the American Nurses Association (ANA). The sample frame consisted of full-time hospital staff nurses (unit based, not working through a temporary agency) with no administrative or educational responsibilities. The study measured the effects of nurse work hours on patient safety by (1) documenting the total scheduled and unscheduled hours worked by nurses; (2) describing the nature of nurses' overtime work hours in terms of what proportion of hours worked were overtime hours, how often nurses worked overtime, and whether overtime was voluntary or mandatory; and (3) determining whether there was an association between errors and near-errors and the numbers and types of hours worked by the nurses.

Study participants recorded information about their scheduled work hours, actual work hours, errors, and near-errors daily in a diary for 28 days. Nurses were also asked to describe all errors and near-errors. The researchers then categorized each error or near-error by type (e.g., medication administration, procedural, transcription) based on the nurse's description. Error rates per hour were calculated according to the number of errors and hours worked, adjusting for multiple work shifts for the same nurse. The associations between error rates and both overtime and scheduled work shift duration (in hours) were estimated using regression models. The p-values for the adjusted incidence rate ratios were constructed based on robust variance estimates, with α = 0.05. Near-errors were examined using the same procedures.

For all study nurses, the overall error rate was 0.00336 errors per hour worked. Working overtime—working longer than scheduled on a given day or working extra shifts ("scheduled overtime")—had no effect on error rates unless shift durations exceeded 12 consecutive hours. Once shift durations exceed 12 consecutive hours, both voluntary and mandated overtime significantly increased error rates (0.00375/hour and 0.00490/hour, respectively) (p = 0.02 for voluntary overtime and 0.03 for mandated overtime). Results remained consistent when outliers (i.e., 54 extremely long shifts of more than 23 hours, nurses with more than 7 errors each) were removed from the analyses. Results were somewhat different for near-errors. Being mandated to work overtime was associated with significant increases in the rate of near-errors for shifts scheduled for 12 hours or more; however, the rate of near-errors associated with working voluntary overtime for periods exceeding 12 consecutive hours was not increased.[4]

Data on Nurse Work Hours

Nursing staff working in in-patient facilities have traditionally worked in 8-hour shifts, but increasingly work longer hours. Reasons for these increases include the desire for increased compensation (elective overtime), requirements by health care organizations to work overtime (mandatory overtime) to compensate for insufficient staffing, and the desire for more flexible work hours (e.g., 10- or 12-hour shifts) to accommodate either facility or individual nurse needs or both. Scheduled shifts may be 8, 10, or 12 hours and may not follow the traditional pattern of day, evening, or night shifts. Nurses working on specialized units, such as the operating room, dialysis units, and some intensive care units, may be required to be on call in addition to their regularly scheduled shifts (Rogers, 2002).

Representative, quantitative data describing the work hours of nurses are scarce. Evidence of the long hours worked by direct-care nurses working in hospitals and nursing homes was obtained from a random sample survey of nurses licensed to work in either Illinois or North Carolina[5] as part of a longitudinal study of nurses' worklife and health funded by the

---

[4]Unpublished study data from Ann Rogers, Ph.D., University of Pennsylvania (personal communications on January 25, 2003, June 29, 2003 and July 18, 2003).

[5]These states were selected because they have large ethnic diversity in their registered nurse (RN) populations and because they renew RN licenses annually, providing up-to-date mailing lists.

National Institute for Occupational Safety and Health (NIOSH) of the U.S. Centers for Disease Control and Prevention (CDC). Of the 674 registered nurse (RN) respondents to this 2002–2003 survey who were employed as a full-time hospital or nursing home general-duty/staff nurse, 27.2 percent reported working more than 13 hours at a stretch one or more times a week, and an additional 18.9 percent reported doing so once a month or every other a week. Only 19.5 percent reporting never doing so, while 34.4 percent reported doing so only a few times per year.[6] Extended work hours also are indicated by their frequently being cited by nurses as a key area of job dissatisfaction (U.S. General Accounting Office [GAO], 2001); by the extent to which nursing organizations have sought legislative, regulatory, and contractual relief from this practice; and by the few studies of hours worked by nursing staff in hospitals and nursing homes.

Work Hours of Hospital Nurses

Data collected from the 2000 National Sample Survey of Registered Nurses indicate that full-time hospital nurses (including direct-care, administrative, and other hospital nurses) worked on average 42.2 hours per week, in contrast to their average scheduled hours of 39.3 hours per week (Spratley et al., 2000). In 2001, 17 percent of a national representative sample of newly licensed RNs surveyed by the National Council of State Boards of Nursing in its twice yearly survey of entry-level nurses reported working (in all settings of care, full- and part-time) an average of 36.5 nonovertime hours per week and an average of 4.6 hours of overtime per week. Likewise, 17 percent of these newly licensed RNs reported working mandatory overtime (Smith and Crawford, 2002).

As the discussion of staffing levels in Chapter 5 indicates, however, averages do not tell the full story. The AHRQ-funded study of the work hours of a sample of members of the ANA documented the variation in the work patterns of full-time, direct-care hospital staff nurses in terms of hours worked, duration of shifts, and amount of overtime hours worked. The study found that although the majority (84.3 percent) of scheduled shifts were 8 or 12 hours in duration, 3.5 percent were for periods greater than 12 hours. Scheduled shift durations ranged from 2 to 22.5 hours (see Figure 6-1).

Furthermore, a comparison of *scheduled* and *actual* work times revealed that all nurses had started work earlier than scheduled, stayed later than scheduled, or both at least once during the 28-day period. Nurses reported working on average 13.4 days (range 1–24) during this 28-day data-gather-

---

[6]Unpublished data from Alison Trinkoff, Ph.D., University of Maryland at Baltimore, NIOSH grant R01OH3702 (personal communication, April 9, 2003).

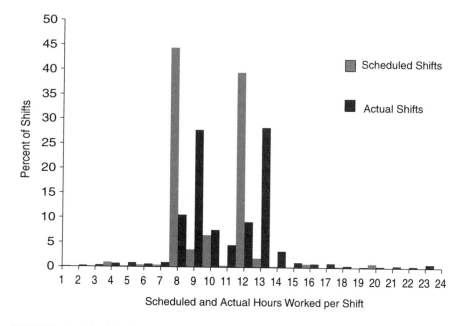

FIGURE 6-1 Scheduled and actual shift durations.
SOURCE: Ann Rogers, Ph.D., University of Pennsylvania (personal communication on July 4, 2003).

ing period, and working beyond their scheduled shift times on average 10.9 days (range 1–24). Nurses started work early, left later than scheduled, or both on 81.4 percent of shifts. As a result, actual (as opposed to scheduled) work shift durations ranged from 1 hour, 15 minutes (an obstetrical nurse who was sent home because of a low census) to 23 hours, 57 minutes (see Figure 6-1). Almost half of the shifts worked (43 percent) exceeded 12 hours (1074 shifts), and one-quarter exceeded 12 hours, 50 minutes. There were 51 double (16-hour) shifts reported, 51 shifts in which participants worked more than 16 but less than 20 hours, and 103 shifts that exceeded 20 consecutive hours. A comparison of actual and scheduled work times revealed that participants worked on average 1 hour, 9 minutes extra per scheduled shift (range 18 minutes–19 hours, 30 minutes).

Work Hours of Nursing Staff in Nursing Homes

Research on the work hours of nursing staff in nursing homes also has revealed extended work hours. In site visits to 17 nursing homes in Ohio, Colorado, and Texas in 2001, researchers found that double shifts (i.e., two consecutive 8-hour shifts totaling 16 hours) and extra shifts were performed in many of these facilities on a regular basis. Double shifts in particular were pervasive. In 13 of the 17 nursing homes, at least one nursing staff member, but frequently more, had worked between one and three double shifts in the previous 7 days. In five nursing homes, at least one staff member had worked between four and seven double shifts in the last 7 days. In one of the facilities, more than a third of the interviewed nursing staff had worked between eight and eleven double shifts in the last 14 days. All direct-care nursing staff (RNs, licensed practical nurses [LPNs]/licensed vocational nurses [LVNs], and nursing assistants [NAs]) were engaged in these work practices; however, double shifts were performed most often by NAs (Centers for Medicare and Medicaid Services [CMS], 2002).

Responses to the Evidence

The committee finds the evidence that prolonged work hours and fatigue affect worker performance to be very strong. We also note that there is no evidence to suggest that any amount of training, motivation, or professionalism is able to overcome the performance deficits associated with fatigue, sleep loss, and the sleepiness associated with circadian variations in alertness (Battelle Memorial Institute, 1998; Dinges et al., 1996; Jha et al. 2001; McCartt et al., 2000). The recent AHRQ-funded study of nurse work hours and health care errors discussed above provides additional compelling evidence of the effect of nurses working long hours on patient safety.

The committee reviewed evidence on how other safety-sensitive industries—nuclear energy production, public and commercial transportation, the military, police, and firefighters—have responded to such evidence. All have placed some restrictions on the work hours of personnel (see Appendix C). The health care industry is notable in that, with few exceptions, it places no such limits on work hours. However, a number of organizations are beginning to respond to the evidence. As of 2002, eight states had enacted legislation or regulations prohibiting facilities from requiring nurses to work certain extended hours (ANA, 2002). Legislation also has been introduced federally and within additional states to ban mandatory overtime for nurses. The Safe Nursing and Patient Care Act of 2003 (HR 745 and SB 373), introduced in the 108th U.S. Congress, would, in part, prohibit mandatory overtime for nurses and other licensed health care providers. As part of the ANA's nationwide state legislative agenda, other state nurses' associations are pressing for prohibitions on mandatory overtime in state statutes and regulations. No proposals address how long nurses may work on a voluntary basis.

Jha et al (2001: 530) note that "in most high-hazard industries the assumption is that fatigue and long, aberrant work hours leads to poor performance, and the burden of proof is in the hands of those who believe that such work practices are safe." They recommend that, "given that medical personnel, like all human beings, probably function suboptimally when fatigued, efforts to reduce fatigue and sleepiness should be undertaken, and the burden of proof should be in the hands of the advocates of the current system to demonstrate that it is safe." Based on the evidence presented above, the committee concurs and makes the following recommendation:

> **Recommendation 6-1.** To reduce error-producing fatigue, state regulatory bodies should prohibit nursing staff from providing patient care in any combination of scheduled shifts, mandatory overtime, or voluntary overtime in excess of 12 hours in any given 24-hour period and in excess of 60 hours per 7-day period. To this end:
>
> - HCOs and labor organizations representing nursing staff should establish policies and practices designed to prevent nurses who provide direct patient care from working longer than 12 hours in a 24-hour period and in excess of 60 hours per 7-day period.
> - Schools of nursing, state boards of nursing, and HCOs should educate nurses about the threats to patient safety caused by fatigue.

The committee calls attention to several parts of this recommendation. First, the recommendation calls for limiting the number of hours nurses spend in providing *direct patient care*. If for example, a nurse completes a 12-hour shift and needs to stay beyond this period to document care or attend a training or education activity, this time would not be included in the 12-hour limit. Rather, the recommendation is intended to limit the amount of time that fatigued nurses will have responsibility for direct patient care. We include clinical supervision in this definition of direct care because such supervision also requires the exercise of clinical judgment and often involvement in clinical care, both of which would be adversely affected by fatigue.

Second, the committee does not distinguish in this recommendation between voluntary and mandatory overtime. We note that personal strength of will and the exercise of free will are not effective countermeasures to the effects of sleep loss and fatigue. Consequently, while the committee believes HCOs might want to limit their use of mandatory overtime in the interest of nurse retention and recruitment, excessive hours endanger patient safety regardless of whether they are worked under a mandate or on a voluntary basis. The committee consequently recommends that working more than 12 hours in any 24-hour period and more than 60 hours in any 7-day period be prevented except in case of an emergency, such as a natural disaster. In the event that nurses are required to work excessive hours because of an emergency, this information should be immediately disclosed to the public so that elective admissions can be postponed and other admissions diverted to different units or facilities. Similarly, in any instance where a nursing shortage prevents an HCO from securing sufficient nurses to prevent work hours in excess of 12 hours in any 24-hour period and more than 60 hours in any 7-day period, this information also should be disclosed to the public, so that elective admissions can be referred to other facilities or delayed until staffing is remedied. If an admission cannot be delayed or referred to another HCO, the patient and their family should be informed about the shortage of staffing and that nursing staff is working under conditions adverse to patient safety. Family members may want to attend to a patient for longer periods of his or her inpatient stay, when nursing staff is working longer work hours and there is a shortage of nursing staff.

Finally, by recommending a regulatory role in encouraging safe work hours, the committee does not intend to encourage the creation of burdensome oversight mechanisms that, for example, would require the submission or inspection of individual nurse time sheets. Rather, the committee encourages HCOs, state boards of nursing, and schools of nursing to educate nurses and themselves about the dangers of fatigue. We also recommend that HCOs, working with their labor partners, develop staffing and work-hour policies designed to prevent fatigue caused by excessive work hours. Such policies and procedures might include, for example:

- Acknowledging the responsibility of nurses who work in more than one facility to ensure that their total patient care hours worked do not exceed the patient safety thresholds identified in the above recommendation.
- Ensuring that any use of mandatory overtime by the facility will not require nurses to provide more than 12 hours of patient care in any 24-hour period or more than 60 hours of patient care in any 7-day period.
- In health care organizations that allow nursing staff to self-schedule, preventing nursing staff from scheduling more than 12 hours of patient care in any 24-hour period or more than 60 hours of patient care in any 7-day period.

The committee anticipates these policies being facilitated by the authority of regulations promulgated by state boards of nursing, which license nurses and regulate the practice of nursing, and by other state agencies that have authority over the work of nurses and unlicensed NAs.

DESIGN OF WORK PROCESSES AND WORKSPACES

This section reviews the evidence on the design of work processes and workspaces, including the inherent risks to patient safety involved in certain nursing work processes, reduced patient safety due to inefficient nursing work processes, and the effect of the physical design of workspaces on both safety and efficiency. The final section examines how work processes and workspaces can be designed to enhance the safety and efficiency of the direct care provided by nursing staff to patients.

Inherent Risks to Patient Safety in Some Nursing Work Processes

Flaws in work or equipment design, equipment failures, and unanticipated interactions in work processes are recognized threats to safety in a many industries, including health care (Hyman, 1994; Senders, 1994). Medication administration and handwashing are two common nursing activities well documented as involving threats to patient safety.

Medication Administration

Medication administration is a high-frequency activity performed by nurses in every setting of care. It also is associated with great risks to patients. More than 770,000 people annually are estimated to suffer injury or death in hospitals as a result of adverse drug events (ADEs) (Kaushal and Bates, 2001). One study of preventable ADEs in hospitals found that 34 percent of such events occurred in connection with administering the drug (a nursing role), as opposed to ordering, transcribing, or dispensing of the drug (Bates et al., 1995). A 6-month study of all ADEs in two tertiary care hospitals found that 38 percent had resulted from administration by nursing staff (Pepper, 1995). The administration of medications is a complex process involving selecting the correct drug, dose, route, patient, and time, while also remaining alert to prescribing or dispensing errors. Consequently, errors in medication administration are enabled and caused by many factors.

Causes of medication administration errors The increasing numbers of new drugs available for administration are frequently cited as a factor in medication errors (O'Shea, 1999). With increased numbers of drugs for administration comes a concomitant increase in nurses' responsibilities for knowledge of drug action, side effects, and correct dosage. Yet studies have documented that lack of knowledge about medications is a persistent problem—and a cause of ADEs. A systems analysis of ADEs occurring in 11 medical and surgical units in two tertiary care hospitals over a 6-month period found that lack of knowledge about the drug was the most common cause of ADEs among both physicians and nurses. At the level of physician ordering, lack of awareness of drug interactions and correct dosing was the most frequent problem; at the nurse level, during administration of medications, overdosing of anti-emetics, mixing drugs in incompatible solutions, and overly rapid infusion of intravenous drugs were the most common errors (Leape et al., 1995).

Mathematical proficiency is a prerequisite for accurately performing many aspects of medication administration, such as intravenous regulation (Ashby, 1997; Calliari, 1995). Nurses' poor mathematical and drug calculation skills have been linked to medication errors (Bindler and Bayne, 1991; O'Shea, 1999). Yet experts in human factors and ergonomics estimate that humans will normally (under conditions that do not involve any time pressures or stresses) make simple arithmetic errors at a rate of 3 per 100 calculations (Park, 1997). When nurses must calculate drug dosages under conditions of stress or time constraints, it is likely that this error rate will be higher.

Other causes of ADEs include stresses in the environment, including interruptions, fatigue, and overwork; miscommunication, including illegibility of written drug orders; lack of information about the patient; and problems with infusion pumps and IV delivery (Pape, 2001).

Potential remedies   A number of strategies have been proposed to address the above problems, including ongoing in-service education, use of reference material as decision support, and medication administration assistance devices. The Institute for Safe Medication Practices and AHRQ have identified three medication administration technologies (in addition to computerized prescriber order entry at the point of prescribing) as important strategies for reducing medication errors at the point of medication administration by nurses: unit dose dispensing, bar-coding of medications, and use of "smart" infusion pumps.[7]

---

[7]Murray (2001) also examined automated medication dispensing systems—drug storage or cabinet dispensing systems that allow nurses to obtain medications at the point of use (some at the bedside) by electronically dispensing the medications at a specified time and tracking their use. However, Murray found that the "limited number of available, generally poor quality studies does not suggest that automated dispensing devices reduce medication errors." Studies of their use observed: nurses waiting at busy administration times, removal of doses ahead of time to circumvent the waiting periods, and overriding of the device when a dose was needed quickly. The author cites these incidents as examples of "an often-raised point with the introduction of new technologies, namely that the latest innovations are not a solution for inadequate or faulty processes or procedures" (Murray 2001: 114). This caution echoes a warning by the Institute for Safe Medication Practices that health care systems should "not place sole emphasis, resources, or reliance on automation while sacrificing or ignoring other safety initiatives . . . automation alone is not the panacea for medication errors that some believe it to be" (Anonymous, 2000).

• *Unit dose dispensing*—Murray and Shojania (2001) review the evidence associated with "unit dose dispensing"—the practice of having hospital pharmacies dispense medications to nursing stations in individually packaged doses ready to be given to the patient. Unit dose dispensing is common on general medical and surgical hospital units, but less so in intensive care units, operating rooms, and emergency departments. In the latter areas, bulk medication stock systems are still found. In a 1999 survey of hospital pharmacy directors, 80 percent reported that unit dose dispensing was used for 75 percent or more of oral doses and 52 percent of medications for injection. Murray and Shojania (2001: 104-105) conclude that although the evidence for the effectiveness of unit dose dispensing is "modest," studies evaluating the practice are "overall relatively consistent in showing a positive impact on error reduction." The Institute for Safe Medication Practices notes, however, that the unavailability of unit dose packaging by manufacturers is becoming more widespread (Young, 2002). Information on the use of unit dose dispensing in nursing homes was not found.

• *Bar code medication administration*—The Veterans Administration (VA) health system has used a bar code medication administration (BCMA) assistance device in almost all of its medical centers since 1999. This device, consisting of a wireless laptop computer atop a medication cart and a bar code reader, enables nurses to administer and document medications online at the point of administration. The nurse logs on to the BCMA computer, scans the patient's ID bracelet, and brings the patient's medication record up on the screen. The nurse then scans the medication bar code (placed there by the pharmacy) and verifies the patient's identity and medications against active orders. If there are any issues, an alert appears. If not, the nurse administers the medication and documents this on the computer. A comparison of errors committed in 1993 (the last full year of completely manual drug administration) and those committed in 2001 at the VA medical center initiating the project revealed a 86 percent reduction in the overall medication error rate (Johnson et al., 2002). Despite similar findings at other VA facilities and endorsement by the Institute for Safe Medication Practices, a survey conducted by the American Society of Health Systems Pharmacists in 1999 found that only 1.1 percent of U.S. hospitals used bar code technology to scan a patient's ID wristband, nurse's badge, and prescribed drug at the bedside (Young, 2002). To encourage more widespread use of this practice, the U.S. Food and Drug Administration (FDA) proposed a new regulation on March 14, 2003, that would require human drug and blood products to be barcoded. "The proposed rule would not require hospitals to introduce the new automated technologies, but the development of consistent bar codes on pharmaceutical and blood products would greatly encourage hospitals to implement bar code based systems to reduce ADEs associated with medication errors."[8]

- *Smart infusion pumps*—Smart infusion pumps allow hospitals to enter various drug infusion protocols into a drug library with predefined limits. If a dose is programmed outside of established limits or clinical parameters, the pump halts or emits an alarm. Some pumps have the capability of integrating patient monitoring and other patient parameters, such as age or clinical condition. Clinical trials will soon be under way to assess the performance of these devices in reducing medication error rates (Institute for Safe Medication Practices, 2002).

In addition to the above remedies, low-tech strategies, such as decreasing interruptions and distractions, providing standardized protocols, and using checklists for drug administration, have been developed and used in efforts to reduce drug errors (Pape, 2003). Ensuring safe staffing levels (see Chapter 5) and preventing nurse fatigue as described earlier in this chapter can also reasonably be expected to help protect against medication administration errors. Effective redesign of medication administration also depends on the creation of a culture of safety and the establishment of a fair and just error-reporting system that is conducive to the discovery of medication errors (as discussed in Chapter 7).

Handwashing

Absence of handwashing is an example of a health care error of omission—an error that results from the failure to take an action, as opposed to an error of commission accompanying the performance of an action. Errors of omission are usually more difficult to detect than those of commission. However, the prevalence of the absence of handwashing is indicated by the tremendous morbidity, mortality, and health care costs resulting from hospital-acquired infections—found in 7–10 percent of hospitalized patients and causing approximately 80,000 deaths per year (Lautenbach, 2001). Infections are also are the major cause of transfer of nursing home residents to hospitals (CMS, 2002). It is also well established that (1) most hospital-acquired pathogens are transmitted from patient to patient via the hands of health care workers, and (2) handwashing is the simplest and most effective, proven method for reducing the incidence of nosocomial infections. Nevertheless, Lautenbach (2001) presents an array of evidence that handwashing by all health care workers is performed at very low rates. In the 11 studies reviewed, rates of handwashing ranged from 16 to 81 percent; only two studies noted compliance levels above 50 percent.

---

[8]Federal Register, Volume 68, No. 50, Friday March 14, 2003, Proposed Rule. Page 12520.

A number of causes have been identified for low rates of handwashing, some of which are a product of the work environment. Studies indicate that workers with the highest workload are the least likely to wash their hands; lack of time is one of the most commonly cited reasons for failure to wash hands. In a survey of health care workers, 75 percent stated that rewards or punishments would not increase handwashing, but 80 percent said that easy access to sinks and handwashing facilities would. Studies also have indicated that rubbing hands with a small amount of fast-acting antiseptic is more effective and takes less time than traditional soap-and-water handwashing. A recent study comparing alcohol hand rubs with soap-and-water handwashing found that hygienic hand rubs could reduce handwashing time by more than 75 percent Lautenbach (2001). A national stakeholders meeting convened in July 2003 by the U.S. Centers for Disease Control and Prevention (CDC) and the American Hospital Association (AHA) reaffirmed that alcohol-based hand rubs are more effective in reducing bacteria on workers' hands, save workers' time, and are associated with improved adherence to guidelines on handwashing. This stakeholder meeting was convened to identify ways that hospitals can fully use alcohol-based hand rubs and not jeopardize fire safety (CDC, 2003). Some also have suggested that the application of behavior theory and human factors approaches to infection control practices might help achieve sustained increases in handwashing rates (Lautenbach, 2001).

Reduced Patient Safety Due to Inefficient Nurse Work Processes

A number of studies provide evidence that nurses spend a significant portion of their time in activities that are inefficient and decrease the amount of time they have available to monitor patient status, provide therapeutic patient care, and educate patients. In a survey of 50 percent of RNs living in Pennsylvania, 34.3 percent of hospital nurses reported performing housekeeping duties, 42.5 percent delivering and retrieving food trays, and 45.7 percent transporting patients. Of these same nurses, 27.9 percent and 12.7 percent, respectively, reported leaving undone patient/family education and patient/family preparation for discharge (Aiken et al., 2001). When delivery of medications, medical equipment or supplies, blood products, or laboratory specimens is needed for the patient and transport staff are not available, this activity often is carried out by the nurse. Such practices occur frequently (Prescott et al., 1991; Upenieks, 1998). In separate studies comparing the efficiency of two different nurse call systems, 50 to 80 percent of calls were found not to require a response from a licensed nurse (Miller et al., 1997, 2001).

More recently, in a work sampling study involving 239 hours of observation of 26 hospital nurses at nine hospitals with a reputation among industry experts for providing "excellent nursing care," failures in the design or execution of hospital work processes were found to be so common that they were considered virtually routine. The nurses shadowed faced an average of one work design problem per hour in five broad categories of work problems: missing or incorrect information, missing or broken equipment, waiting for a (human or equipment) resource, missing or incorrect supplies, and simultaneous demands on their time. Of the problems observed, 39 percent caused, on average, a 90-minute delay in patient care, including delays in medication, treatment, food, transfer and discharge, laboratory results, and surgery. Numerous patients experienced long waits for transfer and had to have laboratory samples redrawn because earlier samples had been processed incorrectly. Researchers found that on average, 33 minutes was lost per 8-hour shift as a result of coping with work system failures (Tucker and Edmondson, 2002, 2003).

As discussed in earlier chapters, there is strong evidence that documenting patient care and large quantities of paperwork also consume very large amounts of nurses' time.

Documentation and Paperwork

Nurses spend much time documenting patient care activities. Documenting patient care and completing other paperwork to meet facility, insurance, private accreditation, state, and federal requirements, as well as to furnish information needed by other providers, is uniformly cited as imposing a heavy demand on nurses' time in hospitals, nursing homes, home health agencies, and community and public health settings. Estimates from work sampling studies and surveys of nurses within individual hospitals of the amount of time spent in patient care documentation range from 13 to 28 percent (Pabst et al., 1996; Smeltzer et al., 1996; Upenieks, 1998; Urden and Roode, 1997), although this proportion has also been shown to differ across shifts (Korst et al., 2003; Scharf, 1997). In a study in which the average time nurses spent in documentation was found to be 15.8 percent, day shift nurses spent 19.7 percent, while night shift nurses spent 12.4 percent (Korst et al., 2003). Completion of all required paperwork is cited as one reason nurses work overtime (see Chapter 5). As discussed earlier, because it cannot be accomplished in an 8-hour shift, it becomes a sort of "unofficial" mandatory overtime (Trossman, 2001).

Home care nurses are estimated to spend a much greater proportion of their time in documenting care. Although no work sampling studies of time spent in documentation among home health nurses were located, some have estimated that these nurses spend twice as much time in documenting patient care as do hospital nurses, in part because of more prescriptive federal regulatory requirements for documentation in home health care than in hospital care (Trossman, 2001).

In addition to being time-consuming, required documentation is often redundant and irrelevant. Documentation redesign initiatives undertaken internally by hospitals have found an excess number of forms and duplication of patient information, such as vital statistics and allergies, in multiple locations throughout patients' charts (Brunt et al., 1999). Moreover, in some HCOs, both nurses and other health professionals state that they rarely read nurses' notes (Brooks, 1998; Brunt et al., 1999).

Multiple sources of demands for documentation and paperwork. The types of required documentation performed by nurses vary. Some may be characterized as "administrative," that is, not treatment-specific (e.g., documentation of advance directives, permission for release of information, informing patients of their rights). Other documentation pertains to nursing care and typically includes patient care plans; progress notes, flow charts, and shift-to-shift documentation or reports; medication administration and treatment records; patient education; admission, discharge, and transfer notes; justification for use of restraints; and patient classification systems (Butler and Bender, 1999; Smeltzer et al., 1996). Nurses in particular settings must also complete setting-specific documentation. For example, home health care nurses utilize CMS' Outcome and Assessment Information Set (OASIS)—a dataset sometimes more than 50 items long that is used in patient assessment. Nursing home nurses must complete CMS' Minimum Data Set (MDS). Finally, nurses sometimes practice lengthy narrative charting as a defense against potential litigation and as a way to document professional practice. "If it isn't charted, it didn't happen," is a well known nursing maxim (Trossman, 2001).

Internal and external solutions are needed. Because documentation demands arise from sources both internal and external to the HCO, strategies for reducing the documentation burden have been undertaken by both HCOs and external parties. Some HCOs have successfully employed work redesign and automation to reduce documentation demands.

With regard to *work redesign*, HCOs have reduced the amount of time nurses spend in documentation activities by eliminating documentation of the same information in multiple locations by multiple clinicians (Brunt et al., 1999; Zerwekh et al., 2000) and by using graphs, flow charts, and clinical algorithms or pathways to minimize the need for more time-consuming narrative notes (Bridgeman et al., 1997; Brunt et al., 1999). Efficient documentation practices also have been achieved by using "exception-based charting," which focuses attention on abnormal or significant findings rather than on documentation of normal findings (Blachly and Young, 1998; Murphy et al., 1988). Exception-based charting does not ignore normal findings; rather, it allows a notation (e.g., a check mark or caregiver initials) that care was provided in accordance with certain hospital-adopted standards of care, such as those found in clinical pathways. Narrative or more detailed notes are written when care and responses deviate from the expected:

> For example, nurses formerly were asked to file an IV site check . . . every hour to "prove" that hourly checks were performed. Such documentation was mechanistic and was often entered all at once at the end of the shift. It did nothing to improve quality of care and provided no advantage. The new [charting by exception] approach allows the nurse to chart once, verifying the IV site was checked hourly . . . (LaDuke, 2001: 285).

Exception-based charting is used more often in acute care settings than in long-term care (Blachly and Young, 1998). In both settings, it is associated with reducing the amount of time nurses spend in documenting care (Blachly and Young, 1998; Stephens and Mason, 1999; Wroblewski and Werrbach, 1999).

Some of the most effective strategies for achieving more-efficient documentation result from multidisciplinary documentation redesign initiatives (Brunt et al., 1999; Mosher et al., 1996; Smeltzer et al., 1996). For example, an interdisciplinary documentation work redesign and performance improvement initiative undertaken by Summa Health System in Akron, Ohio, found at baseline an excess number of forms, duplication of information throughout patient charts, poor use of data and information across disciplines, and large amounts of nursing time dedicated to patient care documentation. After a broad-based interdisciplinary initiative examining the processes and information flow needed to support interdisciplinary practice, Summa reengineered its patient care documentation processes.

Among the positive results of this initiative were the elimination of 80 forms; a decrease in multiple data entry (e.g., allergies were documented in 15 places prior to the redesign and in 2 places following the redesign; diagnoses were listed in 16 versus 4 places); and a decrease in the amount of time nurses spent in documentation from baseline survey reports of 25–40 percent to postimplementation survey reports of 10–20 percent. All these results were achieved by redesigning manual documentation processes; automated documentation was defined as a future goal (Brunt et al., 1999).

With regard to the use of *automation*, evidence exists that automated computer-based data entry, *if carefully designed*, can reduce the time required for documentation (Pabst et al., 1996), improve the quality of documentation (Nahm and Poston, 2000), or both. Some organizations have achieved cost savings as well (Baldwin, 1998; Weiss and Hailstone, 1993;

White and Hemby, 1997), sometimes through decreased use of overtime (Allan and Englebright, 2000; Smith et al., 1998). However, automation alone—without efficient underlying documentation processes and careful design of applications—will not always achieve these results (Allan and Englebright, 2000; Larrabee et al., 2001), as one hospital's efforts illustrate:

> Nurses complained about the length of time it now took them to document. They felt they were charting information that no one was reviewing or that was clinically irrelevant. Many of their complaints focused on the way the software worked, as opposed to the way it had been individualized by the facility. Frustration with . . . the number of screens that had to be traversed to enter the simplest data were often voiced. To reduce aggravation and documentation time, many nurses completely bypassed the structure provided by the care plan and wrote an electronic narrative note. Thus was lost much of the benefit of putting documentation online: clinical information systems do not have the sophistication to analyze a narrative note in a meaningful way.
>
> Physicians were unhappy with the new nursing documentation . . . the medical staff simply could not find the information they wanted. . . .
>
> Medical records staff observed that the nursing documentation, when printed, was many pages long but did not offer a clear picture of the patient . . .
>
> Eventually it was decided that the documentation structure . . . should be revisited . . . (LaDuke, 2001: 284)

As the above case illustrates, carefully reviewing documentation requirements in combination with automating information input and access increases the likelihood of decreasing the time required for documentation while maintaining, if not improving, patient care documentation (Allan and Englebright, 2000; Butler and Bender, 1999). Successful automation initiatives also are associated with the use of computerized patient records (Clayton et al., 2003; Walker and Prophet, 1997).

As noted earlier, however, internal efforts by HCOs alone are not likely to maximize documentation efficiency and utility because many documentation demands are imposed by external entities, including regulators and payors. In recognition of this fact, in 2001 the Joint Commission on Accreditation of Healthcare Organizations (JCAHO) convened a 20-member task force of hospital leaders, clinicians, and other experts to conduct an in-depth review of its hospital standards and requirements for demonstrating compliance. The task force's recommendations for streamlining standards and standards compliance requirements are scheduled to be formally implemented on January 1, 2004 (JCAHO, 2002). Similar actions by governmental regulators could be useful in decreasing the documentation burden on nurses, as several governmentally mandated reporting tools (e.g., OASIS) have been cited by nurses as requiring large amounts of time and not enabling adaptation to individual patient needs (Trossman, 2001).

Finally, nurses are also influenced by practices learned as a part of professional education and training. Yet documentation practices used to demonstrate critical thinking skills and knowledge to a preceptor may not always be necessary for effective documentation in clinical practice. Moreover, as noted above, some nurses practice detailed documentation as a proactive defense against litigation (Fiesta, 1993).

Effect of the Physical Design of Workspace on Efficiency and Safety[9]

The physical features of inpatient facilities can obstruct efficient nursing work and diminish patient safety. Poor layout of patient care units and patient rooms and poor design and deployment of communication technologies reduce the amount of time nurses have available to monitor patient status and provide direct care. The increasing practice of transferring patients to different care units also presents opportunities for inefficiencies, gaps in care, and care errors.

Design of Patient Care Units

The majority of hospital in-patient care is delivered on patient care units (also called "nursing units"), where patients are grouped according to age, diagnosis, or clinical condition (e.g., medical, surgical, pediatric, oncology, intensive care, or cardiology). Smaller community hospitals may have less specialization of patient care units and group more diverse populations into fewer units to respond to fluctuations in census. Although nursing units account for less than half of the total area of most hospital buildings, their size and shape still dictate the overall design of the entire structure.

Nursing units possess three to four distinct spaces: the patient space, the nursing station(s), the "core" space, and the hallway. The design and location of these spaces, the location and storage of equipment, the relationships of the patient rooms to the various supplies, the materials used, and the technology required to deliver care vary greatly from hospital to hospital:

- *Patient rooms*—Patient rooms can be private or semiprivate. In some cases, "semi-private" can mean as many as four to six beds in one large room. In the last 10 years, in response to growing inpatient acuity and

---

[9]This section incorporates content from a paper commissioned by the committee on "Evidence-based Design of Nursing Workspace in Hospitals," written by Ann Hendrich, Ascension Health and Nelson Lee, Rapid Modeling, Inc., Cincinnati, Ohio (March 24, 2003).

scarcity of critical care beds, these four- to six-bed rooms increasingly have been used as "progressive care" rooms for patients with a level of acuity between critical care and medical–surgical to enable better nursing observation. Patient room assignment is guided by the sex of the patient, the presence or absence of an infectious process, and (when possible) patient preference. These factors can greatly decrease the efficiency of patient placement and nurse staffing in any hospital when the right "type" of room has to be located for a specific type of patient. Moreover, features of patient rooms can directly affect patient safety. For example, the majority of falls of hospitalized patients occur in the patient's room, usually in association with elimination needs (Hendrich et al., 1995, 2003).

• *Nursing station*—The nursing station is the hub of the nursing unit for both simple and complex communications in a multitude of care delivery processes. Some refer to it as the "so-called" nursing station, noting that it has become the location for the unit secretary as well as all health professionals who spend any time on the patient care unit, including physicians, pharmacists, respiratory therapists, physical therapists, dieticians, social workers, and pastoral care staff (Hamilton, 1999). The nursing station also is the point where nurses take and receive patient orders on paper or by phones; answer or initiate phone calls and pages; receive faxed reports; view orders and reported results (e.g., laboratory, x-ray); pick up stat pharmacy deliveries; document the care process; and collaborate and socialize with other nurses, physicians, and allied health care workers. The resultant milieu can be a chaotic work environment that introduces environmental factors, including high noise levels and simultaneous conversations, conducive to human errors. The most familiar nursing unit design has a centralized nursing station.

• *Core unit space*—The core of a nursing unit, sometimes referred to as the "nursing space," often consists of clean and dirty utility rooms (equipment/instruments); medication, treatment, and supply rooms; a pantry for food and beverages; staff lounge/locker space; medical equipment storage; a housekeeping closet; and staff and/or patient conference room(s).

• *Hallway*—The hallway of a nursing unit is the necessary space between patient rooms and the nursing station and core unit. The hallway represents the total distance the nurse must travel between spaces, and it is heavily influenced by the size and class of patient rooms (private/semiprivate). The location of the patient rooms, nursing station, and core unit space relative to this hallway is critical to the overall time and distance nurses must travel to deliver patient care. Because of a lack of adequate storage space, medication carts, wheelchairs, isolation carts, and dietary carts are often found in the hallway, blocking travel for both patients and caregivers and introducing safety hazards (falls, fire, public access to medications and supplies) in the environment.

Nursing units have varying geometric designs (Bobrow, 1978; Bobrow and Thomas, 2000; Cox and Groves, 1990; Hamilton, 1990; James and Tatton-Brown, 1986). The most common designs are as follows:

- *Simple open or nightingale form*—Consists of an open ward without individual patient rooms. Patient beds face inward toward a single walkway, with a nursing station located in the middle; support spaces (e.g., supplies) are located off the unit. Some trauma or cardiovascular intensive care units are still configured as open wards for high-acuity surgical patients. Critical-care unit shapes (e.g., circular, linear, horseshoe, triangle) have been developed on the premise that every patient should be observable from a central nursing station (Hamilton, 1999).
- *Corridor or continental form*—Patients are located on one or both sides of a corridor with four to six beds in a room, for a total of up to 30 beds (can be in a "T", "C", or "L" shape).
- *Duplex or nuffield*—Has Corridor characteristics, but is split into two sections containing up to 20 beds each. Each section has its own nursing station. Nursing and ancillary space is shared between the two sections.
- *Racetrack or double corridor*—Patient rooms are farther apart, with support spaces between the two corridors. Cross-over hallways connect the two corridors at the ends and complete the loop or "racetrack." This design can require that nurses spend much of their time traveling, since it utilizes only one clean and dirty utility room and a single nursing station. Travel distance from the nursing station to the utility room to the patient is very high, and visualization of the corridors is poor. A modified version of this unit design is one of the most common types found in acute care hospitals.
- *Courtyard*—Sometimes referred to a "complicated racetrack," this design has an open courtyard for ventilation in the middle of the unit (used in Europe in hospitals without air conditioning). The design creates a need for additional nursing stations with increased travel distances.
- *Cruciform or cluster*—A modern Corridor ward plan that has more barriers, walls, doors, and toilets erected between the nursing station and patients. The shape is manipulated to group as many patients as possible around the nursing station and increase patient privacy.
- *Radial*—A circle design that permits a "fishbowl" view of each patient room from the nursing station. Observation is maximized in a central location.
- *Triangle*—The space in the middle of the triangle balances the support space and the number of beds (usually around 30 beds). Unlike the racetrack, this design attempts to minimize nursing travel distance.

Hybrids of these designs are created by varying their corners and lines.

Each of the above nursing unit designs has advantages and disadvantages depending on which single perspective is considered—the patient, the caregiver, or the hospital. Open ward or "fishbowl' designs can maximize observation and staffing efficiencies, yet a patient's privacy can be greatly decreased (Hamilton, 1999). The racetrack design can maximize the number of beds on a unit but significantly increase nurse travel times. The triangle can provide less travel distance but greatly reduces available square footage in the patient's room, and affects family space and patient–family interaction.

A 1994–1996 time and motion study of more than 1,000 hours of nursing unit time on a medical–surgical unit in a comprehensive tertiary care hospital over an 18-month time period documented how nurses and other health care workers spend their time and provided insight into how the environmental design of the nursing unit can affect nursing workload (Hendrich and Lee, 2003a). Four cameras were installed to capture all nursing unit activities simultaneously in patient rooms, the nursing hallway, and the nursing station. A total of 978 hours was accepted into the study, with 3,690 events being measured in the patient rooms. In addition, a random 24-hour continuous sample of all activities in the nursing station was taken from the 978 hours. The analysis tracked excess motion, inefficiencies, health care worker patterns, ergonomics, workspace organization, safety, and how nurses spent their time. The study found that:

- The total time all health care workers (not just nurses) spent in patient rooms on direct care and assessments ranged from only 1.1 to 3.3 hours (median 1.7) in a 12-hour period.
- The majority of the nurses' time was spent walking between the patient rooms and the nursing unit core, or in the nursing station.

Patient Transfers

The transfer or hand-off of patients from nurse to nurse, shift to shift, unit to unit, and HCO to HCO has also been identified as a potential source of errors and adverse patient events (Cook et al., 2000). These transfers create opportunities for gaps in the continuity of patient care through loss of information or interruptions in the care delivery. Most of these gaps in care are anticipated and addressed by the health care system through such mechanisms as shift-to-shift-reports by nurses, patient care planning and discharge instructions, and discharge summaries. When gaps are unanticipated or not well bridged or when events or conditions overwhelm usually effective bridging mechanisms, patient safety is threatened. Patient hand-offs also result in duplication of effort and waste.

Interunit patient transfers within acute care hospitals in particular are associated with risks to patients and require a significant amount of direct and indirect labor. Such transfers originated with the creation of the first coronary care units in the 1960s and the specialized intensive care units (e.g., neonatal, medical, and surgical) that followed. These higher levels of specialized care created the need to transfer patients to higher- or lower-acuity care units as their clinical condition worsened or improved (Gallant and Lanning, 2001). The number of transfers increased even more with the creation of progressive, step-down, or transition units, which offer an intensity of nursing service between that of an intensive care and a general medical–surgical unit. Thus, it is not unusual to see a patient cared for by five different nursing units—e.g., operating room, postanesthesia care unit, critical care unit, step-down unit, and general–medical surgical unit—during his or her hospital stay. Transferring patients to units with higher staffing levels and greater experience in caring for critically ill individuals offers advantages for the clinical care of patients, but the unintended consequences of these patient transfers are also worthy of study. For example, this increasing specialization of nursing units and the resulting increase in interunit patient transfers introduces disruption in patient care and creates patient flow bottlenecks due to waits and delays in bed assignments.

A 13-month (2000–2001) observational study of 200 patient transfers within a 500-bed tertiary-level hospital tracked time and tasks for each patient transfer between units (other types of transports to procedures or testing off the unit were not included) (Hendrich and Lee, 2003b). Each transport was observed in an effort to collect valid and reliable measures of the time and activities necessary for health care workers to move patients between nursing units. Among the study findings were the following:

- The average elapsed time from the point at which the physician wrote a patient transfer order until the patient arrived in a new bed on another nursing unit was 306 minutes (5.1 hours), with a median of 250 minutes (4.16 hours).
- The actual measured *direct* labor cost (based on the number of caregivers, their job class, and their hourly wage times the number of minutes involved in transport activity) was $35.17 an hour. (Subsequent nursing wage increases will increase this actual cost significantly).
- Additional indirect hospital costs associated with patient transfers included lost nursing productivity, the cost of equipment required for transport, duplication and rework of the patient care process (documentation, forms, and assessments), errors, omissions or events that occurred as a result of the transfer, and laundry/linen and housekeeping expenses.
- Patient length of stay was estimated to increase up to half a day for each transfer due to disruptions in the care process.

Other patient transfers occur between patient rooms in the same unit—sometimes for infection-control purposes, and at other times because of difficulties between roommates in semiprivate rooms. In a new 348-bed facility built by Bronson Methodist Hospital in Kalamazoo, Michigan, savings of about $500,000 per year were noted as a result of the use of all private rooms and not having to transfer patients because of infection control or roommate problems (Rich, 2002).

Other new technologies or work design strategies can create unintended gaps in care. Cook et al. (2000: 792) cite the use of "patient care technicians" as an example of how new work design can actually create new opportunities for error:

> . . . consider the effects of dividing nursing work between nurses and "patient care technicians." The economic benefits of division are substantial: it allows the nurse to spend virtually the entire work shift concentrating on high level tasks that require certain credentials (giving intravenous drugs, for example) while other tasks are given to less skilled personnel. Among the side effects of such a change, however, are restrictions on the ability of the individual nurse to anticipate and detect gaps in the care of the patient. The nurse now has more patients to track, requiring more (and more complicated) inferences about which patient will next require attention, where monitoring needs to be more intensive, and so forth.

All of these patient hand-offs create opportunities for gaps in care, as well as the need for re-work and waste.

Poor Communication Technology

Nursing staff spend a great deal of time hunting down other nurses, physicians, and patient information. One hospital work sampling study of nurses across all hospital inpatient units found that nurses spent 10 percent of their time in patient-related communication. The major problem faced by these nurses was "looking for someone down the long halls to relay a message" (Linden and English, 1994). In a study of communication systems in a 56-bed neurological unit at a Midwest hospital, nurses estimated that they spent 25 percent of their time looking for another person, for example, the nurse with the narcotic keys or staff needed to help turn or transfer a patient or help with procedures (Miller et al., 1997).

Redesign of inefficient nurse call systems has been identified as an opportunity to decrease the amount of "non-value-added" time that nurses spend handling calls that do not require a response from a licensed nurse or responding to mistaken calls (i.e., the patient turned on the nurse call light by mistake). A study of nursing units at two large metropolitan hospitals found that almost 70 percent of nurse calls did not require a licensed nurse to meet the patient's needs (Miller et al., 1997). Design features to make nurse call systems more efficient and effective that have been identified by nurses include providing higher-quality audio, using medical secretaries to serve as the first responder and "triage" calls not requiring the assistance of a nurse, allowing nurse call lights to be turned off at the nursing station instead of requiring someone to go into the patient's room for the purpose, providing room-to-room communication, using such devices as locator badges to locate needed personnel, and enabling hands-free operation of the system (Miller et al., 1997, 2001).

Providing the capability for computerized physician order entry and making patient education material available electronically to nurses also have been identified as strategies to facilitate communication. With computerized physician order entry, nurses do not have to engage in transcription or verification of orders. Electronic patient education materials, unlike printed materials, are easily modifiable to meet clinician and patient needs; it is also possible to track which materials were given and by whom, assess follow-up and comprehension, and link education activities and documentation (Case et al., 2002).

Sensory Interference

Sensory distractions and interference, such as noise, poor lighting, glare-producing surfaces, and clutter, can interfere with nurses' work (Spath, 2000). Some hospitals further report that creating calming, "healing environments" through such design features as softer colors and indirect lighting has decreased patients' use of pain medications and saved hospitalization costs (Rich, 2002).

Noise is recognized as a serious health hazard to hospital patients, but it is also recognized as interfering with worker performance. While most studies of the effects of noise in the work environment have been conducted in non–health care settings, the contribution of noise levels to nurse stress and work distractions is increasingly being documented (Morrison et al., 2003; Topf, 2000). In health care facilities, sources of noise can range from overhead paging systems and equipment alarms to heating, ventilation, and air-conditioning (HVAC) systems, plumbing, and ice machines. Reducing noise by installing materials that absorb sound, such as ceiling and wall materials and carpeting, can be accomplished at modest cost (Walsh-Sukys et al., 2001).

Noise and other sensory interference can be reduced by employing activities, tools, and principles developed by a number of different disciplines, including human factors, ergonomics, and engineering—many of which are already being used by some HCOs. New construction projects especially—whether a new building or an expansion or renovation of existing space—

present opportunities to improve workspace and work design. The effect of these and other design characteristics of nursing workspaces (and other aspects of health care facility design) on patient outcomes and facility performance are being studied under a research project (The Pebble Project) sponsored by The Center for Health Design, a nonprofit research and advocacy organization, and a network of 11 health care providers (The Center for Health Design, 2003a). Among the preliminary findings reported by the project are decreases in patient transfers, nosocomial infections, patient falls, medication usage, and medical errors (The Center for Health Design, 2003b).

Designing Work Processes and Workspaces to Enhance Safety and Efficiency

The Work Design Process[10]

Work design involves examining the various elements or factors that workers use, encounter, and experience in performing their work. In addition to the characteristics of the workers themselves, the elements considered include the nature of the task to be performed; the tools and technologies available for use; the physical environment in which the work is to be carried out (e.g., noise level, lighting, space, sources of distractions and interruptions); and organizational conditions, such as the level of communication and collaboration among the individual(s) who perform or use the work. These five elements are described as a work system because they interact with and influence each other. In examining these elements, questions such as the following are addressed:

• What are the characteristics of the *individual* performing the work? Does the individual have the musculoskeletal, sensory, and cognitive abilities to do the required task? If not, can any of these gaps in ability be accommodated in the design of the task?

• What *tasks* are being performed, and what characteristics of those tasks may contribute to unsafe patient care? What in the nature of the tasks allows the individual to perform them safely or assume risks in the process?

• What *tools and technologies* are being used to perform the tasks, and do they increase or decrease the likelihood of untoward events?

---

[10]This section incorporates content from a paper commissioned by the committee on "Reducing Workload and Increasing Patient Safety Through Work and Workspace Design," prepared by Pascale Carayon, Ph.D.; Carla Alvarado, Ph.D.; and Ann Schoofs Hundt, Ph.D. All are with the Center for Quality and Productivity Improvement, Department of Industrial Engineering, University of Wisconsin-Madison.

- What aspects of the *physical environment* can be sources of error or promote safety? What in the physical environment ensures safe behavior or allows room for unsafe behavior?
- What in the *organization* prevents or allows exposure to hazard, and what promotes or hinders patient safety? What allows for assuming safe or unsafe behavior by the individual?

Because of their interrelatedness, work design needs to consider all these elements. Whenever one work element changes, there will be implications for the other elements (Carayon et al., 2003).

Work design is performed by collecting and analyzing data and information such as that listed above on the task or problem area, synthesizing the information, developing a proposed plan, and evaluating the plan once it has been implemented. Various approaches can be used to collect and analyze data and information: direct measurement, observation, surveys, interviews, review of organizational documents (e.g., position descriptions, organization chart), and analysis of archival data (e.g., patient satisfaction data, error reporting systems). Because each of these approaches has both weaknesses and strengths, multiple approaches provide the greatest confidence in the results obtained.

Several work and error analysis techniques also have been developed that can help individuals involved in work redesign initiatives discover more fully all contributing causes of adverse patient events, especially the latent conditions that contribute to the occurrence of such events.[11] Three commonly used work redesign techniques are work sampling, root-cause analysis, and anticipatory failure analysis. Methods for achieving "LEAN" operations (defined below), widely used in other industries, are also beginning to be applied to work and workspace design in HCOs. These techniques are each discussed below.

Work and Error Analysis Techniques

Work sampling In work sampling studies, workers are observed a specified number of times at random or fixed intervals. For each observation, data are recorded on the task being performed (Carayon et al., 2003). Work sampling has been used to obtain insights into how nursing staff use their time, identify problem areas, and provide information for unit and work redesign (Linden and English, 1994; Pedersen, 1997; Scherubel and Minnick, 1994; Upenieks, 1998; Urden and Roode, 1997). However, work

---

[11]As discussed in Chapter 1, latent conditions are usually less visible at the time an error occurs.

sampling studies are limited in their power to accurately reflect all of nurses' work (Carayon et al., 2003) because the method assumes that the tasks involved are observable, unambiguous, mutually exclusive, and exhaustive—not always the case with much of nursing work.

Root-cause analysis   Root-cause analysis has long been used in engineering to examine organizational or system problems. It is a retrospective, qualitative process aimed at uncovering the underlying cause(s) of an error by looking past the "sharp end" of an error (see Chapter 1) to the enabling latent conditions that contributed to or enabled the occurrence of the error. Root-cause analysis involves a cycle of questions: What happened? Why did it happen? What were the most proximate factors causing it to happen? Why did those factors occur? and What systems and processes underlie those proximate factors? Answers to these questions help identify barriers and causes of problems so similar problems can be prevented in the future.

JCAHO requires that health care organizations perform root-cause analysis in response to all sentinel events. JCAHO also requires that HCOs, based on the results of this root-cause analysis, develop and implement an action plan consisting of improvements designed to reduce risk and monitor the effectiveness of those improvements (JCAHO, 2003). Wald and Shojania (2001) note that root-cause analysis is a labor-intensive process, and that there is not yet evidence that by itself it can improve patient safety. However, they also observe that the technique provides HCOs with a formal structure for learning from past mistakes.

Anticipatory failure analysis   While root-cause analysis is performed in response to an adverse event that has already occurred, anticipatory failure analysis is used to identify and eliminate known and/or potential failures, problems, and errors from a system, design, process, and/or service *before* they occur. Failure modes and effects analysis (FMEA) is one technique used to conduct this type of analysis. Its goal is to prevent errors from occurring by attempting to identify all of the ways a device or process can fail, estimate the probability and consequence of each failure, and then take action to prevent the potential failures from occurring. Failure modes and effects analysis is typically conducted by multidisciplinary teams in an HCO on many different patient care processes, including device design. It is used to assess both existing and new products and processes (Carayon et al., 2003).

"LEAN" operations   Root-cause analysis and anticipatory failure analysis are typically used to help nurses perform desirable, "value-added" nursing activities, such as medication administration, documentation, and patient monitoring, more efficiently or safely. LEAN operation techniques address not the enhancement of desirable, value-added activities, but the elimination of undesirable, often invisible activities—the waste inherent in

all work processes—through continuous improvement in pursuit of perfection (Alukal, 2003). The term is used in this country to refer to techniques pioneered in the Toyota Production System (described in Chapter 4), which are well known to most industrial engineers.

LEAN thinking is based on the premise that all processes are composed of value-added and non–value-added activities and time. In a hospital environment, value-added represents any activity that increases the health, healing, wellness, and satisfaction of the patient. These are activities that are patient-centric, timely, and not wasteful. Non–value-added activities are those that do not increase the health, wellness, and satisfaction of the patient, and thus should be eliminated, simplified, or reduced.

In attempts to increase efficiency and the quality of their products, most organizations typically focus on value-added activities and core competencies. Traditionally, very little consideration is given to the non–value-added activities that occur throughout the organization. The result is that the root causes of waste and inefficiency that result in poor performance are often nurtured by the organization and institutionalized in policies and procedures. LEAN techniques attempt to eliminate sources of waste through the use of such practices as the following:

- **Visual controls**—keeping work processes and indicators in view so everyone can understand the status of the work system at a glance.
- **Streamlined physical plant layout**—designing facility layout to optimize the sequencing of work processes.
- **Standardized work**—using prescribed methods to perform routine tasks.
- **Point-of-use storage**—locating supplies, equipment, information, and procedure rules where they will be used, thus saving the time otherwise involved in locating and obtaining them.

The Toyota Production System identifies seven categories of waste attributable to a manufacturing facility. A brief summary of those seven categories, modified for the hospital environment and design of nursing workspace, is shown in Table 6-1 (Hendrich and Lee, 2003c). LEAN techniques and other work analysis approaches (e.g., total quality management, continuous quality improvement, and six sigma DMAIC [define, measure, analyze, improvement control]) are not mutually exclusive. Rather, they are complementary and can be used together (Alukal, 2003; Smith, 2003).

Work design principles Regardless of the resources, approaches, and sources of expertise an HCO is able to bring to bear on a specific work design effort, principles for effective and safe work design have been identified that can guide all work (re)design initiatives. These principles, detailed

TABLE 6-1   Seven Categories of Waste as Applied to the Hospital Environment

Category	Root Causes of Hospital Waste
Poor Utilization of Resources	People, resources, and supplies are deployed or stored in the hospital at the wrong place, at the wrong time, and in the wrong quantities. Time must be spent in locating and obtaining those items needed to provide care.
Excess Motion	Poorly designed workspaces and units, process complexity, and discontinuous processes contribute to excess caregiver motion in the workspace, patient room, and/or nursing hallway.
Unnecessary Waiting	Delays involving patients, nurses, and resources are caused by process complexity and interdependency, poor execution, organizational misalignment, and inaccessible information. Nurses must wait to provide care because necessary personnel, supplies, authorizations, or patients are not where they need to be.
Transportation	Movement of resources and inventory is inefficient because of policy and process inefficiencies, intra-unit patient transfers, and inefficient layout and unit organization.
Process Inefficiency	Unnecessary steps in the patient care process, poor execution, and unplanned interruptions take health care workers away from the patient.
Excess Inventory	More supplies and inventory are on hand than are needed, creating waste. This includes waste of nursing personnel when, for example, nurses are called in to work, but then sent home because of low census.
Defects/Quality Control	Mistakes, omissions, and accidents are caused by distractions, discontinuous processes, and nonconformance or lack of standardization.

in the following subsections, aim to create reliable and safe patient care processes by:

- *Eliminating errors*—changing work processes so errors cannot be made. While the total elimination of all errors is impossible, work design principles should aim to continuously eliminate errors consistent with principles of continuous quality improvement, the defect-free goals of the Toyota Production System described in Chapter 4, six sigma DMAIC approaches to error reduction, and other improvement approaches that have "zero errors" as their goal.
- *Reducing error occurrence*—redesigning processes so that errors are less likely.

- *Detecting errors early*—catching errors early before patient harm occurs.
- *Containing the effects of errors*—designing features to mitigate the consequences of errors once they occur (Spath, 2000).

Directly involving workers throughout the design process   The workers who currently perform the activity to be redesigned or will perform a new activity are the users, beneficiaries, and consumers of work design. Therefore, their active participation in all aspects and stages of work (re)design is essential. *Active* participation, in which employees are directly involved in the work redesign activity, is distinguished from *passive* participation, whereby the organization communicates with employees regarding the work redesign (Carayon et al., 2003). As discussed in Chapter 4, employee participation is a key ingredient in successful organizational change, improving the outcome of work (re)design, and facilitating its successful implementation. Benefits include more thorough diagnosis of and formulation of solutions for problems and more rapid implementation of technological and organizational change, as well as increased employee motivation, job satisfaction, and performance (Lawler, 1986; Noro and Imada, 1991; Wilson and Haines, 1997).

Nursing units are organized in a variety of ways, reflecting different decision-making, work allocation, communication, and management approaches (Kovner, 2001). Resources and work processes also differ on nursing units, as do patient levels of care and the experience level of nurses (Deutschendorf, 2003). Evidence does not yet exist for identifying any one best model for providing nursing care (Seago, 2001). A unit with highly experienced RNs may need a different structure from one with novice nurses. As the nature of nurses' work changes, new models will need to be developed and deployed (Kimball and O'Neil, 2002). Thus work processes need to be designed with consideration of unit-specific structures and processes (Deutschendorf, 2003), something that is best accomplished through the active involvement of nursing unit staff.

Simplifying and standardizing common work procedures and equipment   Simplifying key work processes can greatly reduce the likelihood of error and facilitate the formulation of solutions when problems occur (IOM, 2000). Standardizing processes reduces the need for workers to rely on memory and allows new workers unfamiliar with a procedure or device to employ it safely. The increasing use of clinical pathways in many hospitals (see Chapter 5) is an example of standardizing patient care to reduce variation in practice and opportunities for error. Simplifying and standardizing routine procedures, such as IV insertion, catheter insertion, dressing changes, care for decubiti, tracheotomy care, and other nursing treatments and procedures, minimizes opportunities for slips and lapses.[12] Standardization also can be used for both facility and room design (e.g., location of electrical outlets, bed controls, and equipment cupboards), medical equipment (e.g., IV pumps, hand disinfection products, and sinks), and location of monitors and other equipment. Standardization of patient care environments and equipment decreases the cognitive load on nurses, making slips and lapses less likely to occur during routine tasks by minimizing decision time and manipulation time.

Avoiding reliance on individual worker memory Given the enormous and expanding body of health care knowledge, and the great variation in patients' health status and needs, as well as the very nature of the human condition, individual nurses cannot be expected to retain all the information necessary to provide state-of-the-science health care. Both automated and hard-copy memory aides, such as procedure checklists and protocols, clinical pathways, drug reference databases, and computerized decision aids, can help compensate for the limitations of human memory (Spath, 2000).

Decreasing interruptions, distractions, and interferences An interruption has been defined as the cessation of a task before its completion as the result of any external factor, and a distraction as an external stimulus causing a human response but not cessation of a task (Flynn et al., 1999). Interference denotes competition for the cognitive resources required for the performance of simultaneous tasks, which often occurs in busy work settings. Errors attributed to interference appear to be more likely with novel or difficult tasks (Dornheim, 2000).

Most evaluations of the effects of interruptions, distractions, and interference on human performance have been conducted in industries other than health care. These factors have been found to be important contributors to nearly one-half of significant aviation flight crew incidents (Dornheim, 2000). When health professionals have been asked to report their perceptions of why medical errors occur, interruptions and distractions have frequently been cited (Ely et al., 1995).

Nurses frequently cite distractions and interruptions as contributing to their commission of medication errors (Wakefield et al., 1998; Walters, 1992). Interruptions and interference are also reported by nurses in nursing

---

[12]"Slips" and "lapses" denote two different types of errors humans make. Slips are observable actions an individual did not intend to take (e.g., slips of the tongue, slips of the pen, slips of surgical techniques). Lapses are generally unobservable errors, such as failures of memory, that are not manifest in the behaviors of an individual and are generally apparent only to the person committing the lapse (Reason, 1990).

homes as occurring frequently and requiring them to repeatedly revise plans, alter directions, and cease activities prior to completion (Bowers et al., 2001). In a random sample survey of nurses licensed to work in Illinois and North Carolina, conducted as part of a longitudinal study of nurses' worklife and health funded by the National Institute for Occupational Safety and Health (NIOSH) of the U.S. Centers for Disease Control and Prevention (CDC), 75 percent of the 674 RN respondents who were currently employed as a full-time hospital or nursing home general-duty/staff nurse agreed or agreed strongly that "my job requires long periods of intense concentration"; 82 percent similarly agreed that "I work very fast"; and 79.6 percent agreed that "tasks are often interrupted without being completed."[13]

Studies of crew resource management in aviation provide insight into how to limit the effects of interruptions and distractions in that setting (Dismukes et al., 1998). Similar strategies have been employed for evaluating errors in operating rooms (Cooper et al., 1984). However, strategies for reducing interruptions and distractions in nursing settings have not been well developed. A quasi-experimental study of two interventions in a medical–surgical unit (an active avoidance protocol for staff and wearing of a color-coded vest with a warning to avoid interrupting a nurse who is administering medications) found that interruptions and distractions could be significantly reduced (Pape, 2003). Other strategies include closing the patient's door while conducting bedside care and using manual or electronic message boards to convey nonurgent requests.

Instilling redundancy and back-up systems   High-reliability organizations and other safety-conscious organizations design redundancy into their production processes to ensure that there are several ways to identify problems before they become catastrophic. For example, the control tower of a navy aircraft carrier, which is responsible for all activity on the flight deck and hangar, uses more than 20 devices to ensure communication with critical parts of the ship. The landing signal officer on the flight deck is connected directly to the air commander in five different ways: a regular telephone, two sound-powered hot lines, two radios, and a public address system. These multiple communication channels are supplemented by the tower's capability to call the deck "foul" or not ready to receive an airplane, which serves as one final way to communicate with the landing signal officer. Similarly, airlines have two qualified pilots on each commercial flight, and air traffic controllers work in pairs. Members of such organiza-

---

[13]Unpublished data from Alison Trinkoff, Ph.D., University of Maryland at Baltimore, NIOSH grant R01OH3702 (personal communication, April 9, 2003).

tions learn what is important by observing where the organization focuses its time, energy, and resources. When an organization spends the money to create redundancy, there is no question in anyone's mind that the organization takes the possibility of errors very seriously (Roberts and Bea, 2001).

In manufacturing industries, a person or machine may be unable to respond to a request on demand because of an unexpected mechanical breakdown. For this reason, surplus stocks of parts and equipment are maintained. When customer needs are so large and unpredictable that it is impossible for a plant to adjust production in a timely manner, "buffer stock" is kept at or near the shipping point as a countermeasure (Spear and Bowen, 1999). In the work environment of nurses, redundant staffing or "slack" in staffing is recommended (see Chapter 5) as one way to ensure the ability to respond to unexpected variations in need for additional staff.

Using constraint and forcing functions   The most unambiguous way to design work so as to prevent a worker from making an error is to render the worker incapable of taking the erroneous action (referred to as a constraint) (Reason, 1990). For example, the design of certain vehicles prevents automatic door devices from being deployed accidentally when the vehicle is in motion. Conversely, a forcing function forces a worker to take a correct action.

Avoiding reliance on individual vigilance   Because of the limits of humans' ability to maintain a high intensity of vigilance over prolonged periods of time, it is important not to rely on a single individual's vigilance to monitor for threats to safety. A good example of how equipment has been engineered to decrease the need for extensive vigilance on the part of a nurse is the use of alarms on automatic IV pumps and other patient care and patient monitoring devices. The patient and family members can provide additional monitoring assistance. When patients and their families are knowledgeable about any treatment protocols and prescribed medications, they can take a more active role in monitoring care, as well as providing self-care.

Reducing and compensating for hand-offs   A number of strategies to address issues associated with patient hand-offs (see the discussion earlier in this chapter) are being implemented today. "Universal rooms," single-stay units, and acuity-adaptable rooms all aim to place a single patient in a care room or nursing unit for his/her entire hospital stay (Gallant and Lanning, 2001). The room or unit adapts to the changing health status of the patient, eliminating the need for patient transfers. However, early testing of acuity-adaptable rooms has indicated that several factors are critical to their appropriate use.

The first of these factors is the environmental design component—an acuity-adaptable headwall (e.g., one that includes additional gas and line outlets). The second is advanced medical–surgical skills on the part of the nurse. The third is identifying the subset of intensive care unit patients appropriate for care in an acuity-adaptable unit. While trauma patients in an intensive care unit typically require highly specialized, intensive interventions, a more hemodynamically stable group, such as coronary care patients, may be able to receive better care on an acuity-adaptable unit that provides both step-down and general medical care. Finally, there needs to be a sufficient number of patients in a like disease state to justify consolidating multiple levels of care into one unit (Gallant and Lanning, 2001).

The committee found only one study that tested the application and safety of acuity-adaptable rooms. This study found significant improvements in quality and operational costs, including a large reduction in clinician hand-offs and transfers, reductions in medication and patient falls, improvements in patient satisfaction, and an increase in patient days per bed on a base of fewer beds (more efficient use of beds) (Hendrich et al., 2004). Further testing is needed on the use of acuity-adaptable rooms as an alternative to transferring patients to a unit staffed with specially trained nurses and other care providers who have benefited from experience with a high volume of intensive care unit interventions.

There are other ways to decrease the risks of hand-offs. They include hospital-wide automated patient records so that there is no temporary loss of patient care information (as can occur when a patient's hard-copy record is transferred to a new unit), and providing ample space in the patient care room for family to accompany the patient.

Improving information access   Good decision making requires good information. This information can best be provided through automated and integrated clinical information systems that provide access to patient information, together with clinical decision support systems (Ball et al., 2003) (see Chapter 5). Information technology used in this way can reduce work errors and inefficiencies.

The increase in safety and efficiency achieved through automated patient records integrated with other clinical information systems is well illustrated by the automated information systems in place at Intermountain Health Care in Salt Lake City (Peck et al., 1997). Access to patient information is facilitated through automated patient records. Patient histories, physical exams, vital signs, and other clinical data are documented on line. When patient records are automated in this way, all patient data are easily accessed and viewed. The nurse can see the patient's longitudinal history. Little time is wasted in calling to see whether a laboratory test or radiology result is available, because the patient record is linked to the laboratory or radiology department, and test results are entered immediately. Allergy information is always accessible, so that caregivers are aware of preexisting conditions. Clinicians need not be physically or temporally co-located to collaborate since they can view and discuss data simultaneously. Providers with a legitimate need to know can access the record anytime, anywhere.

Intermountain Health Care identifies other benefits of automated patient records integrated with automated clinical information systems. These benefits include the following:

- *Data that are organized and legible*—The nurse can see all of the prescribed drugs for a patient in one location; the doses are written clearly, and names are spelled correctly. Data are grouped to ensure that important data are not buried among the more routine. A problem list shows acute and chronic conditions and complete known allergies. Other health care team members can view the nurse's concerns and respond to them. Abnormal findings are highlighted, and trends can be graphed and compared with interventions (e.g., temperature spikes correlated with drug administration). An integrated plan allows all members of the collaborative care process to see what is happening and decide what should occur in the future. Everyone knows who is responsible for the patient and who needs to communicate about the patient's care.

- *Support for ongoing knowledge acquisition*—The patient's clinical data can be linked to reference literature to answer questions about policies, procedures, prognosis, diagnoses, educational material, appropriate drug dose, drug contraindications, and the like.

- *Generation of alerts, reminders, or suggestions when standards of care are not being followed*—Rules can be implemented to address changes in the patient's condition or to remind providers of process issues. For instance, Intermountain Health Care (IHC) manages patients receiving the medication coumadin by having the computer screen show the results of the most recent clotting factor test or the unanticipated absence of such results to see which patients are out of acceptable blood value ranges and need dosage adjustments or another test. Similar messages for ventilator management are sent directly to the provider. Intermountain Health Care also manages populations of people with diabetes by reminding providers which patients have not had glycosalated hemoglobin tests, retinal exams, and so on. Similar reminders are sent about pap smears, mammograms, and immunizations. Process reminders are also used. When documentation is not recorded that a wound dressing has been changed according to schedule, IV tubing has been changed, or drugs have been administered, the automated patient record generates reminders according to rules that are agreed upon by providers. These measures help integrate evidence-based medicine into the process of care.

• *Asynchronous messaging*—This technique allows team members to communicate with one another without each member having to be present at the same exact location at the same point in time. This prevents wasting large amounts of time trying to track down a busy physician during office hours or a nurse on the following shift. Things that should be communicated do not slip between the cracks. At Intermountain Health Care, 2,568 staff voluntarily chose to start using a message log in the first year after the message log application was made available. These users are primarily in the ambulatory arena; application to Intermountain Health Care acute care facilities is now under way. Other applications, such as personal radio transceivers, also facilitate instant messaging.

In general, an electronic information database aids patient care, quality assessment, and research. The hallmark of quality improvement is feedback to users on the results of their activities. With the ability, for example, to assess how often different nursing divisions use restraints for similar populations, one can begin to assess processes that lead to improved outcomes. The degree to which skin breakdowns occur in patients being cared for on different units can be assessed and the results fed back. Ultimately, much of patient safety derives from this process of analysis. Paper abstraction of handwritten charts is highly laborious and prevents large-scale analyses of nursing care. Automated record systems offer the potential to manage and assess the care provided to a much larger population on a routine basis.

As the discussion in earlier chapters on paperwork and documentation practices makes clear, automating patient records and clinical information also can reduce costs. Moreover, the nurse does not spend as much time in the find-and-fetch mode. Inventories are updated when supplies are used, so new supplies can be on hand when needed; charges are generated by the entry of point-of-care documentation rather than by the filling out of billing slips. Filing activities by ward clerks are reduced, allowing more time to help the nurse. Educational materials can be printed for the patient in multiple languages (Clayton, 2001).

Remaining alert to the limitations of and risks created by technology
In searching for ways to improve patient safety, technology is often proposed as a strategy. Despite its potential, however, patient safety experts caution that technology by itself is not a panacea. While able to remedy some problems, technology may also generate new forms of error and failure (Battles and Keyes, 2002; Cook, 2002; Reason, 1990). Fundamental to the successful introduction of technology is a thorough understanding of the work flow and work processes involved in patient care (Cook, 2002; Goldberger and Kremsdorf, 2001). The expected benefits of a new technology may not occur if the technology is not designed appropriately (i.e.,

according to human factors and ergonomic principles) or does not fit with the rest of the work system.

For example, while microprocessor-controlled medication infusion pumps eliminate many cumbersome processes that are often the source of errors, they also introduce new demands, such as complicated set-up and operation procedures, that can lead to new sources of error. Bar coding technology can prevent patient misidentification, but the possibility exists that an error committed during patient registration may be disseminated throughout the information system and may be more difficult to detect and correct than with conventional systems (Wald and Shojania, 2001). Whenever a technology is implemented, then, the human factors characteristics of its design and its potential positive *and* negative influences on other work system elements should be studied.

Paying ongoing attention to work design Successful implementation of work redesign is not a one-time effort. Few changes in complex organizations work perfectly when first introduced; virtually all require modification over time to achieve optimum results. Ongoing monitoring, feedback, and redesign are therefore needed to create and sustain effective change (Goodman, 2001). Work (re)design should be considered a continuous process.

Moreover, it is not unusual for organizations or departments that have implemented innovations most recently to perform worse than those that implemented comparable innovations a year or two before. Macduffie and Pil (1996) point out that in the automobile industry, plants struggle in the first year following adoption of a new work system with the right mix of incentives, managerial supports, and training needs, as well as coordination difficulties with other units. Those that sustain the change into the second year begin to see cost and quality improvements. New practices often initially undermine existing routines and competencies and require ongoing learning, redesign of the change, and creation of support practices to capture the promised benefits.

Workspace Design for Safety and Efficiency

An example: Methodist Hospital, Clarian Health Partners In the mid-1990s, the Methodist campus of Clarian Health had two floors of nursing unit shell space available as the result of a consolidation process. An interdisciplinary planning effort employed continuous quality improvement principles and systems thinking, along with evidence from the literature, to determine how to best use this space. In addition, two work process and patient flow studies were conducted. The first was a 1,000-hour video capture of time and motion on a medical–surgical unit that simultaneously detailed all activities in the patient room, nursing hallway, and nursing station. The second was an observational study of internal patient transfers.

As a result of these efforts, the interdisciplinary team determined that it was possible to redesign workspaces to (1) eliminate resource waste (caregiver and fiscal), (2) improve caregiver work environment and personal satisfaction, (3) improve patient care, (4) employ healing environment concepts, and (5) support future care delivery while solving patient flow problems. To these ends, it would be necessary to shift indirect time back to the nurse and patient care by reducing the steps necessary for nursing staff to obtain supplies, reduce transfers of patients, rework the care delivery model, minimize delays in patient placement and waits in holding areas, eliminate equipment duplication, maximize technology for efficiency, and have patient and caregiver information readily available at the point of care.

In 1999, the resulting Cardiac Comprehensive Critical Care unit was opened. It contains 56 acuity-adaptable, 400-square-foot patient rooms (28 per floor) designed to offer three main zones: the family zone, the patient zone, and the caregiver zone. The patient zone includes patient beds with acuity-adaptable headwalls and advanced computer technology directly at the patient's bed, allowing staff to record weight and other vital data without disturbing the patient. Patients are admitted to and discharged from the same patient room. The family zone (150 square feet) offers such features as a chair-bed for nighttime visitation, a refrigerator, a computer hook-up, voice mail and TV/VCR, and customized educational kiosks and computer-based patient education. The staff zone offers similar conveniences. Because most of the distance traveled by nurses consists of going back and forth to the nursing or supply station, necessary supplies are maintained in the patient room. Nursing stations with computer access and servers for supplies are decentralized just outside the patient room. Corridor design allows for emergency equipment, such as defibrillators, to be hidden behind doors. Additional features for staff include a computerized education center for uninhibited access to e-learning and hospital information. Personal paging and an ID tracking system also pinpoint staff locations.

A comparison of 2 years of predesign baseline data with 3 years of data following the redesign found statistically significant changes in pre and post measures, including:

- A 90 percent reduction in patient transports. The two units had averaged 200+ interunit transfers per month in the 2 years prior to the new design. With the new design, patient days per bed increased, although the units had fewer beds than previously.
- A 70 percent reduction in medication errors.
- A decrease in the cardiac population's fall index to a national benchmark level of two falls per 1,000 patient days.

- A decrease in nurses' walking time and trips to obtain supplies. These and other efficiencies significantly increased available nursing time and permitted a reduction in budgeted staff care hours while increasing direct patient care time.
- A decrease in patient dissatisfaction.

The Cardiac Comprehensive Critical Care Unit has been recognized by the American Association of Critical Care Nurses/Society for Critical Care Medicine/American Institute of Architects as "best design in a critical care nursing unit" (Hendrich et al., 2004).

Potential workspace design elements for safety Workspace design initiatives, such as that of Methodist Hospital and those undertaken by the Pebble Project, aim to improve efficiency, safety, and overall patient and workforce experiences in care delivery. Several workspace design elements (shown in Table 6-2) based on LEAN operation and other work design principles can potentially achieve workload reductions and more efficient and safer care delivery in general patient care rooms (Hendrich and Lee, 2003c; Ulrich, 1991). Similar concepts apply to the design of adult critical care units (Hamilton, 1999) although there are special considerations for neonatal intensive care units (Graven, 1997). The committee notes that little research has been conducted establishing the efficiency and effectiveness of these measures in improving patient safety. However, the committee also notes the evidence in support of their use as LEAN practices, as well as their beneficial effect on patients, and strongly urges further implementation and evaluation of these interventions.

Getting started in work redesign Some of the principles and methods of work design are relatively intuitive and easy to apply. Many HCOs already practice root-cause analysis; others have used work sampling and failure modes and effects analysis to redesign work. Work redesign is sometimes undertaken using quality improvement approaches such as the plan-do-check-act cycle (Carayon et al., 2003). Many of the documentation redesign initiatives described earlier were undertaken by interdisciplinary teams without the use of professional experts in work redesign. Other HCOs, including small community hospitals, have reported the use of internal work teams composed of existing staff to redesign work processes (Doerge and Hagenow, 1995; Fletcher, 1997). However, work design initiatives can be enhanced when individuals with knowledge of different disciplines, such as environmental design, human factors, and industrial relations, are involved. Sometimes this specialized knowledge can be supplied only by experts in work design with these areas of expertise.

TABLE 6-2   Workspace Design Elements for General Patient Care Rooms Based on LEAN Principles

Nursing Unit Design	Elements of Workspace Design	LEAN Principles
The patient room	Divide the room into workspace zones of care (Gallant and Lanning, 2001): • Patient • Caregiver • Family	Maximize zones for order, efficiency, and standardization with an integrated approach. Direct caregivers should determine how this is best accomplished.
Acuity-adaptable headwall	An ambidextrous (each side of the bed) headwall is equipped with gases, lines, and electrical ports to accommodate advanced medical surgical acuity (Gallant and Lanning, 2001; Hendrich et al., 2004). Electrical plug-in locations are provided at varying heights on the wall (low/mid/high) to decrease back strain.	Maximize the flexibility of care levels within the same patient room. Eliminate nursing trips around the bed to access a singular port. Eliminate the need for many intra-unit patient transfers, reduce the workload index; conserve critical care beds; and improve the throughput and capacity of the hospital.
Bed types	Beds with built-in functionality (scales, fall monitors, chair–bed status, motorized drives) can eliminate lifting and transfers and increase nursing efficiency and workload.	Eliminate or reduce redundant devices (scales, restraints). Reduce the opportunity for caregiver injuries.
A staff observation window for each patient room with acuity-adaptable headwalls	This feature supports the acuity-adaptable care model, in which high observation must be balanced with privacy as patient acuity changes. This element is believed to be a requirement if different levels of patient acuity are to be handled in the same patient room. A full or half window on the inboard side of the patient room permits observation of two to three patients at a time when decentralized nursing stations are used. A blind, curtain, or opaque glass can be used for privacy.	Eliminate many interunit transfers, thereby improving the workload index. Reduce the need for low-risk monitored patients to occupy critical care beds.

TABLE 6-2 Continued

Nursing Unit Design	Elements of Workspace Design	LEAN Principles
Family zone	A dedicated space is provided within the room with adequate chair, sofa, or bench seating to permit overnight stays (Gallant and Lanning, 2001; Ulrich, 1991), as well as a small locker or storage space. A mini-refrigerator in the family zone can provide access to nutritional supplements for the patient, and the family/significant other can participate in family-centered care, with the nurse as caregiver.	Social supports tend to decrease stress and improve outcomes (Ulrich 1991). Many nursing call lights meet simple nutrition needs. Through self/family-centered care, nursing time can be preserved for activities requiring advanced skills.
Private, adequate patient room	An ideal room size has not been determined. Private, ample-size rooms ensure family space, adequate caregiver space, and appropriate space for safe patient mobility. The minimum space to meet these requirements, as well as to anticipate emerging, acuity-adaptable technology for the patient room, is probably at least 250 square feet (Hendrich et al., 2004).	Accommodate the family, the acuity-adaptable headwall, and anticipated future technologies. Improve workspace conditions by promoting an organized work area. Potentially reduce patient risk of infection and errors when only one patient is in a room.
Patient beds positioned to enable patients to see out a window, preferably providing visual exposure to everyday nature; exterior windows designed to distribute	Views of nature provide positive distractions that can decrease stress and aid healing. Natural lighting provides a connection with nature. Staff lounges should be a respite for stress reduction and socialization if desired.	Reduce worker stress and errors and promote patient healing and comfort through the provision of natural light and a connection with nature (Ulrich, 1991).

continued

TABLE 6-2   Continued

Nursing Unit Design	Elements of Workspace Design	LEAN Principles
natural light into the patient's room and the nursing workspace and staff lounge whenever possible[a]		
An enlarged door entrance to the patient's toilet	The door should be large enough to accommodate two caregivers and the patient or a patient with an assistive device (walker, cane, wheelchair).	Provide adequate maneuvering space for proper body mechanics to reduce opportunities for caregiver or patient injury. Locate the toilet close enough to the patient's bed to permit patient transfers to the toilet without additional lifting or equipment, thus reducing caregiver injuries and skin friction for the patient. Eliminate or greatly reduce the need for bedside commodes, provide patient privacy in a safer toilet area with appropriate grab bars, and reduce caregiver contact with human waste.
Equipment and supplies	Locate small supplies used most frequently by nurses inside the patient's room.	Reduce workload and improve productivity by using a small equipment cart or built-in cabinetry in the patient's room to safely store supplies that represent 80 percent of caregiver trips outside the room.

TABLE 6-2   Continued

Nursing Unit Design	Elements of Workspace Design	LEAN Principles
Servers	Cabinetry or drawers are designed to be "served" or filled from outside the patient's room by non-nursing personnel (care partners).	Provide immediate access to laundry and linen. Allow for transfer of soiled and clean materials and keep the hallway clear. Conserve scarce nursing resources and time.
Nursing call light system	A multifunctional communication network can optimize communication (Miller et al., 1997, 2001). Nursing unit communication systems utilize voice, phone, and staff tracking capabilities based on digital and infrared technology to enable communication between the patient and nurse and among caregivers.	Reduce travel time and caregiver response times to call lights. Support decentralized nursing stations for maximum efficiency. Eliminate non–value-added nursing time and motion.
Patient education systems	Standardized programming is available on diseases, procedures, and self-care. These programs can be delivered via the hospital intranet or television network.	Use patient/family education to enhance outcomes, enable early discharges, and reduce readmissions. Prepare the patient for discharge planning and self-care. Conserve nursing time for advanced, one-on-one, individualized responses to patient questions. Ensure that all patients have access to fundamental medical information as a standard of care.
Lighting and temperature controls	These should be accessible and controlled by the patient within his/her room.	Enable patients to control their own climate and environmental comfort without depending solely upon the nurse or other caregiver. Control over environment decreases stress and promotes wellness (Ulrich, 1991).

continued

TABLE 6-2   Continued

Nursing Unit Design	Elements of Workspace Design	LEAN Principles
Standardized patient rooms with acuity-adaptable headwall	Acuity-adaptable private rooms are standardized in design, equipment, and supplies. The design provides maximum flexibility for future care needs.	Minimize variation, enhance efficiency, and promote error reduction.
		Support principles of just-in-time inventory, and meet the immediate needs of caregiver and patient.
		Anticipate additional shifts in patient acuity and workforce shortages; potentially may reduce future design needs.
Ergonomics • Noise • Seating • Flooring • Colors • Workstation furniture	Silent paging systems; reduce or eliminate unnecessary bedside alarms; build acoustical characteristics into the environment; use full-spectrum colors found in nature; provide a variety of adequate seating choices to match an aging workforce with individual preferences and needs; anticipate a variety of emergency medical response devices; employ low-resistance carpet in the hallway or flooring with noise and stress reduction qualities; and eliminate or improve noisy carts and vibrations.	Create a safe, pleasant working environment to retain a highly skilled, aging, and scarce workforce. Increase productivity.
Positive distractions for the patient	A positive distraction is an environmental element or situation that increases positive feelings; effectively holds attention or interest; may block or reduce worrisome thoughts; and produces desirable physiologic changes, such as decreased blood pressure (Ulrich, 1997).	Provide scenes of nature, laughter/comedy, human contact, music.
Decentralized nursing stations	Distribute the workstations outside each patient room or set of patient rooms.	Reduce the chaotic milieu often found in the nursing station. Eliminate steps, time, and distance. Place the nurse at the point of patient care. Improve patient safety (enhanced observation/fall reduction/reduced waits and delays).

TABLE 6-2 Continued

Nursing Unit Design	Elements of Workspace Design	LEAN Principles
Learning center	Such a center provides electronic access to hospital policies/procedures/nursing information if possible, as well as access to e-learning and reference material on nursing units.	Improve knowledge among nursing staff, and provide immediate access to reference materials in a timely fashion to reduce errors.
Staff lounge	The staff lounge provides private space with adequate accommodations. When possible, it has a window to the outside. The lounge supports caregivers by providing an "off-stage" area for downtime.	Reduce caregiver stress; offer caregivers privacy.
Physician–nurse collaboration areas	Private areas for consultation and collaboration are needed to promote professional interdisciplinary practice. Decentralized nursing stations can detract from staff privacy; an alternative area is needed for compliance with HIPAA[b] patient privacy provisions as well.	Provide space for team-centered care. Reduce errors and improve care processes through collaboration.
Supplies and equipment	Adequate space for storage of patient equipment should be conveniently located in the core space out of the hallway. Automated supply systems should be standardized and matched against patient populations.	
Medication delivery	Robotic, automated, or mobile carts should be conveniently distributed on the unit with adequate ratios to nursing unit size.	Eliminate the need to stand in line to get drugs. Prevent nurse "pocket storage" from automated systems by eliminating lines for access.

[a]This does not apply to neonatal intensive care units, where exposure to direct sunlight has risks for the pre-term infant (Graven, 1997).
[b]Health Insurance Portability and Accountability Act of 1996.

The role of the ergonomist is the subject of debate in the field of human factors and ergonomics. Drury (1995:66–67) argues that "there is no substitute for the ergonomist's knowledge and understanding of both the system under study and the ergonomics literature." Gosbee (2002: 354) argues that "[human factors engineering] must become a core competency of anyone who has significant involvement in patient safety activities." Corlett (1991:418) states that "[we must] give ergonomics away, . . . transfer our knowledge and methods to others who are closer to the places where changes have to be made, so that they do much of the ergonomics for themselves. . . . Until ergonomics is widely practiced by other than professional ergonomists, it is likely to remain something to be added on at the end."

The committee concludes that the dissemination and application of work design knowledge and skills throughout individual HCOs needs to be achieved through multiple mechanisms, including trial and error, creation of in-house expertise, use of consultants, and various education and training mechanisms. HCOs should undertake efforts to increase the knowledge of end users—the nurses whose work is being redesigned—about work design through, for example, on-the-job coaching or continuing education programs. As the complexity of work design initiatives increases, however, there is likely to be a commensurate increased need for professional consultation. The committee makes the following recommendations:

> **Recommendation 6-2. HCOs should provide nursing leadership with resources that enable them to design the nursing work environment and care processes to reduce errors. These efforts must directly involve direct-care nurses throughout all phases of the work design and should concentrate on errors associated with:**
>
> - **Surveillance of patient health status.**
> - **Patient transfers and other patient hand-offs.**
> - **Complex patient care processes.**
> - **Non–value-added activities performed by nurses, such as locating and obtaining supplies, looking for personnel, completing redundant and unnecessary documentation, and compensating for poor communication systems.**

The committee notes that "resources" should include time and financial and consultant resources, as necessary.

> **Recommendation 6-3. HCOs should address handwashing and medication administration among their first work design initiatives.**

Recommendation 6-4. Regulators; leaders in health care; and experts in nursing, law, informatics, and related disciplines should jointly convene to identify strategies for safely reducing the burden associated with patient and work-related documentation.

REFERENCES

Aiken L, Clarke S, Sloane D, Sochalski J, Busse R, Clarke H, Giovannetti P, Hunt J, Rafferty A, Shamian J. 2001. Nurses' reports on hospital care in five countries. *Health Affairs* 20(3):43–53.

Akerstedt T. 1994. Work injuries and time of day—national data. *Proceedings of a Consensus Development Symposium Entitled Work Hours, Sleepiness, and Accidents.* Stockholm, Sweden.

Alaska Oil Spill Commission. 1990. *Spill: The Wreck of the Exxon Valdez.* [Online]. Available: http://www.oilspill.state.ak.us/facts/details.html [accessed July 29, 2003].

Allan J, Englebright J. 2000. Patient-centered documentation: An effective and efficient use of clinical information systems. *Journal of Nursing Administration* 30(2):90–95.

Alukal G. 2003. Create a lean, mean machine. *Quality Progress* 36(4):29–35.

ANA (American Nurses Association). 2002. *State Legislative Trends and Analysis.* Washington, DC: ANA.

Anonymous. 2000. Automation can reduce errors, but don't jump before looking, ISMP says. *Healthcare Risk Management 59.*

Ashby D. 1997. Medication calculation skills of the medical–surgical nurse. *MEDSURG Nursing* 6(2):90–94.

Babkoff H, Mikulincer M, Caspy T, Kempinski D, Sing H. 1988. The typology of performance curves during 72 hours of sleep loss. *The Quarterly Journal of Experimental Psychology* 324:737–756.

Baldwin D. 1998. Implementation of computerized clinical documentation. *Home Health Care Management & Practice* 10(2):43–51.

Ball M, Weaver C, Abbott P. 2003. Enabling technologies promise to revitalize the role of nursing in an era of patient safety. *International Journal of Medical Informatics* 69:29–38.

Bates D, Cullen D, Laird N, Petersen L, Small S, Servi D, Laffel G, Sweitzer B, Shea B, Hallisey R, Vander Vliet M, Nemeskal R, Leape L. 1995. Incidence of adverse drug events and potential adverse drug events: Implications for prevention. *Journal of the American Medical Association* 274:29–34.

Battelle Memorial Institute, JIL Information Systems. 1998. *An Overview of the Scientific Literature Concerning Fatigue, Sleep and the Circadian Cycle.* Prepared for the Office of the Chief Scientific and Technical Advisor for Human Factors, Federal Aviation Administration. [Online]. Available: http://www.unionepiloti.it/diparti/technico/Documenti_dt/studio_Battelle.pdf [accessed July 29, 2003].

Battles J, Keyes M. 2002. Technology and patient safety: A two-edged sword. *Biomedical Instrumentation and Technology* 36(2):84–88.

Bindler R, Bayne T. 1991. Medication calculation ability of registered nurses. *Image: Journal of Nursing Scholarship* 23(4):221–224.

Blachly B, Young H. 1998. Reducing the burden of paperwork: Modified charting by exception for medications. *Journal of Gerontological Nursing* 24(6):16–20.

Bobrow M. 1978. The Evolution of Nursing Space Planning for Efficient Operations. In: Redston L, ed. *Hospitals and Health Care Facilities: An Architectural Record Book.* New York, NY: McGraw-Hill.

Bobrow M, Thomas J. 2000. Inpatient Care Facilities. In: Kliment S, ed. *Building Type Basics for Health Care Facilities.* New York, NY: John Wiley and Sons.

Bowers B, Lauring C, Jacobson N. 2001. How nurses manage time and work in long term care facilities. *Journal of Advanced Nursing* 33:484–491.

Bridgeman T, Flores M, Rosenbluth J, Pierog J. 1997. One emergency department's experience: Clinical algorithms and documentation. *Journal of Emergency Nursing* 23(4):316–325.

Brooks J. 1998. An analysis of nursing documentation as a reflection of actual nurse work. *MEDSURG Nursing* 7(4):189–198.

Brunt B, Gifford L, Hart D, McQueen-Goss S, Siddall D, Smith R, Weakland R. 1999. Designing interdisciplinary documentation for the continuum of care. *Journal of Nursing Care Quality* 14(1):1–10.

Butler M, Bender A. 1999. Intensive care unit bedside documentation systems: Realizing cost savings and quality improvements. *Computers in Nursing* 17(1):32–41.

Cabri J, De Witt B, Clarys J. 1988. Circadian variation in blood pressure responses to muscular exercises. *Ergonomics* 31:1559–1566.

California Nurses Association. 2003. *Mandatory Overtime Is Detrimental to Patient Care and the Health of Nurses.* [Online]. Available: http://www.calnurse.og/cna/patient/nursespeak.html [accessed June 16, 2003].

Calliari D. 1995. The relationship between a calculation test given in nursing orientation and medication errors. *Journal of Continuing Education in Nursing* 26(1):11–14.

Carayon P, Alvarado C, Hundt A. 2003. Center for Quality and Productivity Improvement and Department of Industrial Engineering, University of Wisconsin-Madison. *Reducing Workload and Increasing Patient Safety through Work and Workspace Design.* Paper commissioned by the Institute of Medicine Committee on the Work Environment for Nurses and Patient Safety

Case J, Mowry M, Welebob E. 2002. *The Nursing Shortage: Can Technology Help?* Oakland, CA: California Heathcare Foundation.

CDC (Centers for Disease Control and Prevention). 2003 (July 22). Hand Hygiene in Healthcare Settings. National Stakeholders Meeting on Alcohol-Based Hand-Rubs and Fire Safety in Healthcare Facilities. Executive summary. [Online]. Available: http://www.cdc.gov/handhygiene/firesafety/aha_meeting.htm [accessed September 30, 2003].

Clayton P. 2001. The state of clinical information systems, after four decades of effort. In: Clayton P. *IMIA Yearbook of Medical Informatics—2001.* Stuttgart, Germany: Shattauer Publishing Company. Pp. 333–337.

Clayton P, Hougaard J, Rhodes J, Narus S, Wilcox A, Wallace J, Miller S, Evans R, Hales R, Rowan B, Johnson K, Boyce J, Calder C. 2003. *Improving the Nursing Environment: Reducing the Documentation Burden.* Unpublished paper.

CMS (Centers for Medicare and Medicaid Services). 2002. *Report to Congress: Appropriateness of Minimum Nurse Staffing Ratios in Nursing Homes—Phase II Final Report.* [Online]. Available: www.cms.gov/medicaid/reports/rp1201home.asp [accessed June 25, 2002].

Cohen C, Muehl G. 1977. Human circadian rhythms in resting and exercise pulse rates. *Ergonomics* 20:475–479.

Cook R. 2002. Safety technology: Solutions or experiments? *Nursing Economics* 20(2):80–82.

Cook R, Render M, Woods D. 2000. Gaps in the continuity of care and progress on patient safety. *British Medical Journal* 320(7237):791–794.

Cooper J, Newbower R, Kitz R. 1984. An analysis of major errors and equipment failures in anesthesia management: Considerations for prevention and detection. *Anesthesiology* 60(1):34–42.

Corlett E. 1991. Some future directions for ergonomics. In: Kumashiro M, Megaw E, eds. *Towards Human Work: Solutions to Problems in Occupational Health and Safety*. London: Taylor & Francis.

Cox A, Groves P. 1990. *Hospitals and Health-Care Facilities: A Design and Development Guide*. London: Butterworth and Company, Ltd.

Dawson D, Reid K. 1997. Fatigue, alcohol, and performance impairment. *Nature* 388:235.

Delafosse J, Leger D, Quera-Salva M, Samson O, Adrien J. 2000. Comparative study of actigraphy and ambulatory polysomnography in the assessment of adaptation to night shift work in nurses. *Revue Neurologique* (Paris) 156(6-7):641–645.

Deutschendorf A. 2003. From past paradigms to future frontiers: Unique care delivery models to facilitate nursing work and quality outcomes. *Journal of Nursing Administration* 33(1):52–59.

Dinges D, Graeber R, Rosenkind M, Samuel A, Wegman H. 1996. *Principles and Guidelines for Duty and Rest Scheduling in Commercial Aviation*. NASA Technical Memorandum 110404. Moffett Field, CA: National Aeronautics and Space Administration, Ames Research Center. [Online]. Available: http://olias.arc.nasa.gov/zteam/PDF_pubs/p-g1.pdf [accessed October 4, 2003].

Dirks J. 1993. Adaptation to permanent night work: The number of consecutive work nights and motivated choice. *Ergonomics* 36:29–36.

Dismukes K, Young G, Sumwalt R. 1998. Cockpit interruptions and distractions: Effective management requires a careful balancing act. *ASRS Directline* 4–9.

Doerge J, Hagenow N. 1995. Patient-centered process of work redesign: Arizona hospital reengineers with no outside help. *Health Progress* 76(8):28–32.

Dornheim M. 2000. Crew distractions emerge as new safety focus. *Aviation Week & Space Technology* 60:153–158.

Drury C. 1995. Methods for direct observation of performance. In: Wilson J, Corlett E, eds. *Evaluation of Human Work* (2nd Edition). London: Taylor & Francis. Pp. 45–68.

Duchon J, Keran C, Smith T. 1994. Extended workdays in an underground mine: A work performance analysis. *Human Factors* 36:258–269.

Ely J, Levinson W, Elder N, Mainous A, Vinson D. 1995. Perceived causes of family physicians' errors. *Journal of Family Practice* 40(4):337–344.

Fiesta J. 1993. Charting: One national standard, one form. *Nursing Management* 24(6):22–24.

Fletcher C. 1997. Failure mode and effects analysis: An interdisciplinary way to analyze and reduce medication errors. *Journal of Nursing Administration* 27(12):19–26.

Florica V, Higgins E, Iampietro P, Lategola M, Davis A. 1968. Physiological responses of man during sleep deprivation. *Journal of Applied Physiology* 24:169–175.

Flynn E, Barker K, Gibson J, Pearson R, Berger B, Smith L. 1999. Impact of interruptions and distractions on dispensing errors in an ambulatory care pharmacy. *American Journal of Health-System Pharmacy* 56(13):1319–1325.

Folkard S. 1996. Effects on performance efficiency. In: Colquhoun W, Costa G, Kolkard S, Knauth P, eds. *Shiftwork: Problems and Solutions*. Frankfurt am Main: Peter Lang Publishing. Pp. 65–87.

Fukuda H, Takahashi M, Airto H. 1999. Nurses' workload associated with 16-h night shifts on the 2-shift system. I: Comparison with the 3-shift system. *Psychiatry and Clinical Neurosciences* 53(2):219–221.

Gallant D, Lanning K. 2001. Streamlining patient care processes through flexible room and equipment design. *Critical Care Nursing Quarterly* 24(3):1–20.

Gander P, McDonald J, Montgomery J, Paulin M. 1991. Adaptation of sleep and circadian rhythms to the Antarctic summer: A question of zeitgeber strength. *Aviation, Space and Environmental Medicine* 62:1019–1025.

GAO (U.S. General Accounting Office). 2001. *Nursing Workforce: Emerging Nurse Shortages Due to Multiple Factors.* GAO-01-944. Washington, DC: GAO.

Gillberg M, Kecklund G, Akerstadt T. 1994. Relations between performance and subjective ratings of sleepiness during a night awake. *Sleep* 17:236–241.

Gold D, Rogacz S, Bock N, Tosteson T, Baum T, Speizer F, Czeisler C. 1992. Rotating shift work, sleep, and accidents related to sleepiness in hospital nurses. *American Journal of Public Health* 82(7):1011–1014.

Goldberger D, Kremsdorf R. 2001. Clinical information systems: Developing a systematic planning process. *Journal of Ambulatory Care Management* 24(1):67–83.

Goodman P. 2001. *Missing Organizational Linkages: Tools for Cross-Level Organizational Research.* Thousand Oaks, CA: Sage Publications.

Gosbee J. 2002. Human factors engineering and patient safety. *Quality & Safety in Health Care* 11(4):352–354.

Graven, S. 1997. Pre-symposium workshop: Clinical research data illuminating the relationship between the physical environment and patient medical outcomes. *Journal of Healthcare Design* IX:15–20. Volume IX contains the proceedings of the Ninth Symposium of Healthcare Design, held on November 14–17, 1996, in Boston, Massachusetts. Copyright 1997 by The Center for Health Design, Inc.

Gravenstein J, Cooper J, Orkin F. 1990. Work and rest cycles in anesthesia practice. *Anesthesiology* 72:737–742.

Hamilton D. 1999. Design for flexibility in critical care. *New Horizons* 7(2):205–217.

Hamilton K. 1990. *Unit 2000: Patient Beds for the Future.* Bel Air, TX: Watkins, Carter, Hamilton Publications.

Hanecke K, Tiedemann S, Nachreiner F, Grzech-Sukalo H. 1998. Accident risk as a function of hour at work and time of day as determined from accident data and exposure models for the German working population. *Scandinavian Journal of Work Environment Health* 24(Supplement 3):43–48.

Hendrich A, Lee N. 2003a. A Time and Motion Study of Health Care Workers: Tribes of Hunters and Gatherers. Unpublished data.

Hendrich A, Lee N. 2003b. The Cost of Intra-unit Hospital Patient Transfers. Unpublished data.

Hendrich A, Lee N. 2003c. *Evidence-Based Design on Nursing Workspace in Hospitals.* Report commissioned by the IOM Committee on the Work Environment for Nurses and Patient Safety.

Hendrich A, Nyhuis A, Kippenbrock T, Soja M. 1995. Hospital falls: Development of a predictive model for clinical practice. *Applied Nursing Research* 8(3):129–139.

Hendrich A, Nyhuis A, Bender P. 2003. Validation of the Hendrich II fall risk model: A large concurrent case/control study of hospitalized patients. *Applied Nursing Research* 16(1):9–21.

Hendrich A, Fay J, Sorrels A. 2004 (forthcoming). Cardiac comprehensive critical care: Effects of acuity-adaptable rooms on flow of patients and delivery of care. *American Journal of Critical Care* 13(1).

Hyman W. 1994. Errors in the use of medical equipment. In: Bogner M, ed. *Human Error in Medicine.* Hillsdale, NJ: Lawrence Erlbaum Associates. Pp. 327–347.

Institute for Safe Medication Practices. 2002. "Smart" infusion pumps join CPOE and bar coding as important ways to prevent medication errors. *ISMP Medication Safety Alert.* [Online]. Available: www.ismp.org/MSAarticles/Smart.htm [accessed June 27, 2003].

IOM (Institute of Medicine). 2000. *To Err Is Human: Building a Safer Health System.* Washington, DC: National Academy Press.

IOM. 2001. *Crossing the Quality Chasm: A New Health System for the 21st Century.* Washington, DC: National Academy Press.

James P, Tatton-Brown W. 1986. *Hospitals: Design and Development.* New York, NY: Van Nostrand Reinhold Co.

JCAHO (Joint Commission on Accreditation of Healthcare Organizations). 2002. *Health Care at the Crossroads: Strategies for Addressing the Evolving Nursing Crisis.* Oakbrook Terrace, IL: JCAHO.

JCAHO. 2003. *2003 Hospital Accreditation Standards.* Oakbrook Terrace, IL: Joint Commission Resources.

Jha A, Duncan B, Bates D. 2001. Fatigue, sleepiness, and medical errors. In: Shojania K, Duncan B, McDonald K, Wachter R, eds. *Making Health Care Safer: A Critical Analysis of Patient Safety Practices.* AHRQ Publication No. 01-E058. Rockville, MD: AHRQ.

Johnson C, Carlson R, Tucker C, Willette C. 2002. Using BCMA software to improve patient safety in Veterans Administration Medical Centers. *Journal of Healthcare Information Management* 16(1):46–51.

Kaushal R, Bates, D. 2001. Computerized physician order entry (CPOE) and clinical decision support systems (CDSSs). In: Shojania K, Duncan B, McDonald K, Wachter R. eds. *Making Health Care Safer: A Critical Analysis of Patient Safety Practices.* Rockville, MD: AHRQ. Pp. 59–69.

Kimball B, O'Neil E. 2002. *Health Care's Human Crisis: The American Nursing Shortage:* The Robert Wood Johnson Foundation. [Online]. Available: www.rwjf.org/news/nursing_report.pdf [accessed October 4, 2003].

Knauth P. 1993. The design of shift systems. *Ergonomics* 36:29–36.

Knauth P, Landau K, Droge C, Schwitteck N, Widynski M, Rutenfranz J. 1980. Duration of sleep depending on the type of shift work. *International Archives of Occupational and Environmental Health* 46:167–177.

Kogi K. 1991. Job content and working time: The scope for joint change. *Ergonomics* 34:757–773.

Korst L, Eusebio-Angeja A, Chamorro T, Aydin C, Gregory K. 2003. Nursing documentation time during implementation of an electronic medical record. *Journal of Nursing Administration* 33(1):24–30.

Kovner C. 2001. The impact of staffing and organization of work on patient outcomes and health care workers in health care organizations. *The Joint Commission Journal on Quality Improvement* 27(9):458–468.

Krueger G. 1994. Fatigue, performance and medical error. In: Mary Sue Bogner, ed. *Human Error in Medicine.* Hillsdale, NJ: Lawrence Erlbaum Associates.

Kruger G. 1989. Sustained work, fatigue, sleep loss and performance. *Work & Stress* 3:287–298.

LaDuke S. 2001. Online nursing documentation: Finding a middle ground. *Journal of Nursing Administration* 31(6):283–286.

Lamond N, Dawson D. 1998. *Quantifying the Performance Impairment Associated with Sustained Wakefulness.* South Australia: The Centre for Sleep Research, The Queen Elizabeth Hospital. [Online]. Available: http://cf.alpha.org/internet/projects/ftdt/backgr/Daw_Lam.html [accessed July 7, 2003].

Larrabee J, Boldreghini S, Elder-Sorrells K, Turner Z, Wender R, Hart J, Lenzi P. 2001. Evaluation of documentation before and after implementation of a nursing information system in an acute care hospital. *Computers in Nursing* 19(2):56–65.

Lautenbach E. 2001. Practices to improve handwashing compliance. In: Shojania K, Duncan B, McDonald K, Wachter R, eds. *Making Health Care Safer: A Critical Analysis of Patient Safety Practices.* Rockville, MD: AHRQ. Pp. 119–126.

Lavie P, Chillag N, Epstein R, Tzischinsky O, Givon R, Fuchs S, Shahal B. 1989. Sleep disturbance in shift workers: A marker for maladaptation syndrome. *Work Stress* 3:33–40.

Lawler III E. 1986. *High Involvement Management: Participative Strategies for Improving Organizational Performance.* San Francisco, CA: Jossey-Bass.

Leape L, Bates D, Cullen D, Cooper J, Demonaco H, Gallivan T, Hallisey R, Ives J, Laird N, Laffel G, Nemeskal R, Petersen L, Porter K, Servi D, Shea B, Small S, Sweitzer B, Thompson B, Vander Vleit M. 1995. Systems analysis of adverse drug events. *Journal of the American Medical Association* 274(1):35–43.

Lee K. 1992. Self-reported sleep disturbances in employed women. *Sleep* 15:493–498.

Linde L, Bergstrom M. 1992. The effect of one night without sleep on problem-solving and immediate recall. *Psychological Research* 54:127–136.

Linden L, English K. 1994. Adjusting the cost-quality equation: Utilizing work sampling and time study data to redesign clinical practice. *Journal of Nursing Care Quality* 8(3):34–42.

Luna T, French J, Mitcha J. 1997. A study of USAF air traffic controller shiftwork: Sleep, fatigue, activity, and mood analyses. *Aviation, Space and Environmental Medicine* 68:18–23.

Macduffie J, Pil F. 1996. "High involvement" work practices and human resource policies: An international overview. In: Kochan T, Lansbury R, Macduffie J, eds. *Evolving Employment Practices in the World Auto Industry*. New York, NY: Oxford University Press.

McCartt A, Rohrbaugh J, Hammer M. 2000. Factors associated with falling asleep at the wheel among long-distance truck drivers. *Accident Analysis and Prevention* 32:493–504.

Miller E, Deets C, Miller R. 1997. Nurse call systems: Impact on nursing performance. *Journal of Nursing Care Quality* 11(3):36–43.

Miller E, Deets C, Miller R. 2001. Nurse call and the work environment: Lessons learned. *Journal of Nursing Care Quality* 15(3):7–15.

Mills M, Arnold B, Wood C. 1983. Core 12: A controlled study of the impact of 12-hour scheduling. *Nursing Research* 32:356–361.

Mitler M, Carskadon M, Czeisler C, Dement W, Dinges D, Graeber R. 1988. Catastrophes, sleep, and public policy: Consensus report. *Sleep* 11:100–109.

Mitler M, Miller J, Lipsitz J, Walsh J, Wylie C. 1997. The sleep of long-haul truckers. *The New England Journal of Medicine* 337:755–761.

Monk T. 1990. Shiftworker performance. In: Scott A, ed. *Occupational Medicine State of the Art Reviews. Volume 5*. Philadelphia, PA: Hanley and Belfus, Inc. Pp. 183–198.

Monk T, Folkard S, Wedderburn A. 1996. Maintaining safety and high performance on shiftwork. *Applied Ergonomics* 27:17–23.

Morrison W, Haas E, Shaffner D, Garrett E. 2003. Noise, stress, and annoyance in a pediatric intensive care unit. *Critical Care Medicine* 31(1):113–119.

Mosher C, Rademacher K, Day G, Fanelli D. 1996. Documenting for patient-focused care. *Nursing Economics* 14(4):218–223.

Mullaney D, Kripke D, Fleck P, Johnson L. 1983. Sleep loss and nap effects on sustained continuous performance. *Psychophysiology* 20:643–651.

Murphy J, Beglinger J, Johnson B. 1988. Charting by exception: Meeting the challenge of cost containment. *Nursing Management* 19(2):56–72.

Murray M. 2001. Automated medication dispensing devices. In: Shojania K, Duncan B, McDonald K, Wachter R, eds. *Making Health Care Safer: A Critical Analysis of Patient Safety Practices*. Rockville, MD: AHRQ. Pp. 111–117.

Murray M, Shojania K. 2001. Unit-dose drug distribution systems. In: Shojania K, Duncan B, McDonald K, Wachter R, eds. *Making Health Care Safer: A Critical Analysis of Patient Safety Practices*. Rockville, MD: AHRQ. Pp. 101–109.

Nahm R, Poston I. 2000. Measurement of the effects of an integrated, point-of-care computer system on quality of nursing documentation and patient satisfaction. *Computers in Nursing* 18(5):220–229.

National Transportation Safety Board. 1994. *A Review of Flight Crew-Involved Major Accidents of U.S. Air Carriers, 1978 Through 1990*. NTSB #SS-94-01/PB94-917001. Washington, DC: National Transportation Safety Board.

Noro K, Imada A. 1991. *Participatory Ergonomics.* London: Taylor and Francis.

Office of Technology Assessment, U.S. Congress. 1991. *Biological Rhythms: Implications for the Worker.* OTA-BA-463. Washington, DC: U.S. Government Printing Office.

Olson L, Ambrogetti A. 1998. Working harder: Working dangerously? Fatigue and performance in hospitals. *Medical Journal of Australia* 168(12):614–616.

O'Shea E. 1999. Factors contributing to medication errors: A literature review. *Journal of Clinical Nursing* 8(5):496–505.

Pabst M, Scherubel J, Minnick A. 1996. The impact of computerized documentation on nurses' use of time. *Computers in Nursing* 14(1):25–30.

Pape T. 2001. Searching for the final answer: Factors contributing to medication administration errors. *Journal of Continuing Education in Nursing* 32(4):152–160, 190–191.

Pape T. 2003. Applying airline safety practices to medication administration. *MEDSURG Nursing* 12(2):77–93.

Park K. 1997. Human error. In: Salvendy G, ed. *Handbook of Human Factors and Ergonomics.* New York, NY: John Wiley & Son, Inc. Pp. 150–170.

Peck M, Nelson N, Buxton R, Bushnell J, Dahle M, Rosebrock B, Ashton C. 1997. LDS Hospital: A facility of Intermountain Health Care, Salt Lake City, UT. *Nursing Administration Quarterly* 21(3):29–49.

Pedersen A. 1997. A data-driven approach to work redesign in nursing units. *Journal of Nursing Administration* 27(4):49–54.

Pepper G. 1995. Errors in drug administration by nurses. *American Journal of Health-System Pharmacy* 52:390–395.

Prescott P, Phillips C, Ryan J, Thompson K. 1991. Changing how nurses spend their time. *Image* 23(1):23–28.

Reason J. 1990. *Human Error.* Cambridge, UK: Cambridge University Press.

Rich M. 2002 (November 27). Healthy hospital designs: Improving decor and layout can have impact on care; fewer fractures and infections. *The Wall Street Journal.* Pp. B-1, B-4.

Roberts K, Bea R. 2001. Must accidents happen? Lessons from high-reliability organizations. *Academy of Management Executive* 15(3):70–78.

Rogers A. 2002. Work Hour Regulation in Safety-Sensitive Industries. Paper commissioned by the Institute of Medicine Committee on the Work Environment for Nurses and Patient Safety. Presented to the Committee on November 19, 2002.

Rosa R. 1995. Extended workshifts and excessive fatigue. *Journal of Sleep Research* 4(Supplement 2):51–56.

Rosa R. 2001. Examining work schedules for fatigue: Its not just hours of work. In: Hancock P, Desmond P, eds. *Stress, Workload, and Fatigue.* Mahwah, NJ: Lawrence Earlbaum Associates. Pp. 513–528.

Rosa R, Colligan M. 1988. Long workdays vs. restdays: Assessing fatigue and alertness with a portable performance battery. *Human Factors* 30:305–317.

Rosenkind M, Gander P, Connell L, Co E. 1999. *Crew Factors in Flight Operations X: Alertness Management in Flight Operations.* NASA/FAA.

Scharf L. 1997. Revising nursing documentation to meet patient outcomes. *Nursing Management* 28(4):38.

Scherubel J, Minnick A. 1994. Implementation of work sampling methodology. *Nursing Research* 43(2):120–123.

Schuster M. 1985. The impact of overtime work on industrial accident rates. *Industrial Relations* 24(2):234–246.

Seago J. 2001. Nurse staffing, models of care delivery, and interventions. In: Shojania K, Duncan B, McDonald K, Wachter R. eds. *Making Health Care Safer: A Critical Analysis of Patient Safety Practices. Evidence Report/Technology Assessment No. 43.* Rockville, MD: AHRQ.

Senders J. 1994. Medical devices, medical errors, and medical accidents. In: Bogner M, ed. *Human Error in Medicine.* Hillsdale, NJ: Lawrence Erlbaum Associates.

Smeltzer C, Hines P, Beebe H, Keller B. 1996. Streamlining documentation: An opportunity to reduce costs and increase nurse clinicians' time with patients. *Journal of Nursing Care Quality* 10(4):66–77.

Smith B. 2003. Lean and six sigma: A one-two punch. *Quality Progress* 36(4).

Smith D, Rogers S, Hood E, Phillips D. 1998. Overtime reduction with the press of a button: An unexpected outcome of computerized documentation. *Nursing Case Management* 3(6):266–270.

Smith J, Crawford L. 2002. *Report of Findings from the Practice and Professional Issues Survey—Spring 2001.* NCSBN Research Brief 2. Chicago, IL: National Council of State Boards of Nursing, Inc.

Smith L, Folkard S, Poole C. 1994. Increased injuries on the night shift. *Lancet* 344:1137–1139.

Spath P. 2000. Reducing errors through work system improvements. In: Spath P, ed. *Error Reduction in Health Care.* San Francisco, CA: Jossey Bass. Pp. 199–234.

Spear S, Bowen H. 1999. Decoding the DNA of the Toyota Production System. *Harvard Business Review* 77(5):97–106.

Spratley E, Johnson A, Sochalski J, Fritz M, Spencer W. 2000. *The Registered Nurse Population: Findings from the National Sample Survey of Registered Nurses:* DHHS, HRSA. [Online]. Available: http://bhpr.hrsa.gov/healthworkforce/reports/rnsurvey/rnss1.htm [accessed October 4, 2003].

Stephens S, Mason S. 1999. Putting it together: A clinical documentation system that works. *Nursing Management* 30(3):43–47.

Takahashi M, Arito H, Fukuda H. 1999. Nurses' workload associated with 16-h night shifts. II: Effects of a nap taken during the shifts. *Psychiatry and Clinical Neurosciences* 53(2):223–225.

The Center for Health Design. 2003a. *What Is the Pebble Project?* [Online]. Available: http: www.pebbleproject.org/pebble_faq.php [accessed July 5, 2003].

The Center for Health Design. 2003b. *Pebble Project: Selected Preliminary Data.* [Online]. Available: http://www.pebbleproject.org/pebble_data.php [accessed July 5, 2003].

Topf M. 2000. Hospital noise pollution: An environmental stress model to guide research and clinical interventions. *Journal of Advanced Nursing* 31(3):520–528.

Trossman S. 2001. The documentation dilemma: Nurses poised to address paperwork burden. *The American Nurse* 33(5):1, 9, 18.

Tucker A, Edmondson A. 2002. Managing routine exceptions: A model of nurse problem solving behavior. *Advances in Health Care Management* 3:87–113.

Tucker A, Edmondson A. 2003. Why hospitals don't learn from failures: Organizational and psychological dynamics that inhibit system change. *California Management Review* 45(2):1–18.

Tucker P, Barton J, Folkard S. 1996. Comparison of eight and 12 hour shifts: Impacts on health, wellbeing, and alertness during the shift. *Occupational and Environmental Medicine* 53:767–772.

Ugrovics A, Wright J. 1990. 12-hour shifts: Does fatigue undermine ICU nursing judgments? *Nursing Management* 21:64A–64G.

Ulrich R. 1991. Effects of interior design on wellness: Theory and recent scientific research. *Journal of Health Care Interior Design* 3:97–109.

Ulrich R. 1997. Pre-symposium workshop: A theory of supportive design for healthcare facilities. *Journal of Healthcare Design* Volume IX:3-7. Volume IX contains the proceedings of the Ninth Symposium of Healthcare Design, held on November 14–17, 1996, in Boston, Massachusetts. Copyright 1997 by The Center for Health Design, Inc.

Upenieks V. 1998. Work sampling: Assessing nursing efficiency. *Nursing Management* 29(4):27–29.

Urden L, Roode J. 1997. Work sampling: A decision-making tool for determining resources and work redesign. *Journal of Nursing Administration* 27(9):34–41.

Van-Griever A, Meijman T. 1987. The impact of abnormal hours of work on various modes of information processing: A process model on human costs of performance. *Ergonomics* 30:1287–1299.

Wagenaar A, O'Malley P, LaFond C. 2001. Lowered legal blood alcohol limits for young drivers: Effects on drinking, driving, and driving-after-drinking behaviors in 30 states. *American Journal of Public Health* 91(5):801–804.

Wakefield B, Wakefield D, Uden-Holman T, Blegen M. 1998. Nurses' perceptions of why medication administration errors occur. *MEDSURG Nursing* 7(1):39–44.

Wald H, Shojania K. 2001. Root cause analysis. In: Shojania K, Duncan B, McDonald K, Wachter R, eds. *Making Health Care Safer: A Critical Analysis of Patient Safety Practices.* Evidence Report/Technology Assessment No.43. AHRQ Publication Number: 01-E058. Rockville, MD: AHRQ.

Walker K, Prophet C. 1997. Nursing documentation in the computer-based patient record. *Studies in Health Technology & Informatics* 46:313–317.

Wallace M, Greenwood K. 1995. Twelve-hour shifts [editorial]. *Work and Stress* 9:105–108.

Walsh J, Tepas D, Moss P. 1981. The EEG sleep of night and rotating shift workers. In: Johnson L, Tepas D, Colquhon W, Colligan M, eds. *Biological Rhythms, Sleep, and Shift Work.* New York, NY: Spectrum. Pp. 371–381.

Walsh-Sukys A, Reitenbach A, Hudson-Barr D, DePompei P. 2001. Reducing light and sound in the neonatal intensive care unit: An evaluation of patient safety, staff satisfaction and costs. *Journal of Perinatology* 21:230–235.

Walters J. 1992. Nurses' perceptions of reportable medication errors and factors that contribute to their occurrence. *Applied Nursing Research* 5(2):86–88.

Weiss D, Hailstone S. 1993. Hospital saves with bedside point-of-care system. *Computers in Healthcare* 14(1):28–32.

White C, Hemby C. 1997. Automating the bedside. *Healthcare Informatics* 14(2):68–70.

Williamson A, Gower C, Clarke B. 1994. Changing the hours of shiftwork: A comparison on 8 and 12-hour shift rosters in a group of computer operators. *Ergonomics* 37:287–298.

Wilson J, Haines H. 1997. Participatory ergonomics. In: Salvendy G, ed. *Handbook of Human Factors and Ergonomics.* New York, NY: John Wiley and Sons. Pp. 490–513.

Wojtczak-Jaroszowa J, Banaszkiewicz A. 1974. Physical work capacity during the day and at night. *Ergonomics* 17:193–198.

Wroblewski M, Werrbach K. 1999. Nurses gain more time with patients. *Nursing Management* 30(9):35.

Wylie C, Schultz T, Miller J, Mitler M, Mackie R. 1996. *Commercial Motor Vehicle Driver Fatigue and Alertness Study.* FHWA Report number: FHWA-MC-97-001, TC Report Number TP12876E. Montreal, Canada: Transportation Development Center. Prepared for the Federal Highway Administration, U.S. Department of Transportation; Trucking Research Institute, American Trucking Associations Foundation; and the Transportation Development Centre, Safety and Security, Transport Canada.

Young D. 2002. Health care industry informs FDA of bar-code needs. *American Journal of Health Systems Pharmacists* 59:1592, 1594, 1600.

Zerwekh J, Thibodeaux R, Plesko R. 2000. Chart it once: Innovation in public health documentation. *Journal of Community Health Nursing* 17(2):75–83.

7

Creating and Sustaining
a Culture of Safety

Employing a nursing workforce strong in numbers and capabilities and designing the work of nursing to prevent errors are critical patient safety defenses. Regardless of how strong and how well designed such measures may be, however, they will not by themselves fully safeguard patients. The largest and most capable workforce is still fallible, and the best-designed work processes are still designed by fallible individuals. Moreover, as discussed earlier, each introduction of new health care technology brings a host of unanticipated opportunities for errors. Thus, improving patient safety requires more than relying on the workforce and well-designed work processes; it requires an organizational commitment to vigilance for potential errors and the detection, analysis, and redressing of errors when they occur.

A variety of safety-conscious industries have made such a commitment and achieved lower rates of errors by doing so. These organizations place as high a priority on safety as they do on production; all employees are fully engaged in the process of detecting high-risk situations before an error occurs. Management is so responsive to employees' detection of risk that it dedicates organizational resources—time, personnel, budget, and training— to bring about needed changes, often recommended by staff, to make work processes safer. Employees also are empowered to act in dangerous situations to reduce the likelihood of adverse events. The environment is fair and just—appropriately recognizing the relative contributions of individuals and systemic organizational features to errors, supportive of staff, and fosters continuous learning by the organization as a whole and its employees. These attitudes and employee engagement are so pervasive and observable in the behaviors of such organizations and their employees that an actual *culture of safety* exists within the organization.

The Institute of Medicine (IOM) report *To Err Is Human* calls attention to the need to create such safety cultures within all health care organizations (HCOs) (IOM, 2000). The committee finds that while some progress has been made to this end, a safety culture is unlikely to reach its full potential without years of substantial commitment. The committee reaffirms the importance of the creation and maintenance of cultures of safety and recommends ongoing action by all HCOs to achieve this goal. Action also is needed from state boards of nursing and Congress to enable strong and effective cultures of safety to exist.

This chapter begins by reviewing the essential elements of an effective safety culture, and then addresses the need for a long-term commitment to create such a culture. Barriers to safety cultures found in nursing and external sources are examined next. The chapter then presents examples of the progress being made by some organizations in creating cultures of safety. The final section addresses the need for all HCOs to measure their progress in the creation of such cultures.

ESSENTIAL ELEMENTS OF AN EFFECTIVE SAFETY CULTURE

Conceptual models of organizational safety and empirical studies of organizations widely noted for low levels of errors and accidents (high safety) identify a number of structures and processes essential to effective cultures of safety. Cultures of safety result from the effective interplay of three organizational elements: (1) environmental structures and processes within the organization, (2) the attitudes and perceptions of workers, and (3) the safety-related behaviors of individuals (Cooper, 2000). Chapters 4 through 6 address the contributions of three major environmental structures and processes (i.e., managerial personnel practices, workforce capability, and work design) to patient safety. The focus here is on the safety management systems and psychological and behavioral readiness and ability of all workers necessary for the creation and maintenance of safety cultures.

Commitment of Leadership to Safety

The commitment of leadership to safety is critical to the development of a culture of safety within an organization (Carnino, undated; Manasse et al., 2002; Spath, 2000). Although management has the strongest ability to influence and unite all groups in the organization (by articulating values, reinforcing norms, and providing incentives for desired behaviors), this commitment is needed from all organizational leaders—governing boards and clinical leaders as well as management.

Words alone are an ineffective leadership tool. Leadership commitment must be expressed through actions observable to employees (Carnino, undated; Spath, 2000). Boards of directors can demonstrate this commitment by regular and close oversight of patient safety in the institutions they oversee (IOM, 2000). Leadership actions that management can take include the following:

- Undergoing formal training to gain an understanding of safety culture concepts and practices (Carnino, undated).
- Ensuring that safety is addressed as a priority in the strategic plans of the organization (Carnino, undated; Shrivastava, 1992).
- Having facility-wide patient safety policies and procedures that delineate clear plans for supervisor responsibility and accountability and enable each employee to explain how his or her performance affects patient safety (Spath, 2000).
- Regularly reviewing the safety policies of the organization to ensure their adequacy for current and anticipated circumstances (Carnino, undated).
- Including safety as a priority item on the agenda for meetings (Carnino, undated).
- Encouraging employees to have a questioning attitude on safety issues (Carnino, undated).
- Having personal objectives for directly improving aspects of safety in managers' areas of responsibility (Carnino, undated).
- Monitoring safety trends to ensure that safety objectives are being achieved (Carnino, undated; Spath, 2000).
- Taking a genuine interest in safety improvements and recognizing those who achieve them—not restricting interest to situations in which there is a safety problem (Carnino, undated).
- Reviewing the safety status of the organization on a periodic (e.g., yearly) basis and identifying short- and long-term safety objectives (Pizzi et al., 2001; Spath, 2000).

Finally, leadership's commitment to safety is evidenced by a willingness to direct resources for improved safety, as reflected in the organization's budget (Pizzi et al., 2001; Shrivastava, 1992).

All Employees Empowered and Engaged in Ongoing Vigilance

Organizations with higher rates of accidents tend to believe that managers and system designers will anticipate potential problems in production systems and to assume that workers will always perform in accordance with performance expectations. In contrast, high-reliability organizations and other organizations committed to a safety culture know that system designers, managers, and organizational planners, as well as workers "at the sharp end" (see Chapter 1), are fallible. They know that system designers and managers cannot plan for the infinite variations that can occur within work systems, and that bad things sometimes happen in spite of best efforts to design a "fail-safe" system. Consequently, organizations with a strong safety culture encourage all employees to be on the lookout for any odd or unusual events instead of assuming that the odd or unusual is insignificant (Roberts and Bea, 2001). While management may set the tone, responsibility for safety is acknowledged as the responsibility of all employees. In a safety culture, all who work within the organization are actively involved in identifying and resolving safety concerns and are empowered to take appropriate action to prevent an adverse event (Spath, 2000).

Creating such attitudes and behaviors in workers requires many of the same practices recommended in the preceding chapters—ongoing, effective, multidirectional communication; the adoption of nonhierarchical decision-making practices; empowering of employees to adopt innovate practices to enhance patient safety; and a substantial commitment to employee training)—as well as alignment of employee incentives and rewards to promote safety.

Communication

Communication must accomplish multiple goals. First, leadership needs to convince employees of the organization's commitment to ensuring patient safety and to building a culture of safety. It can do so by the actions described above, but first and foremost by openly acknowledging to employees the high-risk, error-prone nature of the organization's activities (Pizzi et al., 2001) and the need to make fundamental changes in organizational policies and procedures to reduce errors and risks to safety. On an ongoing basis, management must be open to problems and warnings detected by staff that indicate possible degradation of quality (Carnino, undated).

Moreover, in effective safety cultures, patterns of communication are not hierarchical. Hierarchical communication typically reflects an organization's "authority gradient"—the interpersonal dynamics present in situations of real or perceived power (Manasse et al., 2002). Hierarchical lines of communication with steep authority gradients can negatively affect a safety culture. They often involve waiting for orders, unquestioning compliance with directives, and disincentives to questioning or relaying "bad news" up the chain of command. In contrast, in organizations with a strong safety culture, communication is free and open up and down the chain of command and across organizational divisions. Regardless of rank or level of authority, staff are encouraged to speak up if they identify a risk or uncover an error. Workers feel empowered to report observed system or process vulnerabilities that could lead to an accident (Manasse et al., 2002).

Nonhierarchical Decision Making

Like communication patterns, decision making in organizations with a strong safety culture is made at the lowest level appropriate. High-reliability organizations have malleable structures that allow them to expand and contract given the complexity and volatility of the task at hand. Within these expanding or contracting structures, authority migrates to the point in the organization at which specific expertise about the decision exists. Decision makers either work with or are the people who implement the decision. Portions of decisions often come together across groups or individuals within a group. This principle also is essential to the creation of "learning organizations" as described in Chapter 4.

Constrained Improvisation

In organizations with strong safety cultures, employees have permission and indeed are encouraged to engage in "constrained improvisation" (Moorman and Miner, 1998; Weick, 1993) when doing so furthers the goals of the organization. Employees typically improvise three things: tools, rules, and routines. Tools can be and often are used for doing things they were not designed to do; rules are bent in the interest of safety; and routines are altered when they do not work (Bigley and Roberts, 2001). There is an expectation of collaboration across ranks to seek solutions for risks and vulnerabilities as they arise. All employees believe they have the necessary authority and resources to rectify safety hazards as they are identified (Pizzi et al., 2001). It is important to note that, for an organization to be nimble enough to engage in this process appropriately, employees must have a great deal of training and experience.

Training

Safety orientation and recurrent training are essential. Organizations that have fewer accidents teach their people how to recognize and respond to a variety of problems and empower them to act to this end. Staff are trained in safety practices, and education is used to motivate them to anticipate all types of adverse events, eradicate them when possible, and mitigate their effects if they cannot be prevented. When problems are identified, retraining is available without penalty or stigma if safety is involved. Staff who operate equipment or new technology are trained in its use and can recognize maintenance problems and request timely maintenance (Pizzi et al., 2001).

Research on high-reliability organizations shows that they are better than other organizations at training their employees to look for anomalies and potential problems and, most important, to intervene when problems are detected. They also spend more money on training workers to recognize and respond to problems. For example, operators at Diablo Canyon Nuclear Power Plant work their regular shifts 3 weeks of every month. During the fourth week, they train for a wide range of unusual and potentially dangerous reactions. This training keeps them alert to all the things that can go wrong, and reinforces the idea that the organization is taking the likelihood of errors seriously and needs the ongoing vigilance and action of employees to detect errors before they can result in adverse events (Roberts and Bea, 2001).

Rewards and Incentives

In a culture of safety, people are rewarded for their involvement in safety improvements, whether as individuals or as members of safety improvement teams, safety committees, or participants in safety meetings (Carnino, undated; Spath, 2000). Recognition can be formal (e.g., salary increases and promotions based on staff performance criteria related to safety) or informal, but the value of safety permeates the organization's reward system. Safety results are clearly displayed and rewarded at all levels (Pizzi et al., 2001).

Pay and reward systems have received a great deal of attention in the psychological and organizational literatures. It is well known, for example, that rewards and punishment function differently. Rewards convey information about performance the organization wants repeated. Punishment, on the other hand, conveys only information about what the organization does not want. Thus, the use of rewards is a powerful learning mechanism, whereas the use of punishment is less powerful unless it is followed up with information about what the organization desires.

The problem with rewards is that they often are not aligned with desired behavior. Attempts to improve the organization's performance by modifying individual or group incentives often end up rewarding outcomes that actually worsen performance. Such misaligned incentives can undermine important behaviors. For example, rewarding increased productivity can reduce product or service quality, a phenomenon known as the "folly of rewarding A while hoping for B" (Kerr, 1975).

Organizational Learning from Errors and Near Misses

In organizations with strong safety cultures, all errors are considered learning opportunities. Any event related to safety, especially a human or organizational error, is viewed as a valuable opportunity to improve the safety of operations through feedback. High-reliability organizations use accident analysis to:

- Build organizational memory of what happened and why.
- Develop an understanding of accidents that can happen in that particular organization.
- Communicate organizational concern about accidents to reinforce the cultural values of safety.
- Identify parts of the system that should have redundancies (Roberts and Bea, 2001).

This attitude toward safety is one of the hallmarks of knowledge management and is possessed by "learning organizations" (DeLong and Fahey, 2000) as described in Chapter 4. Learning in this way requires a fair and just reporting system of near-misses as well as errors, analysis of reported events, and feedback.

Confidential Error Reporting and Fair and Just Responses to Reported Errors

Trust is a critical factor in developing an effective error-reporting system (Manasse et al., 2002). Evidence indicates that approximately three of every four errors are detected by those committing them, as opposed to being detected by an environmental cue or another person (Reason, 1990). Therefore, employees need to be able to trust that they can fully report errors—particularly human errors—without fear of being wrongfully blamed, thereby providing the opportunity to learn how to further improve the process (Spath, 2000). This point cannot be overemphasized. When such reporting has been introduced in health care work environments, reporting of errors and near-misses has increased dramatically, and improvements in the safety of care delivery have been enabled (Tracy, 1999). Just 16 months after the piloting of the Veterans Administration's (VA) Patient Safety Improvement Initiative, the VA observed a 30-fold increase in reported events and a 900-fold increase in reported near misses for events designated as "high priority." This increase was attributed, in part, to the VA's emphasis on a nonpunitive approach to error reporting (Bagian et al., 2001). Examination of error-reporting systems in 25 nonmedical industries found immunity from reprisals to be one of three factors important in determining the quality of incident reports and the success of incident-reporting systems. The other two were confidentiality or data deidentification on reports of errors—making the reported data untraceable to caregivers, patients, or institutions—and ease of reporting (Barach and Small, 2000).

Without an understanding and acceptance of human fallibility, personal shame also is a disincentive to error reporting. In a pretest of a survey of employee attitudes at five VA facilities prior to implementation of a near-miss reporting system, 49 percent of the 87 respondents admitted "they are ashamed when they make a mistake in front of others." Those who reported feeling ashamed also were more likely to report that they did not tell others about their mistakes (Augustine et al., 1999).

To counteract "blame and shame," the personnel or team involved in an error should be encouraged to propose corrective and preventive measures (Carnino, undated). A fair and just environment extends beyond the attitudes and behaviors of management to those of coworkers. Training in the underlying concepts and principles of human error also can help counteract judgmental attitudes about peers who report errors, which is essential to prepare the work environment for the more fundamental, critical relationship changes that must be employed to ensure long-term safety (Jones, 2002; Pizzi et al., 2001).

The most obvious way to ensure the confidentiality of data on reported errors is to have reports filed anonymously. This approach has drawbacks as well as benefits. In some situations, it may be difficult to guarantee anonymity. When reports are filed anonymously, analysts cannot contact the reporters for more information. Anonymous reports also may be unreliable. Moreover, anonymity is susceptible to criticism that it threatens accountability and the transparency of health care. Despite these drawbacks, some experts studying reporting systems in a variety of industries conclude that it may be important to provide anonymity early in the evolution of an incident-reporting system, at least until trust has been built and reporters see practical results (Barach and Small, 2000). Another strategy, employed by the Federal Aviation Administration's error-reporting system, is to deidentify the reported data after they have been reported.

Reporting Near Misses as Well as Errors

Experts who have studied accident- and error-reporting systems also assert the benefits of reporting not just errors and accidents that have occurred, but near misses as well (Bagian and Gosbee, 2000; Barach and Small, 2000). A near miss is an event that could have had adverse consequences but did not; it is indistinguishable from a full-fledged adverse event in all but outcome. Examples of near misses are a nurse giving a patient an incorrect medication from which the patient suffered no adverse consequences, and a nurse programming the wrong rate of flow for an intravenous infusion, but the error being detected by a nurse taking over care of the patient so that again the patient suffers no adverse consequences.

Near misses offer effective reminders of system hazards and help counteract the tendency to forget to be afraid. For example, data on near misses in aviation have been used effectively to redesign aircraft, air traffic control systems, airports, and pilot training programs (Barach and Small, 2000). Reports of near misses are also likely to be more candid than error reports, and provide the opportunity to learn without first having to experience an adverse event (Bagian and Gosbee, 2000). Collecting and analyzing data on near misses offers several other advantages: (1) near misses occur 3–300 times more often than adverse events, offering the opportunity for more powerful quantitative analysis; (2) there are fewer barriers (e.g., shame and fear of reprisals) to data collection; (3) recovery strategies can be studied to assist in developing effective defense mechanisms to prevent future errors; and (4) hindsight bias is reduced (Barach and Small, 2000).

Data Analysis and Feedback

Once errors and near misses have been reported, the organization needs to have procedures for analyzing the data and feeding back the results to reporters. The use of root-cause analysis (described in Chapter 6) and the existence of a corrective action program are positive indications of a good safety culture (Carnino, undated; Spath, 2000). Injury-producing incidents and significant near misses are investigated for their root causes, and effective preventive actions are taken (Pizzi et al., 2001). Such research and analysis should not be considered luxuries, but essential to the effective design of safe systems of care because analysis provides the information needed for preventive measures (IOM, 2000).

An examination of error-reporting systems in 25 nonmedical industries found that independent outsourcing of report collection and analysis to peer experts and the provision of rapid, meaningful feedback to reporters and all interested parties are important in determining the quality of error reports and the success of error-reporting systems (Barach and Small, 2000). Staff should be given timely feedback on the results of analysis of their reports, and told how the data were used to improve systems and prevent future errors.

Overall Features of an Effective Error-Reporting System

The above characteristics underscore the recommendations of an Expert Advisory Panel on Patient Safety System Design convened by the Veterans Administration to identify and examine alternative procedures for internal reporting and reviewing of adverse events (Bagian and Gosbee, 2000). These experts conclude that, to be effective, any internal organization reporting system needs to possess the following features:

- First and foremost, it should not be perceived as part of a punitive system; people will not openly report to a system if they believe doing so could result in punitive action.
- Confidentiality mechanisms should be in place so people will be confident that they will not be placing themselves in jeopardy by reporting.
- The reporting mechanism should stress capturing a description of what happened through the use of narratives, not just "checking off boxes" in a structured format.
- The reports need to be analyzed by people who have practical, hands-on knowledge of the subject matter under consideration. Moreover, that analysis should be performed by more than one individual, since a fresh eye often produces more meaningful results.
- Voluntary rather than mandatory reporting systems are more likely to uncover events because they reduce the disincentive of fear of punishment.
- The reporting system should not be a "counting effort" because there will always be underreporting for a host of reasons. The experts note that the real purpose of a reporting system is to ferret out and correct vulnerabilities, not to count them. This point is particularly important because of the potential misconception that increased reporting represents increased danger.
- Timely and appropriate feedback to reporters is essential to the ongoing trust and effectiveness of the reporting system.

To Err Is Human reiterates that reporting systems within organizations should be voluntary and confidential, have minimal restrictions on acceptable content, include descriptive accounts and stories, and be accessible for contributions from all clinical and administrative staff (IOM, 2000).

NEED FOR A LONG-TERM COMMITMENT TO CREATE A CULTURE OF SAFETY

Instituting the structures and processes described above requires changes in attitudes, beliefs, and behaviors. It is not easily accomplished. Some have estimated that it can take 5 years to develop a culture of safety that permeates the entire organization (Manasse et al., 2002).

The International Atomic Energy Agency, which has monitored and studied safety and cultures of safety across many countries' nuclear energy installations, likewise observes that cultures of safety develop over time. Their development occurs in three stages (Carnino, undated):

- Stage 1—Safety management is based on rules and regulations.
- Stage 2—Good safety performance becomes an organizational goal.
- Stage 3—Safety performance is seen as dynamic and continuously improving.

In **Stage 1**, the organization sees safety as an external requirement imposed by governmental or other regulatory bodies. There is little awareness of the behavioral and attitudinal aspects of safety; safety is viewed primarily as a technical issue. Mere compliance with rules and regulations is considered adequate, and the following characteristics may be observed:

- Problems are not anticipated; the organization reacts to them as they occur.
- Communication between departments is poor.
- Departments and functions behave as semiautonomous units, evidencing little collaboration and shared decision making.
- The decisions taken by departments and functions focus on little more than the need to comply with rules.
- People who make mistakes are simply blamed for their failure to comply with the rules.
- Conflicts are not resolved; departments and functions compete with one another.
- The role of management is perceived as endorsing the rules, pushing employees, and expecting results.
- Little listening or learning occurs within or outside of the organization, which adopts a defensive posture when criticized.
- Safety is viewed as a required nuisance.
- Regulators, customers, suppliers, or contractors are treated cautiously or in an adversarial manner.
- Short-term profits are regarded as all-important.
- People are viewed as "system components"; they are defined and valued solely in terms of what they do.
- An adversarial relationship exists between management and employees.
- There is little or no awareness of work processes.
- People are rewarded for obedience and results, regardless of long-term consequences.

In **Stage 2**, good safety performance becomes an organizational goal, perceived by management as important even in the absence of regulatory pressure. Although there is a growing awareness of behavioral issues, this aspect is largely missing from the safety management methods employed, which comprise technical and procedural solutions. Safety performance is addressed, like other aspects of the business, in terms of targets or goals. The organization begins to examine the reasons why safety performance reaches a plateau, and is willing to seek the advice of other organizations. In this stage, the following characteristics may be observed:

- The organization concentrates primarily on day-to-day matters; there is little in the way of strategy.
- Management encourages cross-departmental and cross-functional teams and communication.
- Senior managers function as a team and begin to coordinate departmental and functional decisions.
- Decisions are often centered on cost and function.
- Management's response to mistakes is to institute more controls through procedures and retraining; somewhat less blaming occurs.
- Conflict is disturbing and discouraged in the name of teamwork.
- The role of management is perceived as applying management techniques, such as management by objectives.
- The organization is somewhat open to learning from other companies, especially with regard to techniques and best practices.
- The cost of safety and productivity are viewed as detracting from one another; safety is perceived as increasing costs and reducing production.
- The organization's relationships with regulators, customers, suppliers, and contractors are distant rather than close, reflecting a cautious approach whereby trust must be earned.
- It is important to meet or exceed short-term profit goals. People are rewarded for exceeding goals regardless of the long-term results or consequences.
- The relationship between employees and management is still adversarial, with little trust or respect demonstrated.
- There is growing awareness of the impact of cultural issues in the workplace. People do not understand why added controls fail to yield the expected results in safety performance.

In this stage, the organization establishes a vision of the desired safety culture and communicates it throughout the organization. A systematic effort is made to gather input regarding the culture's strengths and weaknesses. The organization develops a strategy for realizing desired changes by allocating budgetary resources, personnel, training, and time to the program, implementing the strategy and holding people accountable for meeting objectives.

In **Stage 3,** safety performance is viewed as dynamic and always amenable to improvement. The organization has adopted the idea of continuous improvement and has applied the concept to safety. There is a strong emphasis on communication, training, management style, and improving efficiency and effectiveness. Everyone in the organization can contribute. Some behaviors and attitudes are understood to either enable or obstruct safety. Consequently, the level of awareness of behavioral and attitudinal issues is high, and measures are taken to effect improvements in these areas. Progress is made one step at a time and never stops. The organization also asks how it might help other companies. In this stage, the following characteristics may be observed:

- The organization begins to act strategically, with a focus on the longer term as well as an awareness of the present. It anticipates problems and deals with their causes before they occur.
- People recognize and state the need for collaboration among departments and functions. They receive management support, recognition, and the resources they need for collaborative work.
- People are aware of work or business processes in the company and help managers manage them.
- Decisions are made with full knowledge of their safety impact on work or business processes, as well as on department and functions.
- There is no goal conflict between safety and production performance, so safety is not jeopardized in pursuit of production targets.
- Almost all mistakes are viewed in terms of variability in work processes. The important thing is to understand what has happened rather than to find someone to blame. This understanding is used to modify the processes as necessary to avoid similar errors in the future.
- The existence of conflict is recognized and addressed through an attempt to create mutually beneficial solutions.
- Management's role is perceived as coaching people to improve business performance.
- Learning from other sources both within and outside of the organization is valued. Time is made available for the purpose and devoted to adapting such knowledge to improve business performance.
- Safety and production are viewed as interdependent.
- Collaborative relationships are developed between the organization and regulators, suppliers, customers, and contractors.
- Short-term performance is measured and analyzed so changes can be made to improve long-term performance.
- People are respected and valued for their contributions.

- The relationship between management and employees is respectful and supportive.
- Awareness of the impact of cultural issues is reflected in key decisions. The organization rewards not just those who produce, but also those who support the work of others. People are rewarded for improving processes as well as results.

The characteristics of all three stages can serve organizations as a basis for self-diagnosis. They can also be used by an organization to give direction to its development of a safety culture by identifying its current position and the position to which it aspires. It should be noted that an organization at any given point in time may exhibit a combination of the characteristics listed under each stage and that different departments or other components of an organization may be at different stages.

The time required for an organization to progress through the three stages cannot be predicted. Much will depend on the circumstances of an individual organization and the commitment and effort it is prepared to devote to effecting change. However, sufficient time must be taken in each stage to allow the benefits from changed practices to be realized and to mature. People must be prepared for such change. Too many new initiatives in a relatively short period of time can be organizationally destabilizing. The important point to note is that any organization interested in improving its safety culture should start and not be deterred by the fact that progress will be gradual (Carnino, undated). HCOs should also expect to face a number of barriers unique to health care and the work environment of nurses.

BARRIERS TO EFFECTIVE SAFETY CULTURES FROM NURSING AND EXTERNAL SOURCES

As HCOs undertake the creation of a culture of safety, they must dedicate the internal personnel and other resources required to effect the needed changes. They must also deal with two barriers that must be overcome if they are to achieve the maximum benefit from their efforts—one that originates in the nursing profession (and also is found among other health professionals) and one that is found in the external legal/regulatory environment.

A Nursing Culture That Fosters Unrealistic Expectations of Clinical Perfection

Nurses are trained to believe that clinical perfection is an attainable goal (Jones, 2002) and that "good" nurses do not make errors (Banister et al., 1996). Like the general public, they perceive errors to be due to careless-ness, inattention, indifference, or uninformed decisions. Requiring high stan-dards of performance for nurses is both appropriate and desirable, but be-comes counterproductive when it creates an expectation of perfection. Because they regard clinical perfection as a professional goal, nurses feel shame when they make an error (Leape, 1994), which in turn creates pres-sure to hide or cover up errors (Osborne et al., 1999; Wakefield et al., 1996) (see the example presented at the beginning of Chapter 1).

It is difficult to transform thinking associated with the blame and shame mentality (Banister et al., 1996; Manasse et al., 2002). In a study conducted to assess safety culture transformation over time at six VA medical centers, the first change noted was the realization that errors are the result of a systemic rather than an individual problem. Within a year, health care pro-viders were reporting that they would not think less of coworkers who made errors. One of the last changes to occur was that providers did not think worse of themselves when an error occurred.[1] Such a transformation requires extensive education and training and support at all levels of the organization.

Litigation and Regulatory Barriers

Unfortunately, regulatory boards and litigation practices reinforce the myth of clinical perfection, as illustrated by the two cases presented in Box 7-1.

These two cases (Cook et al., 2000; Grant, 1999; Knox, 2000; Schnei-der, 1999; Senders, 1999) illustrate a persisting focus on individuals rather than systems as the sources of error among licensing boards in medicine, nursing, and pharmacy; regulatory bodies, such as health departments; and sometimes the judicial system (Grant, 1999; Manasse et al., 2002). Mal-practice litigation reinforces this perception. One result of this situation is that the consequences of litigation for the nurses involved in these and simi-lar adverse events, in which nurses were fined, fired, sued, or otherwise punished (Serembus et al., 2001; Sexton, 1995), create serious disincentives to disclosure of errors or near misses on the part of nurses and other health professionals. The threat of legal liability is a strong barrier to voluntary reporting of errors (Schneider, 1999) and to the design of measures to pre-vent additional errors in the future.

The IOM report *To Err Is Human* speaks directly to these disincentives and identifies two steps HCOs can take to counteract them when designing

---

[1]Personal communication, Gail Powell-Cope, Ph.D., Veterans Integrated Service Network 8, Patient Safety Center, and James A Haley Veterans Hospital, Tampa, Florida, July 30, 2003.

their internal error-reporting systems: pledging the confidentiality of the reporter and the information contained in the report, and obtaining and maintaining data in a manner that prevents identification of the reporter or the specific event even if access to the report is obtained. This latter strategy can be pursued by adopting anonymous reporting of adverse events and near misses, or by deidentifying information once reported, as discussed earlier (IOM, 2000).

To Err Is Human also cites the need for federal legislation to extend peer review protections to data collected and analyzed by HCOs for purposes of improving safety and quality. It notes that all but one of the states have passed such legislation, but that these state laws vary in scope and strength. Federal legislation could remedy this situation, providing uniform national protection for the creation of cultures of safety in HCOs (IOM, 2000). This concept also has been endorsed by the Medicare Payment Advisory Commission, which has recommended that Congress enact legislation to protect the confidentiality of individually identifiable information relating to errors in health care delivery when that information is reported for quality improvement purposes (Medicare Payment Advisory Commission, 1999). Australia and New Zealand currently offer such legal protection for reporters of health care errors (Barach and Small, 2000).

To Err Is Human suggests that a combination of federal legislation and internal protections for the reporter and reported data is best. Each alone is imperfect, but together they offer stronger assurance of confidentiality (IOM, 2000).

Another strategy is being tested in the United Kingdom to guide decisions regarding culpability in unsafe acts in which health care professionals are involved. An "incident decision tree," based on the decision tree in Reason's (1997) publication *Managing the Risks of Organizational Accidents* (see Figure 7-1), has been developed to help health care organizations to discriminate fairly and justly among willful acts of wrongdoing, inadvertent human error, and system contributions to error. Doing so can help a health care organization determine the appropriate response to an error in which an individual "at the sharp end" is involved.

The incident decision tree is based on the premise that while the vast majority of unsafe acts involve "honest" or nonculpable errors, a small minority of individuals commit reckless unsafe acts, and will continue to do so if left unchecked. To create a just culture, it is necessary to reach a collective agreement on where the line should be drawn between acceptable and unacceptable errors. To assist in differentiating between blameworthy and blameless acts, the model incorporates the following "substitution" test:

> Substitute the individual involved in the adverse event or near miss with another individual possessing comparable qualifications and experience. Then

BOX 7-1 Litigation and Regulatory Barriers to Effective Safety Cultures: Two Case Examples

In the investigation of a widely publicized fatal chemotherapy overdose in 1994 of a health columnist for the *Boston Globe*, the state department of public health, the Joint Commission on Accreditation of Healthcare Organizations, and the National Institutes of Health found no fault on the part of any of the nurses involved in the administration of the medication. The nurses had checked the patient's name, medication, dosage and route, frequency of administration, and specific directions for administration against the physician's order. The investigation of the incident revealed that the error had been caused by a number of system problems, including that the patient was being treated according to an investigational protocol and that the only reference source for confirming the drug, dosage, frequency, and route (apart from the physician's order) was the protocol document itself. Moreover, the research protocol document was found to be flawed and confirmed the physician's mistaken order. Finally, there was no computerized pharmacy check system. Despite these findings, 4 years after the overdose, the state board of nursing proposed sanctions against the nurses involved (Grant, 1999) and subsequently reprimanded or placed on probation 16 nurses involved in the administration of the medication (Knox, 2000).

In 1996, a woman with a prenatal history of syphilis gave birth to a baby boy. Because of the absence of documentation of treatment for syphilis, neonatology and pediatric infectious disease experts agreed that the baby should be treated with a dose of penicillin G, 150,000 units/kg by intramuscular (IM)

ask the following question: "In light of how events unfolded and were perceived by those involved in real time, is it likely that this new individual would have behaved any differently?"

If the answer is "probably not," blaming the individual at the sharp end of the error is an inappropriate response. Similarly, blame is not assigned to the individual if his/her peers respond "probably not" to the question "Given the circumstances that prevailed at that time, could you be sure that you would not have committed the same or similar type of unsafe act?" (Reason, 1997: 208).

Ensuring confidential reporting of errors, using fair and just procedures for assessing causation, and extending peer review protections to data collected by HCOs together can reduce the disincentives to error reporting that thwart the detection and prevention of error-producing situations.

injection. In preparing the medication, the pharmacist misread the dose and, because the hospital had no unit dose system, sent the medication to the nursing unit in two syringes containing more medication than the (miscalculated) dose.

Because the volume of the medication would have required the baby to receive five IM injections, the nurses investigated the possibility of giving the drug intravenously. The three nurses (one who cared for both mother and baby, one providing more intensive care to the baby, and a neonatal nurse practitioner) consulted a drug reference book, which indicated that the drug could be given by slow intravenous push. The nurses did not know that there were two different forms of the penicillin: aqueous and viscous. Aqueous penicillin can be given intravenously; viscous penicillin must be given IM. When the dose was administered, the baby suffered a cardiac arrest and died (Schneider, 1999).

This event resulted in indictments against all three nurses on charges of criminal negligence. At trial, the Institute for Safe Medication Practices presented its analysis of the incident showing more than 50 different system failures contributing to the error, including that the drug was seldom used; the pharmacist had miscalculated the dose; the hospital lacked a unit dose medication dispensing system, which required the pharmacist to dispense an amount even greater than the miscalculated dose; the manufacturer's warning on the syringe that it was for IM administration only was difficult to see; and available reference materials were ambiguous about acceptable routes of administration (Cook et al., 2000).

PROGRESS IN CREATING CULTURES OF SAFETY

JCAHO provided a key stimulus for the creation of cultures of safety in HCOs when in 2001 it adopted new patient safety accreditation standards for health care facilities. These standards encourage the development of cultures of safety by, in part, requiring HCO leaders to ensure implementation of an integrated patient safety program throughout the organization (Standard LD.5) (JCAHO, 2003a). In 2003, JCAHO also began requiring accredited organizations to meet annually specified patient safety goals. Each year the goals and associated recommendations will be reevaluated to determine whether they should be continued or replaced (JCAHO, 2003b).

Some HCOs have made great strides in creating cultures of safety. Two examples are described below.

304

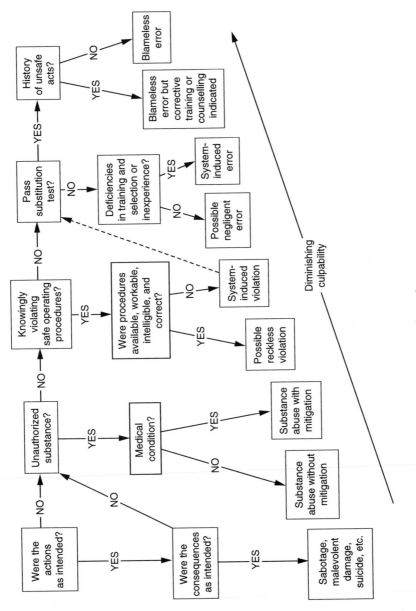

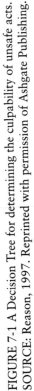

FIGURE 7-1 A Decision Tree for determining the culpability of unsafe acts.
SOURCE: Reason, 1997. Reprinted with permission of Ashgate Publishing.

Good Samaritan Hospital, Dayton, Ohio

In early 2000, Good Samaritan Hospital's (GSH) Vice President of Clinical Effectiveness and Performance Improvement, an early champion of patient safety, began an initiative to create a culture of safety within the hospital. This leader, as well as the director of the hospital's Center of Outcomes Research and Clinical Effectiveness, presented to the quality committee of the hospital's board of trustees a summary of the significance of patient safety and recommendations to institutionalize the vision that safety is essential to the hospital's mission. The vice president also engaged in one-on-one and group discussions with hospital leaders on the importance and benefits of being a safety-reliable organization. Through this consensus process, key hospital leaders committed their support to and agreed to guide the initiative.

To implement this initiative, GSH modified organizational structures and committed resources to the effort. Rather than assigning the project to a preexisting committee, it added a new Safety Board to its administrative infrastructure. This board is composed of physician, nursing, and administrative leaders, including the chief executive officer (CEO) and hospital communications staff. It serves as an oversight body to ensure the advancement of the safety program and to create the policies and procedures needed to implement the program. The Safety Board is also responsible for medical management, risk management, and quality management.

GSH adopted three early aims for its initiative:

- Demonstrate that patient safety is a top leadership priority.
- Promote a nonpunitive culture for sharing information and lessons learned.
- Implement an integrated patient safety program throughout the organization.

GSH evaluates its progress in meeting these aims on a bimonthly basis using a self-assessment tool adapted from such a tool developed as part of a Voluntary Hospital Association collaborative. The Safety Board formulated criteria for each aim. Specific actions undertaken by GSH to achieve these aims have included the following:

- Educational programming for all hospital staff on sentinel events, root-cause analysis, incident reporting, the hospital's safety initiative, and the roles of all employees in patient safety.
- Initiation of an incident and near miss reporting system, supported by automated database software to facilitate the tracking, aggregation, and analysis of incident data.

- Creation of a policy to forego corrective action against an employee if an error is reported within 48 hours.
- Initiation of specific safety improvement projects in such areas as medication safety, blood transfusions, and the transport of critically ill patients.
- Participation in state and local initiatives in patient safety, which has led to the exchange of ideas for improved practice and research.

As a result of this initiative, the hospital has experienced a significant increase in reported errors that has guided system improvements. It further reports a growing awareness that "committing resources to support patient safety initiatives is not in conflict with cost-effective practices. Eliminating rework and errors reduces the cost of providing care and the costs of resolving litigation . . ." (Wong et al., 2002: 372).

Kaiser Permanente

Kaiser Permanente, the largest not-for-profit health maintenance organization (HMO) in the United States, undertook the creation of a culture of safety throughout the organization as part of a Patient Safety Plan initiated in 2001. This initiative is aimed at:

- Creating a strong patient safety culture, with patient safety embraced as a shared value.
- Creating an environment that encourages responsible reporting of near misses and errors and that focuses on fixing systems and not assigning blame.
- Implementing strategies for improvement in patient safety performance.
- Identifying, sharing, and implementing best practices from other parts of the organization and other industries.
- Providing routine patient safety and error prevention training and education for individuals and groups.
- Developing new knowledge and understanding of safety in the delivery system.
- Identifying, assessing, and implementing indicators and measures of safety.

The above activities are focused on instituting the following six strategic themes:

- Safe culture—Creating and maintaining a strong patient safety culture, with patient safety and error reduction embraced as shared organizational values.

- Safe care—ensuring that the actual and potential hazards associated with high-risk procedures, processes, and patient care populations are identified, assessed, and controlled in a way that demonstrates continuous improvement and ultimately ensures that patients are free from accidental injury or illness.

- Safe staff—Ensuring that staff possess the knowledge and competence to perform required duties safely and improve system safety performance.

- Safe support systems—Identifying, implementing, and maintaining support systems—including knowledge-sharing networks and systems for responsible reporting—that provide the right information to the right people at the right time.

- Safe place—Designing, constructing, operating, and maintaining the environment of health care to enhance its efficiency and effectiveness.

- Safe patients—Engaging patients and their families, as appropriate, in reducing medical errors, improving overall system safety performance, and maintaining trust and respect.

Kaiser Permanente formed an internal National Patient Safety Advisory Board to guide this initiative, provide a forum for information sharing, and help integrate safety into the fabric of the organization. Membership includes a representative of Kaiser Permanente's labor–management partnership with the Coalition of Kaiser Permanente Unions. Kaiser Permanente has engaged and educated its labor partners in patient safety through a number of mechanisms, including their participation in patient safety executive walkarounds. In a survey of unit personnel at one facility 6 months following visits from senior executives, 90 percent of respondents stated that things related to patient safety were being done differently, 44 percent indicated that their reporting or discussion of errors and near misses had increased, and 90 percent indicated that they had a better understanding of patient safety. Human factors training and projects have also been launched in the medical center operating room, neonatal intensive care unit, perinatal units, and emergency department to integrate human factors into the provision of care. A National Patient Safety website is available to all Kaiser Permanente employees to increase their knowledge about patient safety.

NEED FOR ALL HCOS TO MEASURE THEIR PROGRESS IN CREATING CULTURES OF SAFETY

As discussed in Chapter 4, achieving any systemic organizational change is not easy. Objective measurement and feedback is needed to manage planned change successfully, and efforts to create cultures of safety are no exception. To this end, initial baseline assessment of each organization's safety culture and ongoing measurement of its progress in achieving the desired cultural shift are required.

Benchmarking Organizational Safety Culture

A number of health care organizations have surveyed themselves to benchmark their culture-of-safety status (Pizzi et al., 2001), using a variety of surveys and checklists that assess the attitudes and perceptions of workers (Cooper, 2000; Pizzi et al., 2001; Spath, 2000). The Agency for Healthcare Research and Quality and the federal government's Quality Interagency Coordination Task Force are developing a public-domain instrument for assessing issues of patient safety, medical error, and event reporting as they relate to an organization's safety culture. This instrument—the Hospital Survey on Patient Safety—is in the final stages of testing and validation and is scheduled to be available in the public domain in early in 2004. It will allow health care institutions to understand the varying safety cultures within their own institutions, how staff view the commission of errors and error reporting, and the extent to which staff perceives the institution to be a safe place for patients.[2]

By themselves, however, surveys of the safety climate (i.e., the aggregation of individuals' attitudes and perceptions about safety) within organizations are believed to be inadequate in evaluating the extent to which a culture of safety has been created (Cooper, 2000). While appraisal of the products or outcomes of the safety culture in operating organizations is a challenge, measurable indicators of the culture's effectiveness are viewed as essential (Cooper, 2000; Spath, 2000).

Measuring Progress

Although measuring the incidence rate of accidents and other adverse safety-related events as patient safety indicators may appear straightforward, it has serious drawbacks. Negative indicators can be demoralizing to employees, as well as misleading. Reported numbers of errors can decline for reasons having little to do with safety, such as underreporting resulting from other organizational incentives (e.g., production incentives) (Cooper, 2000).

In contrast, positive measures of the observable degree of effort expended by organizational members have been identified as a more effective approach to measuring the degree to which an organization has implemented a safety culture. These measures include the degree to which organi-

---

[2]Personal communication, Jim Battles, Ph.D., Agency for Healthcare Research and Quality, July 10, 2003.

zation members report unsafe conditions and the speed with which the organization initiates remedial actions (Cooper, 2000). Other possible indicators include the following (Carnino, undated).

- Percentage of employees who have received safety refresher training during the previous month/quarter.
- Percentage of safety improvement proposals implemented during the previous month/quarter.
- Percentage of improvement teams involved in determining solutions to safety-related problems.
- Percentage of employee communication briefs that include safety information.
- Number of safety inspections conducted by senior managers during the previous week/month.
- Percentage of employee suggestions that relate to safety improvement.
- Percent of routine organizational meetings with safety as an agenda item. (Carnino, undated)

The value of positive safety indicators is that they serve as a mechanism for recognizing employees who are endeavoring to improve safety by their thoughts, actions, or commitment. Recognition of achievement is a powerful motivating force to encourage continued improvement (Carnino, undated).

RECOMMENDATIONS

In light of the findings and principles set forth in this chapter, the committee makes the following recommendations:

Recommendation 7-1. HCO boards of directors, managerial leadership, and labor partners should create and sustain cultures of safety by implementing the recommendations presented previously and by:

- **Specifying short- and long-term safety objectives.**
- **Continuously reviewing success in meeting these objectives and providing feedback at all levels.**
- **Conducting an annual, confidential survey of nursing and other health care workers to assess the extent to which a culture of safety exists.**
- **Instituting a deidentified, fair, and just reporting system for errors and near misses.**

- Engaging in ongoing employee training in error detection, analysis, and reduction.
- Implementing procedures for analyzing errors and providing feedback to direct-care workers.
- Instituting rewards and incentives for error reduction.

Recommendation 7-2. The National Council of State Boards of Nursing, in consultation with patient safety experts and health care leaders, should undertake an initiative to design uniform processes across states for better distinguishing human errors from willful negligence and intentional misconduct, along with guidelines for their application by state boards of nursing and other state regulatory bodies having authority over nursing.

Recommendation 7-3. Congress should pass legislation to extend peer review protections to data related to patient safety and quality improvement that are collected and analyzed by HCOs for internal use or shared with others solely for purposes of improving safety and quality.

REFERENCES

Augustine C, Weick K, Bagian J, Lee C. 1999. Predispositions toward a culture of safety in a large multi-facility health system. *Proceedings of Enhancing Patient Safety and Reducing Errors in Health Care Conference* held at Rancho Mirage, CA. Chicago, IL: National Patient Safety Foundation. Pp. 138–141.

Bagian JP, Gosbee JW. 2000. Developing a culture of patient safety at the VA. *Ambulatory Outreach* Spring:25–29.

Bagian JP, Lee C, Gosbee J, Derosier J, Stalhandske E, Eldridge N, Williams R, Burkhardt M. 2001. Developing and deploying a patient safety program in a large health care delivery systems: You can't fix what you don't know about. *The Joint Commission Journal on Quality Improvement* 27(10):522–532.

Banister G, Butt L, Hackel R. 1996. How nurses perceive medication errors. *Nursing Management* 27(1):31–34.

Barach P, Small S. 2000. Reporting and preventing medical mishaps: Lessons from non-medical near miss reporting systems. *British Medical Journal* 320:759–763.

Bigley G, Roberts K. 2001. Structuring temporary systems for high reliability. *Academy of Management Journal* 44:1281–1300.

Carnino A, Director, Division of Nuclear Installation Safety, International Atomic Energy Agency. Undated. *Management of Safety, Safety Culture and Self Assessment.* [Online]. Available: http://www.iaea.org/ns/nusafe/publish/papers/mng_safe.htm [accessed January 15, 2003].

Cook R, Render M, Woods D. 2000. Gaps in the continuity of care and progress on patient safety. *British Medical Journal* 320(7237):791–794.

Cooper M. 2000. Towards a model of safety culture. *Safety Science* 36:111–136.

DeLong D, Fahey L. 2000. Diagnosing cultural barriers to knowledge management. *Academy of Management Executive* 14(4):113–127.

Grant S. 1999. Who's to blame for tragic error? *American Journal of Nursing* 99(9):9.

IOM (Institute of Medicine). 2000. *To Err Is Human: Building a Safer Health System.* Washington, DC: National Academy Press.

JCAHO (Joint Commission on Accreditation of Healthcare Organizations). 2003a. *2003 Hospital Accreditation Standards.* Oakbrook Terrace, IL: JCAHO.

JCAHO. 2003b. *2003 National Patient Safety Goals.* [Online]. Available: http://www.jcaho. org/accredited+organizations/patient+safety/npsg/index.htm [accessed July 19, 2003].

Jones B. 2002. Nurses and the Code of Silence. *Medical Error.* San Francisco, CA: Jossey-Bass.

Kerr S. 1975. On the folly of rewarding A while hoping for B. *Academy of Management Journal* 18:769–783.

Knox R. 2000, March 16. State board clears two nurses in 1994 chemotherapy overdose, a third nurse receives reprimand for role. *The Boston Globe.* Metro/Region. P. B2.

Leape L. 1994. Error in medicine. *Journal of the American Medical Association* 272:1851–1857.

Manasse H, Turnbull J, Diamond L. 2002. Patient safety: A review of the contemporary American experience. *Singapore Medical Journal* 43(5):254–262.

Medicare Payment Advisory Commission. 1999. *Report to the Congress: Selected Medicare Issues.* Washington, DC: Medicare Payment Advisory Commission.

Moorman C, Miner A. 1998. Organizational improvisation and organizational memory. *Academy of Management Review* 23:698–723.

Osborne J, Blais K, Hayes J. 1999. Nurses' perceptions: When is it a medication error? *Journal of Nursing Administration* 29(4):33–38.

Pizzi L, Goldfarb N, Nash D. 2001. Promoting a culture of safety. In: Shojania K, Duncan B, McDonald K, Wachter R, eds. *Making HealthCare Safer: A Critical Analysis of Patient Safety Practices.* Rockville, MD: AHRQ.

Reason J. 1990. *Human Error.* Cambridge, UK: Cambridge University Press.

Reason J. 1997. *Managing the Risks of Organizational Accidents.* Aldershot, England: Ashgate Publishing Company.

Roberts K, Bea R. 2001. Must accidents happen? Lessons from high-reliability organizations. *Academy of Management Executive* 15(3):70–78.

Schneider P. 1999. Part one: The anatomy of an event. *Proceedings of Enhancing Patient Safety and Reducing Errors in Health Care Conference* held at Rancho Mirage, CA. Chicago, IL: National Patient Safety Foundation.

Senders J. 1999. Part two: Theory and remedy. *Proceedings of Enhancing Patient Safety and Reducing Errors in Health Care Conference* held at Rancho Mirage, CA. Chicago, IL: National Patient Safety Foundation.

Serembus J, Wolf Z, Youngblood N. 2001. Consequences of fatal medication errors for health care providers: A secondary analysis study. *MEDSURG Nursing* 10(4):193–201.

Sexton J. 1995 (July 28). Three resign after an error in transfusion. *New York Times.* P. B4.

Shrivastava P. 1992. Preventing and coping with industrial crises. In: Shrivastava P, ed. *Bhopal: Anatomy of a Crisis.* London: Paul Chapman Publishing Ltd.

Spath P. 2000. Does your facility have a "patient-safe" climate? *Hospital Peer Review* 25:80–82.

Tracy E. 1999. Evolving practice and a culture of safety. *QRC Advisor* 15(10):10–12.

Wakefield D, Wakefield B, Uden-Holman T, Blegen M. 1996. Perceived barriers in reporting medication administration errors. *Best Practices & Benchmarking in Healthcare* 1(4): 191–197.

Weick K. 1993. Organization redesign as improvisation. In: Huber G, Glick W, eds. *Organizational Change and Redesign.* New York, NY: Oxford University Press.

Wong P, Helsinger D, Petry J. 2002. Providing the right infrastructure to lead the culture change for patient safety. *Joint Commission Journal on Quality Improvement* 28(7):363–372.

8

Implementation Considerations and Needed Research

A call for change is persistent throughout this report. The committee's recommendations call primarily for change on the part of health care organizations (HCOs), but also on the part of the federal government, state boards of nursing, educational institutions, professional associations, labor organizations, and nurses themselves across all settings of health care delivery—acute and long-term, and inpatient and outpatient care. All of these entities have long-standing track records of concern for the welfare and safety of patients, and all have continued to pursue this agenda in the face of the tumultuous changes in the U.S. health care system that have taken place over the last two decades.

The turbulence faced by the health care industry is not unique. All sectors of the U.S. economy have faced the threat of reduced revenue, if not from decreases in reimbursement, then from downturns in the economy or increasing competition. Rapid growth in beneficial technological innovations has occurred in all industries and has sometimes brought unanticipated risks to consumer safety, ranging from identity theft to new sources of environmental pollution and occupational or consumer injury. All industries are affected by changes in the workforce, such as its declining size and aging as the baby boomers reach retirement age. And all industries are forced to address the flood of information from and for consumers, the marketplace, and the external environment that forces them to cope with faster and more layered flows of information (Stacey, 1996).

The ubiquitous nature of this turmoil is helpful in that it provides lessons from a variety of industries about how successful organizations respond in times of challenge. One hallmark of successful, thriving enterprises is their capacity to learn and change (Quinn, 1992). This is an important reminder. When considering the recommendations for change presented in this report, the reader may have any one of a number of different responses, ranging from wishing to jump right in, to wanting to wait to undertake new changes until things settle down a bit, to seeking to determine what recommendations are most important and which can be deferred. However, the committee calls attention to evidence that should influence how HCOs and the other entities addressed in this report respond to its recommendations:

• The turbulence experienced by the health care industry is not predicted to lessen. HCOs and other entities that have roles to play in protecting patient safety should not wait to make necessary changes.

• None of the committee's recommendations are of lesser importance; entities will need to act on all of the recommendations to keep patients safe.

• While some recommendations may have immediate cost implications for some organizations, their implementation also is likely to produce benefits (some financial) for all organizations in addition to enhancing patient safety.

• Organizations and individuals need to maintain the capacity for ongoing change and adoption of new work strategies and processes as further research provides additional information on how to increasingly improve support for and deployment of nursing staff to maximize patient safety.

HEALTH CARE ORGANIZATIONS AND OTHER PARTIES SHOULD NOT WAIT TO ACT

The health care system continues to evolve, responding to pressures and opportunities:

• Health care spending in the United States grew 9.6 percent in 2002, nearly four times faster than the overall economy. However, while this increase is very high, it represented the first slowing of the growth rate in 5 years, a slowdown that occurred in all four categories of health care spending—inpatient and outpatient care, prescription drugs, and physician services (Center for Studying Health System Change, 2003).

• Although the transition to less-restrictive managed care has eased financial pressures on providers, declining Medicare and Medicaid payments continue to squeeze hospitals and physicians. Providers are pressing health plans for better payment rates and contract terms, and hospitals and physicians are increasingly competing for profitable specialty medical and ancillary services, resulting in a continued buildup of capacity and technology. In Indianapolis, for example, six new specialty hospitals have opened or are under development. In Seattle, medical groups are opening ambulatory surgery and diagnostic centers and adding capacity to deliver radiology, laboratory, and imaging services in their practices (Lesser and Ginsburg, 2003).

• Private health insurance premiums increased an average of 15 percent in 2003—the largest increase in at least a decade (Center for Studying Health System Change, 2003). Consequently, employers are shifting more costs to employees. In some communities, malpractice premiums are continuing to rise (Lesser and Ginsburg, 2003).

• Fully 80 percent of consumers say they want to receive personal medical information via the Internet. Currently, only 13 percent of physicians report communicating with patients by e-mail, although 39 percent said they would do so if security and privacy issues could be resolved (The Henry J. Kaiser Family Foundation, 2002).

Because of such developments, as well as the rapid growth of diagnostic and therapeutic technologies and biomechanical advances in knowledge,

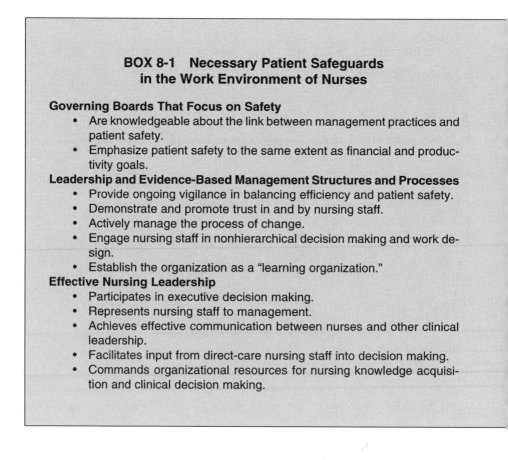

BOX 8-1 Necessary Patient Safeguards in the Work Environment of Nurses

Governing Boards That Focus on Safety
- Are knowledgeable about the link between management practices and patient safety.
- Emphasize patient safety to the same extent as financial and productivity goals.

Leadership and Evidence-Based Management Structures and Processes
- Provide ongoing vigilance in balancing efficiency and patient safety.
- Demonstrate and promote trust in and by nursing staff.
- Actively manage the process of change.
- Engage nursing staff in nonhierarchical decision making and work design.
- Establish the organization as a "learning organization."

Effective Nursing Leadership
- Participates in executive decision making.
- Represents nursing staff to management.
- Achieves effective communication between nurses and other clinical leadership.
- Facilitates input from direct-care nursing staff into decision making.
- Commands organizational resources for nursing knowledge acquisition and clinical decision making.

the U.S. healthcare system, like many sectors of the economy, is unlikely to reach a steady state in the foreseeable future. Therefore, HCOs should not wait for things to settle down before acting of this report's recommendations. Indeed, increasing cost pressures may make these safety practices even more imperative.

MULTIPLE, MUTUALLY REINFORCING SAFEGUARDS ARE NEEDED

As the evidence in the preceding chapters attests, there is no silver bullet, or shortcut for achieving patient safety. The work environment of nurses contains the basic organizational production processes and opportunities for human error well described by experts in organizational safety, as captured in the framework presented in Chapter 2. Using this framework, the committee identified the bundles of safeguards needed in nurses' work environments to safeguard patients, which are summarized in Box 8-1.

Adequate Staffing
- Is established by sound methodologies as determined by nursing staff.
- Provides mechanisms to accommodate unplanned variations in patient care workload.
- Enables nursing staff to regulate nursing unit work flow.
- Is consistent with best available evidence on safe staffing thresholds.

Organizational Support for Ongoing Learning and Decision Support
- Uses preceptors for novice nurses.
- Provides ongoing educational support and resources to nursing staff.
- Provides training in new technology.
- Provides decision support at the point of care.

Mechanisms That Promote Interdisciplinary Collaboration
- Use interdisciplinary practice mechanisms, such as interdisciplinary patient care rounds.
- Provide formal education and training in interdisciplinary collaboration for all health care workers.

Work Design That Promotes Safety
- Defends against fatigue, and unsafe and inefficient work design.
- Tackles medication administration, handwashing, documentation, and other high-priority practices.

Organizational Culture That Continuously Strengthens Patient Safety
- Regularly reviews organizational success in achieving formally specified safety objectives.
- Fosters fair and just error-reporting, analysis, and feedback system.
- Trains and rewards workers for safety.

Each of these safeguards is a defense against the occurrence of errors. As the work of experts in organizational safety attests, error-producing events can arise at any organizational level, within any organizational component, and within any work process. Safeguards are needed for each of these sources of patient safety errors; isolated defenses will be insufficient.

Redesigned work practices will still be unsafe if the number of nurses available to perform the work as designed is insufficient. Moreover, an apparently sufficient number of nurses will not perform as needed if they are suffering from the effects of fatigue, inexperienced in a given work process, or unfamiliar with the HCO's work processes because they are secured from a temporary or travel nurse agency. And errors will still occur even when the most capable workforce provides care using the best-designed work processes, because neither the nurse nor the work process is perfect. Defenses against human errors can be developed and put in place only if nursing staff are not afraid of reporting the errors and are involved in designing even stronger defenses. Finally, instituting all of these defense strategies can be accomplished only by individuals who have a vision of and command resources for the organization as a whole—that is, an organization's leadership and management. The actions of these leaders are the essential precursor to the creation of safer health care environments. They must be motivated by a passion to maximize the safety of all patients served by their institution. When implementing the committee's recommendations, however, they may also observe some additional benefits to their institution.

BENEFITS IN ADDITION TO PATIENT SAFETY ARE LIKELY

The costs of implementing the committee's recommendations will vary by facility and by recommendation. Some of the recommendations (e.g., establishment of a strong nursing leadership position, education and attention of governing boards with regard to safety, and adoption of management practices that are supportive of patient safety) are not likely to have significant immediate cost implications; other recommendations, such as limiting nurse work hours and ensuring safe staffing levels, may have such implications.

It is not possible to predict the costs that individual HCOs will face in implementing all of the committee's recommendations. Costs will vary to the extent that organizations have already embraced these practices. Many of the recommendations (e.g., better work design and the creation of cultures of safety) echo those made in two prior Institute of Medicine (IOM) reports—*To Err Is Human* (IOM, 2000) and *Crossing the Quality Chasm* (IOM, 2001). As noted throughout the present report, a number of facilities have already undertaken many of those recommendations. Actions of the federal government to fund more research on why errors occur and how to prevent them, to collect data on patient safety, to support the acquisition of information technology, and to disseminate patient safety information to consumers and providers (Clancy and Scully, 2003) have been a key stimulus for these efforts. Significant improvements in the safety of patients have also been spurred by health care purchasers' preferentially selecting HCOs based on their adoption of certain patient safety actions (e.g., computerized physician order entry), accreditation standards on patient safety adopted by the Joint Commission on Accreditation of Healthcare Organizations [JCAHO], continued public attention to patient safety from the media, and the internal commitment to patient safety made by many HCOs. However, adoption of patient safety practices has been uneven (Boodman, 2002; Millenson, 2003). HCOs that have been slower to respond to past IOM recommendations will have more work to do in implementing those contained in this report.

The committee adhered strictly to its charge to identify "potential improvements in health care working conditions that would likely increase patient safety." The committee did not address working conditions that would increase *worker* safety, nurse retention or recruitment, or patient satisfaction with care. Yet we repeatedly noted how often patient safety practices identified from the evidence reviewed for this study were the same as those recommended by organizations studying the nursing shortage, worker safety, and patient satisfaction. We note that retention of nurses and other health care workers in short supply, increased patient satisfaction with care, and potentially some return on financial investment may also result from undertaking the recommendations of this report.

Better Retention of Nurses and Other Health Care Workers in Short Supply

The nursing shortage discussed in Chapter 3 has been the subject of much study. Many expert panels and organizations have identified the need for HCOs to undertake actions to retain the nurses they already employ as an essential strategy for addressing this shortage (AHA Commission on Workforce for Hospitals and Health Systems, 2002; GAO, 2001; JCAHO, 2002; Kimball and O'Neil, 2002). It has been observed that even if the nursing education pipeline can be stimulated to increase the supply of new nurses, hospitals and other HCOs will still face shortages in nursing staff if work environments are so inhospitable that nurses leave to work in other places or abandon the practice of nursing altogether. Indeed, some have asserted that there is not a shortage of nurses, only a shortage of nurses who want to work in hospitals under today's working conditions (Lafer et al., 2003).

Strategies consistently recommended by experts to increase nurse recruitment and retention by HCOs include the following (AHA Commission on Workforce for Hospitals and Health Systems, 2002; JCAHO, 2002; Kimball and O'Neil, 2002):

- Strengthen nursing leadership within HCOs.
- Employ management practices that support staff involvement in care design and organizational decision making.
- Decentralize decision making for patient care and resource deployment decisions.
- Ensure appropriate nurse staffing levels.
- Provide ongoing support for nurses' education and training after they are hired.
- Provide decision support.
- Limit nurses' work hours so as not to create undue fatigue.
- Redesign work to increase safety and decrease inefficiency.
- Reduce the burden of paperwork and documentation.
- Implement and reward collaborative and multidisciplinary approaches to accomplishing work.

Moreover, the research that led to the creation of the magnet hospital designation—denoting hospitals that have higher levels of nurse retention and recruitment in the face of nurse shortages and an environment competing for the available nurse workforce—found the following workplace characteristics to be associated with better nurse recruitment and retention (McClure et al., 2002):

- Participatory management that involves nursing staff at all levels in decision making.
- Able, qualified and effective nursing leadership.
- Decentralized decision making, providing nursing staff with control over nursing work processes.
- Adequate staffing and, with few exceptions, low employment of nurses from temporary agencies.
- Strong postemployment education and training, including long orientation periods, use of preceptors and mentors for novice nurses, and ongoing education and training support.
- Strong interprofessional collaboration with physicians (Hinshaw, 2002; Kramer and Schmalenberg, 2002).

Because of the substantial similarities between the patient safety practices recommended by the committee and those recommended by experts and supported by research as promoting nurse retention and recruitment, we believe that implementation of the patient safety practices recommended in this report is likely to yield benefits to HCOs in the recruitment and retention of nurses. Moreover, we note that nurses are not the only group of health care workers in short supply. The hospital industry has documented shortages in imaging/radiology technicians; pharmacists; laboratory technicians; speech, physical, and occupational therapists; and respiratory therapists, among others (AHA Commission on Workforce for Hospitals and Health Systems, 2002; First Consulting Group, 2001; JCAHO, 2002). If work environments are constructed in a way that fosters better retention and recruitment of nurses, it is reasonable to expect that these practices will also permeate the work environments of other health care professionals. (The committee believes it unlikely—and undesirable—that HCOs will adopt work environment practices that apply only to nursing staff.) We note that a substantial amount of the evidence underpinning the recommendations contained in this report was obtained from industries other than health care. It is therefore reasonable to believe that these work practices are appropriate and beneficial not only to the nursing workforce, but to all health care workers. In implementing these recommendations across all workers, economies of scale should be achieved, and better retention and recruitment of all health care workers may result.

Increased Patient Satisfaction

Many of the practices recommended by the committee may also increase patients' satisfaction with their care. While variables not related to nurses' work environment (e.g., institution size [Young et al., 2000]), have been linked to patient satisfaction, findings from a study of magnet hospitals and hospital units with similar organizational traits suggest that features of nurses' work environment found in magnet hospitals also influence patient satisfaction (Aiken, 2002). Moreover, increased patient satisfaction is linked to adequate nurse staffing levels (Luther and Walsh, 1999) and to the physical design and layout of patient care units (Fowler et al., 1999).

Potential Financial Advantages

Increased retention of nurses is likely to be cost-beneficial for HCOs. There is also evidence that redesigning work processes to produce safer health care can yield cost savings for HCOs.

A 2001 survey of directors of nursing of all U.S. nonfederal acute care hospitals found that (for the 14.7 percent of hospitals responding), on average, 21.3 percent of all full-time hospital registered nurses (RNs) had resigned or been terminated during the preceding year. While most hospitals reported turnover rates of 10–30 percent, some reported much higher rates.

For example, 2 percent of responding hospitals reported turnover rates of 50 percent or higher (The HSM Group, 2002). Turnover rates among nursing staff in nursing homes are even greater. A national survey conducted in 2001 by the American Health Care Association (AHCA) revealed annual turnover rates of 78 percent for nursing assistants (NAs), 56 percent for staff RNs, 54 percent for licensed practical nurses (LPNs)/licensed vocational nurses (LVNs), and 43–47 percent for directors of nursing and RNs with administrative duties (AHCA, 2002).

Turnover of nursing staff exacts a high price on HCOs. Estimates of the replacement cost per nurse range from "a conservative estimate" of $10,000 per RN (The HSM Group, 2002) to approximately 100 percent of a nurse's salary ($42,000–$46,000 per year for medical–surgical and other non–intensive care unit nurses to $64,000 for critical care and other specialty care nurses (Kosel and Olivo, 2002) VHA Inc. estimates that, assuming an average cost of $64,000 to replace a nurse, an HCO with an RN workforce of 600 full-time equivalents (FTEs) and an annual turnover rate of 20 percent would spend $5.52 million a year to support its turnover. Cutting the turnover rate to 15 percent (a 25 percent reduction) would result in direct savings of $1.38 million per year (Kosel and Olivo, 2002). The Advisory Board estimates $800,000 in savings to a 500-bed hospital from reducing RN turnover from 13 to 10 percent (Advisory Board Company, 2000 as cited in Aiken et al., 2001). Likewise, a 2001 study conducted by VHA Inc.'s Consulting Services showed that organizations with higher turnover rates (21 percent or greater) had a 36 percent higher cost per discharge than those with a turnover rate of 12 percent or less. In a separate study of 235 hospitals, low-turnover organizations (those with turnover rates of 4–12 percent) were found to average a 23 percent return on assets, compared with a 17 percent return for organizations with turnover rates of more than 22 percent (Kosel and Olivo, 2002). JCAHO (2002) has concluded that there is a strong business case for actions that increase nurse retention.

There also is evidence that adopting health care practices that increase safety can decrease some HCO costs. Increased patient safety has obvious advantages to society and the economy at large, but the financial (business) advantage to an HCO is not always as visible. In case studies of the business case for four medical interventions (i.e., use of a lipid clinic, diabetes management programs, a smoking cessation program, and a workplace wellness program), favorable benefits were estimated to accrue to patients and society at large, but effects on the provider of care generally were judged to be financially unfavorable (Leatherman et al., 2003). However, these case studies did not analyze the costs to HCOs due to errors in health care that might have taken place in the absence of these interventions (i.e., lipid clinic, diabetes management programs, a smoking cessation program, and a workplace wellness program).

Costs to HCOs resulting from medical errors include operating, legal, and marketing costs. When preventable medical errors occur, the organization incurs the immediate cost of staff resources involved in reporting the error to internal (and external, if required) entities and in intervening to prevent recurrence and mitigate the effect of the error. Risk managers and providers expend time in generating reports and designing and carrying out error analyses. An HCO also may incur additional patient care costs created by the error, such as costs associated with transfer to higher level of care, use of additional diagnostic resources, or an extended hospital stay.[1] If legal claims are made, direct costs incurred include legal fees, settlements and payments, and the time expended by risk management personnel. Indirect litigation costs include time spent by providers and others in litigation and depositions, which not only decreases productivity, but also can impair morale. Long-term legal costs include higher premiums. Marketing costs are also increased in efforts to contain "bad press" and loss of market share (Weeks et al., 2001).

A review by the Agency for Healthcare Research and Quality (AHRQ) of practices used by hospitals to decrease adverse drug events (ADEs) found that costs to hospitals (excluding malpractice and litigation costs) increased as a result of the ADEs occurring within their facility. These increased costs resulted in part from extended lengths of stay. Patients who experienced an ADE were hospitalized an average of 8 to 12 days longer than those who did not experience such an event. AHRQ estimates that, depending on facility size, hospital costs for all ADEs can be as high as $5.6 million per hospital. AHRQ notes that before the advent of managed care, hospitals would have shifted a large portion of these costs to the patient or the insurer. Today, hospitals are more likely to have to absorb the added expense (AHRQ, 2001).

LDS Hospital in Salt Lake City, for example, found in a 4-year, matched case-control, severity-adjusted study that the occurrence of the ADE resulted in an average increased cost to the facility of $2,013 (p < 0.001), with a range of $677 to $9022. In 1992, direct hospital costs for ADEs were $1,099,413; over the 4-year study period, the excess hospital costs attributable to ADEs totaled $4,482,951 (not including liability costs or the costs associated with injuries to the patient). The authors estimate that, at the time of the study, if 50 percent of the ADEs had been potentially preventable, successfully targeted programs could have saved more than $500,000 annually (Classen et al., 1997). AHRQ notes that a 50 percent reduction in

---

[1]Although, perversely, organizational costs associates with errors may be offset through increased reimbursement for treatment of complications resulting from the error (Weeks et al., 2001).

ADEs is realistic; a number of studies have indicated that between 28 and 95 percent of ADEs are preventable (AHRQ, 2001).

Tracking patient safety errors also can result in cost savings. At LDS Hospital in Salt Lake, such tracking identified 25 ADEs related to a new brand of the drug vancomycin. This brand was being used because it cost $5,000 per year less than the brand used previously. However, LDS discovered that treating the patients who suffered these ADEs cost $50,000 in extra care expenses. Without its error-tracking system, the hospital would have assumed it was saving $5,000 per year when it was actually spending an additional $45,000 per year (Classen et al., 1997).

However, HCOs should not wait for proof of the financial advantage that will accrue to them before pursuing the patient safety recommendations contained in this report. The committee believes that pursuit of patient safety is an ethical and professional obligation of those who work in a health care system that aims to "first, do no harm." A number of HCO chief executive officers (CEOs) who are investing in high-cost patient safety systems and information technology infrastructure agree (Kinninger and Reeder, 2003; Solovy, 2003).

ADDITIONAL RESEARCH IS REQUIRED TO FURTHER INCREASE PATIENT SAFETY

Changing health care delivery practices to increase patient safety must be an ongoing process. Research findings and dissemination of practices that individual HCOs have found successful in improving patient safety will help HCOs as learning organizations add to their repertoire of patient safety practices. The committee calls attention to several areas in which, at present, information is limited about how to design nurses' work and work environment to make them safer for patients.

Information on Nurses' Work

As noted in Chapter 3, because data are not collected routinely on the activities performed by nurses and how nurses spend their time, it is difficult to measure the effects of interventions aimed at redesigning care to improve safety or efficiency or to understand the implications of policy changes for nursing practice. Research is needed on how to collect information on nurses' work on an ongoing basis.

Better Information on Nursing-Related Errors

Because medication errors constitute a large share of all health care errors, medication administration by nurses has received a great deal of attention from researchers and system designers aiming to develop safer medication administration processes. Handwashing and nosocomial infections have similarly received attention. However, other nursing activities that might offer the potential for high-yield increases in patient safety are unknown. Analysis of data from state and other error-reporting systems might help identify such procedures or nursing actions and attract the attention of multiple HCOs, offering a critical mass of initiatives for identifying safer patient care practices.

Safer Work Processes and Workspace Design

Similarly, research is needed in how to increase the safety of other specific nursing work processes, such as patient monitoring. Moreover, although Chapter 6 identifies a number of strategies for improving the layout of nursing units and patient care rooms to increase nursing time and the ease of patient hospitalization, these strategies have to date been identified primarily through focus groups and ad hoc user input. Research comparing different layouts of nursing units and patient rooms would help identify principles and practices of safer workspace design.

A Standardized Approach to Measuring Patient Acuity

As discussed in Chapter 5, HCOs use a variety of tools to measure patient acuity as a basis for allocation of nursing staff and other managerial decision making. Nursing research, such as research on staffing levels, often needs to adjust for or otherwise address the acuity levels of patients. However, there is no standard method used across all hospitals for measuring the severity of illness of all hospital patients. This lack of a standardized approach hampers interpretation of research results in the aggregate.

Safe Staffing Levels at the Level of Different Nursing Units

The committee finds evidence for the effect of nurse staffing levels on patient safety to be highly convincing. As discussed in Chapter 5, however, generalizing the results of hospital-wide staffing studies that combine data from all nursing units to the diverse patient care units within hospitals is inappropriate. More studies are needed on the effect of staffing levels within certain types of nursing units (e.g., medical–surgical, labor and delivery), as has been done for intensive care. (The committee believes additional studies of intensive care unit staffing are also needed). The committee notes that such research will be challenging because the smaller number of patients found in individual care units will make statistical analysis difficult. We reiterate that, to best interpret the aggregate findings of such staffing studies, a standardized approach to measuring and adjusting for patient acuity will be needed.

Strategies to Help Night Shift Workers Compensate for Fatigue

The evidence reviewed in Chapter 6 clearly shows that workers, regardless of the degree to which they are rested, are affected by work hours that are in opposition to the body's normal circadian rhythms—that is, night shift work hours. Research is needed to identify strategies that can help nurses combat the effects of such work hours.

Research on the Effects of Successive Days of Working Sustained Work Hours

Continued research is needed on the effects of sustained work hours. In particular, such research needs to address the number of successive days that should be worked without a day or days off.

Research on Collaborative Models of Care

Chapter 5 and Appendix B review the benefits to patient safety that are likely to accrue as a result of effective interprofessional collaboration, including approaches to team care. Based on the evidence presented in Appendix B, the committee concludes that there is a need to better understand the mechanisms that produce effective collaboration and team processes:

• What interpersonal and group interaction processes contribute to effective collaboration and delivery of safe care? A number of theories exist concerning how teams perform and how their behaviors contribute to safe or unsafe practices. Additional information is needed about which of these theories are most applicable to the delivery of quality health care and which approaches in health care and other industries demonstrate the most potential for favorable effect.

• How can effective collaboration among groups of health care practitioners with differing characteristics—such as different skill levels (novice nurses versus competent, proficient, or expert nurses) and different duration of employment (e.g., rotating residents and float nurses)—be achieved? What other factors influence effective collaboration, and what strategies are effective in addressing them?

• How do environmental influences affect team performance? For example, what are the effects of stress, organizational culture, and leadership in facilitating or structuring collaborative care?

- How applicable are crew resource management principles and other non–health-related strategies in achieving collaboration and error reduction?
- How can more-productive interpersonal interactions be fostered across the multiple ways in which health care workers interact (e.g., in dyads, small groups, and unit-based teams)? What interpersonal behaviors facilitate effective interaction, decision making, and error prevention? How can these behaviors best be taught?

RECOMMENDATION

In light of the above research needs, the committee makes the following recommendation:

Recommendation 8-1. Federal agencies and private foundations should support research in the following areas to provide HCOs with the additional information they need to continue to strengthen nurse work environments for patient safety:

- Studies and development of methods to better describe, both qualitatively and quantitatively, the work nurses perform in different care settings.
- Descriptive studies of nursing-related errors.
- Design, application, and evaluation (including financial costs and savings) of safer and more efficient work processes and workspace, including the application of information technology.
- Development and testing of a standardized approach to measuring patient acuity.
- Determination of safe staffing levels within different types of nursing units.
- Development and testing of methods to help night shift workers compensate for fatigue.
- Research on the effects of successive work days and sustained work hours on patient safety.
- Development and evaluation of models of collaborative care, including care by teams.

REFERENCES

Advisory Board Company. 2000. *Reversing the Flight of Talent: Nursing Retention in an Era of Gathering Shortage.* Washington, DC: Advisory Board Company.

AHA Commission on Workforce for Hospitals and Health Systems. 2002. *In Our Hands: How Hospital Leaders Can Build a Thriving Workforce.* Chicago, IL: AHA.

AHCA (American Health Care Association). 2002. *Results of the 2001 AHCA Nursing Position Vacancy and Turnover Survey.* Washington, DC: AHCA.

AHRQ (Agency for Healthcare Research and Quality). 2001. *Reducing and Preventing Adverse Drug Events to Decrease Hospital Costs.* Publication number 01-0020. Rockville, MD: AHRQ. [Online]. Available: http://www.ahrq.gov/qual/aderia/aderia.htm [accessed July 14, 2003].

Aiken L. 2002. Superior outcomes for magnet hospitals: The evidence base. In: McClure M, Hinshaw A, eds. *Magnet Hospitals Revisited: Attraction and Retention of Professional Nurses.* Washington, DC: American Nurses Publishing. Pp. 61–81.

Aiken L, Clarke S, Sloane D, Sochalski J. 2001. An international perspective on hospital nurses' work environments: The case for reform. *Policy, Politics, and Nursing Practice* 2(4):255–263.

Boodman S. 2002 (December 3). No end to errors: Three years after a landmark report found pervasive medical mistakes in American hospitals, little has been done to reduce death and injury. *The Washington Post.* Health Section. P. F1.

Center for Studying Health System Change. 2003. Tracking health care costs: Trends stabilize but remain high in 2002. *Data Bulletin 25.*

Clancy C, Scully T. 2003. A call to excellence. *Health Affairs* 22(2):113–115.

Classen D, Pestotnik S, Evans R, Lloyd J, Burke J. 1997. Adverse drug events in hospitalized patients. Excess length of stay, extra costs, and attributable mortality. *Journal of the American Medical Association* 277:301–306.

First Consulting Group. 2001. *The Healthcare Workforce Shortage and Its Implications for America's Hospitals.* [Online]. Available: http://www.fcg.com/webfiles/pdfs/FCG WorkforceReport.pdf [accessed May 19, 2003].

Fowler E, MacRae S, Stern A, Harrison T, Gerteis M, Edgman-Levitan S, Ruga W. 1999. The built environment as a component of quality care: Understanding and including the patient's perspective. *The Joint Commission Journal on Quality Improvement* 25(7):352–362.

GAO (General Accounting Office). 2001. *Nursing Workforce: Emerging Nurses Shortages Due to Multiple Factors.* GAO-01-944. Washington, DC: GAO.

Hinshaw A. 2002. Building magnetism into health organizations. *Magnet Hospitals Revisited: Attraction and Retention of Professional Nurses.* Washington, DC: American Nurses Publishing.

IOM (Institute of Medicine). 2000. *To Err Is Human: Building A Safer Health System.* Washington, DC: National Academy Press.

IOM. 2001. *Assessing the Quality Chasm: A New Health System for the 21st Century.* Washington, DC: National Academy Press.

JCAHO (Joint Commission on Accreditation of Healthcare Organizations). 2002. *Health Care at the Crossroads: Strategies for Addressing the Evolving Nursing Crisis.* JCAHO.

Kimball B, O'Neil E. 2002. *Health Care's Human Crisis: The American Nursing Shortage.* The Robert Wood Johnson Foundation. [Online]. Available: www.rwjf.org./news/nursing_report.pdf [accessed October 4, 2003].

Kinninger T, Reeder L. 2003. The business case for medication safety. *Healthcare Financial Management* February:46–51.

Kosel K, Olivo T. 2002. *The Business Case for Workforce Stability.* Volume 7: VHA Inc. VHA Research Series 2002. Irving, TX: Center for Research and Innovation, VHA Inc.

Kramer M, Schmalenberg C. 2002. Staff nurses identify essentials of magnetism. In: McClure M, Hinshaw A, eds. *Magnet Hospitals Revisited: Attraction and Retention of Professional Nurses.* Washington, DC: American Nurses Publishing. Pp. 25–59.

Lafer G, Moss H, Kirtner R, Rees V, Labor Education and Research Center, University of Oregon. 2003. *Solving the Nursing Shortage.* A report prepared for the united Nurses of

America, AFSCME, AFL-CIO: American Federation of State, County and Municipal Employees (AFSCME). [Online]. Available: http://www.afscme.org/una/snstc.htm [accessed July 30, 2003].

Leatherman S, Berwick D, Iles D, Lewin L, Davidoff F, Nolan T, Bisognano M. 2003. The business case for quality: Case studies and an analysis. *Health Affairs* 22(2):17–30.

Lesser C, Ginsburg P. 2003. *Health Care Cost and Access Problems Intensify.* Issue Briefing 63. Washington, DC: Center for Studying Health System Change.

Luther K, Walsh K. 1999. Moving out of the red zone: Addressing staff allocation to improve patient satisfaction. *The Joint Commission Journal on Quality Improvement* 25(7):363–368.

McClure M, Poulin M, Sovie M, Wandelt M. 2002. Magnet hospitals: Attraction and retention of professional nurses (The Original Study). In: McClure M, Hinshaw A, eds. *Magnet Hospitals Revisited.* Washington, DC: American Nurses Publishing. P. 124.

Millenson M. 2003. The silence. *Health Affairs* 22(2):103–112.

Quinn J. 1992. *Intelligent Enterprise: A Knowledge and Service Based Paradigm for Industry.* New York, NY: The Free Press, a division of Macmillan, Inc.

Solovy A. 2003. *Most Wired 2003: Hospitals and Health Networks.* [Online]. Available: http://www.hospitalconnect.com [accessed July 20, 2003].

Stacey R. 1996. *Complexity and Creativity in Organizations.* San Francisco, CA: Berrett-Koehler Publishers.

The Henry J. Kaiser Family Foundation. 2002. *Trends and Indicators in the Changing Health Care Marketplace—Chartbook.* Washington, DC: The Henry J. Kaiser Family Foundation.

The HSM Group. 2002. *Acute Care Hospital Survey of RN Vacancy and Turnover Rates.* Chicago, IL: American Organization of Nurse Executives.

Weeks W, Waldron J, Foster T, Mills P, Stalhandske E. 2001. The organizational costs of preventable medical errors. *The Joint Commission Journal on Quality Improvement* 27(10):533–539.

Appendix A

Committee Membership and Study Approach

COMMITTEE COMPOSITION

The Committee on the Work Environment for Nurses and Patient Safety included the following members.

Donald M. Steinwachs, Ph.D. (*Chair*), is Professor and Chair of the Department of Health Policy and Management in The Johns Hopkins University Bloomberg School of Public Health. He is Director of The Johns Hopkins University Health Services Research and Development Center and Director of the Johns Hopkins and University of Maryland Center for Research on Services for Severe Mental Illness. Dr. Steinwach's current research includes studies of (1) medical effectiveness and patient outcomes for individuals with specific medical, surgical, and psychiatric conditions; (2) the impact of managed care and other organizational and financial arrangements on access to care, quality, utilization, and cost; and (3) the development of better methods for measuring the effectiveness of systems of care, including case mix (e.g., Ambulatory Care Groups), quality profiling, and indicators of outcome. He has a particular interest in the role of routine management information systems as a source of data for evaluating the effectiveness and cost of health care. Dr. Steinwachs is past President of the Association for Health Services Research (now AcademyHealth) and is Chair of the Board of Directors, Coalition for Health Services Research. He serves as a consultant to federal agencies and private foundations, and is on the Board of Directors of Mathematica, Inc. and the Foundation for Accountability.

Ada Sue Hinshaw, Ph.D, R.N., F.A.A.N. (*Vice Chair*), is Professor and Dean of the School of Nursing at the University of Michigan. She was the first Director of the National Institute of Nursing Research at the National Institutes of Health. Her research interests include (1) professionals who function in bureaucracies, job satisfaction, job stress, anticipated turnover, and patient outcomes; (2) quality of patient caregiving; and (3) instrument development and testing, including measures of patient satisfaction, job satisfaction of nurses, and anticipated turnover of nursing staff. In addition, she has studied the use of ratio measurement techniques in building and testing the nurse and patient measures. Dr. Hinshaw is involved in a number of health policy activities. In addition to the Committee on the Work Environment for Nurses and Patient Safety, she has served on the Institute of Medicine's (IOM) Nursing Research Panel Parent Committee on Monitoring the Changing Needs for Biomedical and Behavioral Research Personnel. She has also served on a number of national review committees and policy commissions, including the Advisory Council for the Agency for Healthcare Research and Quality. She is past President of the American Academy of Nursing, and a member of the IOM and its Governing Council. Dr. Hinshaw coauthored the first *Handbook for Clinical Nursing Research* and a text on *Magnet Hospitals Revisited: Attraction and Retention of Professional Nurses*. She has received numerous honors, awards, and honorary degrees.

Joy Durfee Calkin, R.N., Ph.D., is Professor Emeritus of Nursing, University of Calgary, Canada, and a health care consultant. She practiced pediatric and adult nursing in Canada, the United States, and the United Kingdom and held faculty positions in the former two countries. Dr. Calkin served as President and Chief Executive Officer (CEO) of Extendicare Inc. in Canada and the United States. Her areas of consulting have included workplace design, staffing patterns, development of clinical administrator programs in medicine and nursing, health systems design, operational and productivity analysis, workforce shortages, and performance improvement. Her research interests include the effect of work and structures for work on worker performance and satisfaction. Dr. Calkin served as a member of the Premier's Commission on Future Health Care for Albertans, the Ontario Minister of Health Task Force on the Nursing Shortage, and the Governor of Florida's Task Force on Accessibility and Affordability of Long-Term Care. She serves on the Board of the Canadian Stroke Network and a Canadian charitable foundation.

Marilyn P. Chow, D.N.S., R.N., F.A.A.N., is Vice President, Patient Care Services, for the Program Office of Kaiser Permanente. She is also Program Director for The Robert Wood Johnson Executive Nurse Fellows Program. A graduate of the University of California, San Francisco School of Nursing, she has held positions in acute care settings, academia, and state and national nursing organizations and has served on numerous local, state, and national committees and boards. She is the At-Large Nursing Commissioner on the Joint Commission on Accreditation of Healthcare Organization Board, a member of the Joint Commission Resources Board, and a member of the Editorial Advisory Board of *Nurse Week*, and is currently serving a 2-year appointment as Senior Fellow of the Center for the Health Professions at the University of California, San Francisco. She also serves as a member of the Hartford Institute for Geriatric Nursing and is a fellow of the American Academy of Nursing. Dr. Chow has coauthored four books, including the award-winning *Handbook of Pediatric Primary Care*. Her awards include the American Nurses Association (ANA) Ethnic Minority Women's Honors in Public Health and the University of California at San Francisco School of Nursing Distinguished Alumni Award.

Paul D. Clayton, Ph.D., is Chief Medical Informatics Officer at Intermountain Health Care, Professor of Medical Informatics at the University of Utah, and Professor Emeritus at Columbia University. Dr. Clayton developed and implemented information systems in cardiology, radiology, and surgery at LDS Hospital and the University of Utah. He joined Columbia University and Presbyterian Hospital in 1987 as director of the Center for Medical Informatics and Professor of Medical Informatics. He became Chair of the newly created Department of Medical Informatics in 1994. When Dr. Clayton joined Columbia Presbyterian, he led efforts to build an integrated information system for the medical center, an effort supported by an Integrated Advanced Information Management System grant from the National Library of Medicine. He was also active in creating an advanced clinical information system with decision-making capability now widely used at Columbia Presbyterian. In 1998, he returned to Salt Lake City to work with Intermountain Health Care in establishing the information underpinnings for an integrated health delivery system. As Chief Medical Informatics Officer, he is interested in creating and implementing systems that use a clinical information system and external sources of knowledge to prompt providers and patients in ways that will improve the quality and cost of health care. Dr. Clayton is an elected fellow of the American College of Medical Informatics and the IOM. He chaired a National Research Council committee addressing issues of confidentiality of health records on the national information infrastructure, and served on the Board of Directors of the American Medical Informatics Association and as President of that organization during 1998 and 1999.

Mary Lou de Leon Siantz, R.N., Ph.D., F.A.A.N., is Professor and Associate Dean for Research at the Georgetown University School of Nursing and Health Studies and Director of the Milagros Center of Excellence in Migrant Health in Washington, D.C. She also serves as a faculty affiliate in the School of Nursing, Department of Family and Child Nursing, University of Washington, Seattle, Washington. She is past President of the National Association of Hispanic Nurses and of the Advocates for Child and Adolescent Psychiatric Nursing. Dr. de Leon Siantz received her bachelor of science degree in nursing from Mount Saint Mary's College, Los Angeles, California; her master's degree from the University of California, Los Angeles; and her doctorate in human development from the University of Maryland, College Park. She is known internationally for her seminal research in child development and mental health with Mexican migrant farm worker children and families in the migrant stream of the United States. She is the author or coauthor of numerous publications on the mental health and development of Hispanic children and their families. She has published many scholarly papers and research abstracts and contributed to numerous books. She consults with the Strategic Planning Committees for the Pacific Northwest Hispanic Health Agenda and the East Coast Migrant Council, developing research initiatives. Her research has focused on the effects of stress on the mental health and parenting behaviors of Mexican migrant mothers, and on factors that influence the successful outcomes of migrant preschool children (funded by the U.S. Department of Health and Human Services). She was a member of the IOM Committee on the Health and Adjustment of Immigrant Children and Families and the Social Policy Committee for the Society for Research in Child Development, cochairing the Subcommittee on Poverty. She has been on the Advisory Council of the National Institutes for Nursing Research. She has been honored by the Texas Migrant Council, San Diego State University, and the National Association of Hispanic Nurses. She serves on numerous review panels, editorial boards, and advisory committees, including the Secretary's Committee on Infant Mortality. Internationally, she has served on the Pan American Health Organization's psychiatric nursing initiative in the Southern Cone of South America.

Charlene A. Harrington, Ph.D., R.N., F.A.A.N., is Professor of Sociology and Nursing in the Department of Social and Behavioral Sciences, School of Nursing, University of California, San Francisco. Her primary work has been in the area of long-term care; she has directed a number of research projects on state long-term care policies, funded by the U.S. Centers for Medicare and Medicaid services (CMS), the Agency for Healthcare Research and Quality (AHRQ), and others. She recently conducted a study of Medicare beneficiary consumer quality complaints with California Medical Review Inc. and a large study of the Medicaid home and community-based service programs in all the states in 1999 for the Health Care Financing Administration. She continues to study state long-term care programs and policies. Dr. Harrington developed a model Nursing Home Consumer Information System (funded by the AHRQ) that was used in developing the

CMS Medicare Nursing Home Compare website. She led a team of researchers in designing a state-of-the-art California Internet-based consumer information system for nursing homes, initiated in 2002. As part of this project, she conducted studies on the relationship between nurse staffing and quality measures, nursing home bankruptcies and closures, nurse staffing and turnover rates, and other quality indicators. She has also been studying the extent of paid and unpaid long-term care services in the home and estimating the costs of expanding these programs across the country. She has published a number of papers on nurse staffing levels and annual state data books on all 16,000 U.S. nursing homes since 1991. She is Director of a new National Center for Personal Assistance Services, funded by the National Institute on Disability and Rehabilitation Research. She has written more than 125 articles and chapters and coedited five books. She has lectured widely in the United States, as well as in other countries.

David H. Hickam, M.D., M.P.H., is Professor in the Department of Medicine of the Oregon Health and Science University and a staff physician at the Portland Veterans Affairs Medical Center. He is board certified in internal medicine and completed a fellowship in health services research. He has maintained both a primary care clinical practice and inpatient attending responsibilities for more than 20 years. He has an active health services research program that has focused on clinical care outcomes, primary care practice variation, and patient safety. He is principal investigator on a contract to prepare an evidence report for the Agency for Healthcare Research and Quality on the effect of health care working conditions on patient safety.

Gwendylon E. Johnson, M.A., R.N.C., is a Staff Nurse in women's health at Howard University Hospital. A diploma hospital graduate, she received a bachelor of science degree from St. Joseph's College in Maine and a master's with a health care administration concentration from the University of Maryland. With nearly 30 years of experience in obstetrical and gynecological nursing, her nursing career has always involved a direct-care commitment. She also has served as an adjunct professor in the graduate programs at Trinity College in Washington, D.C., and as an independent consultant on various projects, including a U.S. Department of Health and Human Services study that examined comprehensive care delivery services for HIV-infected women and their children. She is currently active in the Sigma Theta Tau International Honor Society for Nursing, Chi Eta Phi Sorority, Inc., and the Nurses Ministry and Board of Trustees of New Dawn Baptist Church. She has served on a number of committees and in many representative capacities for the ANA, including serving on the Advisory Board to the ANA Center for Ethics and Human Rights, the ANA Board of Directors, and the editorial board of the *American Journal of Nursing*. She also serves as health and safety officer in her workplace for the District of Columbia Nurses Association.

David A. Kobus, Ph.D., is a Certified Professional Ergonomist with Pacific Science and Engineering Group in San Diego, California, and has been involved in human performance research and project management for over 19 years. His work on the analysis of medical errors currently places him in the forefront of the field of identifying, categorizing, and quantifying errors in health care delivery. Recently, he was one of four psychologists asked by the American Psychological Association to brief congressional committees regarding human factors efforts to reduce error in medicine. In addition, he was asked by the Food and Drug Administration to serve on an expert panel at a public hearing on medical device labeling and as a member of a panel for the safe design of home care medical devices. He is also the Cochair of the Human Factors Task Force on Medical Error for the Human Factors and Ergonomic Society (HFES), past Chair of the Medical Systems and Rehabilitation Technical Group of the HFES, and past President of the San Diego Chapter of the Human Factors and Ergonomic Society. Dr. Kobus has published more than 75 peer-reviewed papers and technical reports and has presented over 50 papers at national and international conferences on human factors, errors in medicine, and medical system design. He has extensive teaching experience at both the graduate and the undergraduate levels in the areas of experimental design, advanced statistics, cognition, biological psychology, and sensory systems. He has also served as principal investigator or as program manager on over 25 research projects related to human factors performance, many of which concerned human–computer interaction of medical systems.

Andrew M. Kramer, M.D., is Professor of Medicine and Head of the Division of Health Care Policy and Research in the Department of Medicine at The University of Colorado. The first recipient of an endowed chair in Health Policy, Dr. Kramer is also Director of the Hartford/Jahnigen Center of Excellence in Geriatric Medicine. Previously, he was Research Director for the Center on Aging and Geriatric Medicine Research Training Program Director. He has over 20 years of experience in health services research, with particular emphasis on quality of care in nursing homes, subacute settings, and home health care. Among his many research studies, he directed analyses of the association between staffing levels and quality of care in the Report to Congress on the Appropriateness of Minimum Nursing Staffing Ratios in Nursing Homes. Recently, he was principal investigator for a study to develop quality measures for use across postacute settings. His current projects include a national study of stroke outcomes across settings and a study to use quality indicators in the nursing home survey process. Dr. Kramer received his medical degree from Harvard Medical School.

Pamela H. Mitchell, Ph.D., R.N., F.A.A.N., is Associate Dean for Research and Professor of Biobehavioral Nursing and Health Care Systems at the University of Washington School of Nursing, where she holds the Elizabeth S. Soule Distinguished Professorship of Health Promotion. She is also adjunct professor of health services at the University of Washington School of Public Health and Medicine and has been engaged in advanced nursing practice, clinical research, and interprofessional clinical education for over 30 years. Her practice and research are in the areas of neuroscience and critical care nursing, and features of health care delivery systems that affect clinical outcomes. She is currently developing and testing a national faculty leadership program in interprofessional education to promote patient safety. She is the founding Director of the Center for Health Services Interprofessional Education and Research at the University of Washington, chairs the American Academy of Nursing Expert Panel on Quality Care, and serves on the Steering Committee for the Agency for Healthcare Research and Quality's Patient Safety Research Coordinating Center. She also has studied organizational work environment issues in multisite studies of the critical care work environment and was a member of the technical advisory board of the recent national study of nurse staffing and patient outcomes in hospitals, funded by the U.S. Department of Health and Human Services. She also is coinvestigator on a new Veterans Administration study to investigate nursing work environments and patient outcomes.

Audrey L. Nelson, Ph.D., R.N., F.A.A.N., has over 26 years of experience as a staff nurse, nurse administrator, and nurse researcher. Dr. Nelson is nationally known for her expertise in patient safety. Currently, she is Center Director for three research centers: the Veterans Health Administration (VHA) Patient Safety Center of Inquiry, VHA Health Services Research Enhancement Program on Patient Safety Outcomes, and Suncoast Development Evaluation Research Center on Safe Patient Transitions, funded by the Agency for Healthcare Research and Quality. Dr. Nelson has joint faculty appointments at the University of South Florida in the Colleges of Public Health and Nursing, where she serves as Associate Director for Clinical Research. Her program of research focuses on safe environments for patients and nurses in the areas of falls and safe patient handling and movement. She has established four research laboratories: Patient Safety Simulation, Gait and Balance, Biomechanics Research, and Patient Safety Engineering. Dr. Nelson also is nationally known in spinal cord injury nursing. She is past President of the American Association of Spinal Cord Injury Nurses, past Chair of the Rehabilitation Research Foundation for the Association of Rehabilitation Nurses, and Steering Committee member for the Consortium for Spinal Cord Medicine Clinical Practice Guidelines. Administratively, she participated in the VHA National Expert Panel on Nursing Staffing Methodologies, chaired a national VHA Task Force on Patient Care

Ergonomics, and chaired a national Veterans Administration task force on Patient Fall Prevention.

Edward H. O'Neil, Ph.D., M.P.A., is Professor of Family and Community Medicine and Dental Public Health at the University of California, San Francisco. He also serves as Director of the Center for the Health Professions, a research, advocacy, and training institute he created to stimulate change in health professions education. The Center for the Health Professions houses a number of initiatives designed to understand and address the issues facing health care and health professionals. Dr. O'Neil is principal investigator for the Pew Scholars Program in the Biomedical Sciences, The Robert Wood Johnson Executive Nurse Fellows Program, the California Workforce Initiative, and the Future Leaders Program, funded by the California HealthCare Foundation. From 1989 through 1999, Dr. O'Neil served as Executive Director of the Pew Health Professions Commission—a nationally recognized advocacy group focused on reform in health workforce issues. He has published numerous articles, chapters, and books on this and other work. He is or has served as a consultant to the World Health Organization, the Government of New Zealand, the Rockefeller Foundation, the Pew Charitable Trusts, the W. K. Kellogg Foundation, the Fetzer Institute, The Robert Wood Johnson Foundation, and the California HealthCare Foundation, as well as a number of federal, state, and institutional agencies. He holds undergraduate and masters degrees from the University of Alabama, a masters of public administration and doctorate in history from Syracuse University, and an honorary degree from New York Medical College.

William P. Pierskalla, Ph.D., is Professor in the Department of Operation and Technology Management in the Anderson Graduate School of Management at the University of California, Los Angeles. He is former Dean of The Anderson School, 1993 to 1997. His current research interests include the management aspects of health care delivery, operations research, operations management, and issues of global competition. He is former President of the International Federation of Operational Research Societies, and serves in an editorial capacity on *Production and Operations Management, International Transactions in Operational Research, Encyclopedia of Operations Research and Management Science, Health Services Management Research*, and the *Health Care Management Sciences Journal*. Dr. Pierskalla is currently Vice President for Publications for the Institute for Operations Research and Management Sciences. He is former President of the Operations Research Society of America and past Editor of *Operations Research*. He previously was Deputy Dean for Academic Affairs, Director of the Huntsman Center for Global Competition and Leadership, and Chairman of the Health Care Systems Department at the Wharton School and

Executive Director of the Leonard Davis Institute of Health Economics at the University of Pennsylvania. He has given numerous lectures and seminars at universities and organizations in the United States, Europe, South America, and the Far East, and has authored over 50 refereed articles in mathematical programming, transportation, inventory and production control, maintainability, and health care delivery. Dr. Pierskalla has served as a consultant to the American Red Cross, analyzing blood supply management, including delivery, testing, and inventory.

Karlene H. Roberts, Ph.D., is Professor in the Haas School of Business at the University of California, Berkeley, where she researches and consults on organizational behavior and industrial relations as they pertain to safety issues. Her areas of expertise include high-reliability organizations and human and organizational error. She has published extensively on such topics as research and management strategies to improve patient safety, the causes and prevention of catastrophic organizational errors, systems theory and how it can be applied to maximizing patient safety, patient safety as an organizational systems issue—lessons from a variety of industries, design and management of high-reliability organizations, risk mitigation in large-scale systems, decision support, the development of technology over time, and the relationship of technology to organizational structure and other organizational processes.

Denise M. Rousseau, Ph.D., is H. J. Heinz II Professor of Organizational Behavior at Carnegie Mellon University, serving jointly in the Heinz School of Public Policy and Management and the Graduate School of Industrial Administration. She has been a faculty member at Northwestern University, the University of Michigan, and the Naval Postgraduate School (Monterey), and visiting faculty member at Chulalonghorn University (Bangkok), Renmen University (Beijing), and Nanyang Technological University (Singapore). Her research addresses the impact of work group processes on performance and the changing psychological contract at work. Dr. Rousseau has authored more than 110 articles that have appeared in academic journals, such as the *Journal of Applied Psychology, Academy of Management Review, Journal of Organizational Behavior*, and *Administrative Science Quarterly*. Her books include *Relational Wealth: Advantages of Stability in a Changing Economy* (Oxford), with Carrie Leana; *Psychological Contracts in Employment: Cross-National Perspectives* (Sage), with Rene Schalk; the *Trends in Organizational Behavior* series (Wiley), with Cary Cooper; *Developing an Interdisciplinary Science of Organizations* (Jossey-Bass), with Karlene Roberts and Charles Hulin; and *The Boundaryless Career* (Oxford), with Michael Arthur. *Psychological Contracts in Organizations* (Sage) won the Academy of Management's best book award in 1996. Professor Rousseau has consulted in diverse organizations and written numerous articles for managers and executives, including "Teamwork: Inside and Out" (*Business Week/Advance*), "Managing Diversity for High Performance" (*Business Week/Advance*), and "Two Ways to Change (and Keep) the Psychological Contract" (*Academy of Management Executive*). She has taught in executive programs at Northwestern (Kellogg), Cornell, and Carnegie Mellon Universities and in industry programs for health care, journalism, and manufacturing, among others. She is a Fellow in the Academy of Management, the American Psychological Association, and the Society for Industrial/Organizational Psychology, and is Editor-in-Chief of the *Journal of Organizational Behavior*. Her current and past editorial board memberships include *Administrative Science Quarterly*, *Journal of Applied Psychology*, and *Journal of Management Inquiry*.

William C. Rupp, M.D., is President/CEO of Immanuel St. Joseph's—Mayo Health System and Vice Chair of Mayo Health System. Previously, Dr. Rupp was President and CEO of Luther Midelfort in Eau Claire, Wisconsin. He led that institution's integration with Mayo Health System and Luther Midelfort's nationally recognized efforts and innovations in patient safety. He is a frequent speaker at Institute for Healthcare Improvement meetings regarding medical practice innovations. He is Vice Chair for Planning of Mayo Health System and has served in multiple community leadership roles in Eau Claire. Dr. Rupp is a practicing oncologist.

STUDY APPROACH

The committee began its work in June 2002. It convened four times during September 2002, November 2002, February 2003, and April 2003 to review evidence and deliberate. Additional deliberations between meetings were held through conference calls.

The committee invited testimony from multiple nursing, labor, health care delivery, quality oversight, advocacy, and other organizations. Those providing testimony included Barbara Blakeney, President, American Nurses Association; Linda Burnes Boltin, Dr.P.H., American Academy of Nursing; Kathleen Long, Ph.D., President, American Association of Colleges of Nursing; Phil Authier, President, American Organization of Nurse Executives; Eileen Zungolo, Ed.D., President, National League for Nursing; Jeanne Surdo, Secretary-Treasurer of United American Nurses; Martha Baker, President, Service Employees International Union, Local 1991; Katherine Cox, Policy Analyst, American Federation of State, County, and Municipal Employees; Gerry Shea, Assistant to the President for Government Affairs, AFL-CIO; Jim Bentley, Senior Vice President for Strategic Policy Planning, American Hospital Association; Steven Chies, Vice Chair, American Health Care Association; Robyn Stone, Ph.D., Executive Director, Institute for the Future of Aging Services, an affiliate of the American Association of Homes and Services for the Aging; Tim Flaherty, M.D., of the American Medical Association and National Patient Safety Foundation; Steven Edelstein, J.D., of the Paraprofessional Institute; Donna Lenhoff, Esq., Executive Director, National Citizens Coalition for Nursing Home Reform; Dennis O'Leary, President, and Margaret van Amringe, Vice President for External Relations, Joint Commission on the Accreditation of Healthcare Organizations; Cathy Rick, Chief Nursing Officer, U.S. Department of Veterans Affairs; Sean Clarke, R.N., Ph.D., of the University of Pennsylvania Center for Health Outcomes and Policy Research; Caryl Lee, R.N., Program Manager, National Center for Patient Safety, U.S. Department of Veterans Affairs; Joyce Berger, Senior Advisor, Health Technology Center; Daved van Stralen, M.D., Medical Director, Totally Kids© Specialty Healthcare, The American Association of Critical Care Nurses; Philip Greiner, Past Chair, and Sonda Oppewal, Chair, Public Health Nursing Section, American Public Health Association; Laurence Wellikson, Executive Director, and Janet Nagamine, National Association of Inpatient Physicians; John Hoff, Deputy Assistant Secretary, and Jennie Harvel, Policy Analyst, U.S. Department of Health and Human Services; and Paul Ginsburg, Ph.D., President, Center for Studying Health System Change.

The committee also commissioned nine papers to provide background information for its deliberations and to synthesize the evidence on particular issues. The authors and their papers were as follows: Julie Sochalski, Ph.D., "The Nursing Workforce: Profile, Trends, Projections"; Barbara Mark, Ph.D., "The Work of Registered Nurses, Licensed Practical Nurses, and Nurses Aides in Acute Care Hospitals"; Barbara Bowers, Ph.D., "The Work of Nurses and Nurse Aides in Long Term Care Facilities"; Karen Martin, "The Work of Nurses and Nursing Assistants in Home Care, Public Health, and Other Community Settings"; Ann Rogers Ph.D., "Work Hour Regulation in Safety-Sensitive Industries"; Gail Ingersoll, EdD, and Madeline Schmitt, Ph.D., "Interdisciplinary Collaboration, Team Functioning, and Patient Safety"; Ann Hendrich, "Evidence-based Design of Nursing Workspace in Hospitals"; Pascale Carayon, Ph.D., Carla Alvarado, Ph.D., and Ann Hundt, Ph.D., "Reducing Workload and Increasing Patient Safety Through Work and Workspace Design"; and Murat Bayiz, "Work and Workload Measurements in Nurse Staffing Models."

In undertaking its work, the committee focused predominantly on nursing care delivered in acute care hospitals and inpatient nursing facilities, because these are the settings in which the greatest amount of evidence exists about the nature of threats to patient safety and possible remedies in the work environment of nurses. The committee noted a number of issues related to, but not part of, its charge, including the nursing shortage, *nurse* safety in the work environment, and problems with nurse retention. It also noted issues with respect to the varying educational paths to licensure as a registered nurse that may have implications for nurse performance in the workplace. As tempting, important, and deserving of study as these issues were, they were beyond the considerable charge given to the committee by the Agency for Healthcare Research and Quality. The committee calls attention to the need for further study in these areas.

Appendix B

Interdisciplinary Collaboration, Team Functioning, and Patient Safety[1]

As concern over the number of health care errors has risen, so has interest in the development of care delivery processes that minimize the potential for error. Among the strategies proposed by experts is the creation, training, and support of highly developed interdisciplinary teams and collaborative work groups (Chassin et al., 1998; Disch et al., 2001; Palmersheim, 1999). The desire for effective team performance has been mentioned in the health care literature for years. What has been less evident is what constitutes effective team performance, how it is created and nurtured, and how it directly or indirectly influences care delivery outcomes. These unknown attributes and products of work teams should be explored thoroughly to enable sound recommendations concerning the promotion of interdisciplinary teams and collaborative work groups as a measure for assuring safe patient care.

This appendix is divided into three main sections. The first contains an extensive review of the literature concerning interdisciplinary teams and their impact on care delivery and safety outcomes. Included in the review are summaries of relevant research from health care, industry, and other work groups involved in error-prone and high-risk team behaviors. The second section provides evidence-based recommendations for strategies to develop, train, and assess the performance of interdisciplinary teams. The final section delineates needs for further research.

---

[1]This appendix was prepared for the committee to inform its deliberations by Gail L. Ingersoll, Ed.D., R.N., F.A.A.N., F.N.A.P., and Madeline Schmitt, Ph.D., R.N., F.A.A.N., F.N.A.P., of the University of Rochester Medical Center.

341

TEAMS AND PERFORMANCE OUTCOMES

The importance of understanding and maximizing team performance has been discussed by several authors, who note that 70 to 80 percent of health care errors are caused by human factors associated with interpersonal interactions (Schaefer et al., 1994). Others stress the increasing numbers of professionals directly involved in care delivery processes and the relationship between the resulting importance of cooperative working relationships and the complexity of patient needs (Headrick et al., 1998). Addressing this demand is hindered by a number of factors, including the wide variation in team makeup, which ranges from those composed of senior clinicians overseeing residents and fellows (Posner and Freund, 1999) to those involving representatives of multiple professions from multiple organizations (Green and Plesk, 2002; Kosseff and Niemeier, 2001; Stone et al., 2002). Clear differences exist in those situations in which team makeup is driven by hierarchical learning or reporting mechanisms and those in which the team members have equal influence on team performance and outcome. In addition, health professionals interact in a variety of ways, ranging from loosely coordinated collaborative relationships at one end of the continuum to more tightly organized work teams at the other, often within the same day (Headrick et al., 1998). Difficulties also arise when determining whether the failure of a team's performance is the cause or the result of poor team member behavior. In a study of deteriorating team performance, a back-and-forth pattern developed between member performance and overall team performance as top management teams began to fail (Hambrick and D'Aveni, 1992).

Theories of Work Team Effectiveness

A number of theories exist concerning the ways in which teams work and how they produce favorable outcomes. Some of the more prominent theories relevant to the discussion of decision making for patient safety and for the creation of desirable care delivery outcomes are reviewed below.

Early Theories of Team Behavior

Early theoretical efforts to conceptualize the group processes operating in teams drew heavily upon sociological studies of hierarchical differentiation. In these investigations, the social structure of the group was examined for its impact on team communication and problem solving (Feiger and Schmitt, 1979). In summarizing the basic research in this field, Feiger and Schmitt note that status-driven hierarchical processes undermine analysis and problem-solving activities in teams. These same processes may facilitate coordination and synthesis activities, however. Feiger and Schmitt also examined the relationship between degree of hierarchy and patient outcomes in four teams in a long-term care setting. They found that better outcomes were perfectly rank-correlated with less hierarchy in the interaction patterns of team members.

In focusing on other group processes that can undermine the effectiveness of team performance, Heinemann and colleagues (1994a) summarize several sociological theories relevant to group decision making and apply them to geriatric interdisciplinary health care teams. Groupthink (Janis, 1972, 1982)—a process theorized to affect highly cohesive teams in which efforts are made to control the input of information that challenges the team's thinking—is more likely to occur in situations of high stress where there is pressure to act. The theory was first used to examine the dynamics of what went wrong in political fiascoes, such as the Bay of Pigs invasion of Cuba under the leadership of President Kennedy and the Challenger disaster. In tests of the theory, directive leadership was found to increase the likelihood of groupthink processes.

Theories of framing and group polarization have been used to refine ideas developed in groupthink theory. Framing theory focuses on the interpersonal context of decision making, while group polarization theory emphasizes how group discussion exaggerates initial preferences of team members for risk taking or caution. Discussions also have focused on the linkages between the stage of development of group/team cohesiveness and the potential for groupthink behavior (Longley and Pruitt, 1980). In addition, Farrell and colleagues have examined how conditions in geriatric teams may approximate conditions required for groupthink processes and illustrate these processes in a case study description (Farrell et al., 1986, 1988, 2001). They offer the following guidelines for minimizing poor decision making related to these team processes: (1) emphasizing open, honest, and direct communication; (2) facilitating team development, which includes writing a mission statement, formulating goals and procedures for operating, clarifying roles, and orienting new team members; and (3) helping teams identify team processes that predispose to poor decision making, such as overreliance on directive leaders and team isolation. They emphasize the importance of retreats, administrative or process meetings, and acknowledgment of effective work.

Group development theory has provided the theoretical context for a number of studies of health care teams (Farrell et al., 1986, 1988, 2001). This theory posits that teams pass through a series of developmental stages prior to reaching their maximum work effectiveness. Few efforts have been made to measure team development and examine factors that influence team development. Consequently, the usefulness of this theory for understanding team safety behavior is uncertain. One study of researcher-designed and/or

-adapted measures of team development and team functioning has been conducted. This investigation explored a variety of factors affecting team development and team functioning and the impact of team functioning on team member burnout (Heinemann et al., 1994b).

Theories of Team Behavior and Error

Sasou and Reason (1999) have created a taxonomy of team errors, which they believe highlights the essential components of error detection in group processes. The dimensions of this taxonomy include (1) a determination of how the team made the error, (2) an appreciation for whether the team recognized the error and corrected it, and (3) an understanding of the human relations that contributed to the error. Sasou and Reason expanded the work of Reason (1990), who categorized human errors into three types—mistakes, lapses, and slips. According to the original conceptualization, mistakes and lapses arise in the planning and thinking process, whereas slips occur primarily in the execution phase. Mistakes and lapses are more likely to occur during team processes, whereas slips are caused primarily by individuals (Sasou and Reason, 1999).

Team errors consist of an error-making process and an error-recovery process. In the error-making process, errors occur as a result of individual or shared decision making. Individual errors are subdivided into independent and dependent errors according to the extent of information available during the decision-making process. Independent errors occur when the information available to the individual team member is correct; dependent errors occur when some part of the information is incomplete, absent, or incorrect. Shared errors are errors shared by some or all of the team members, regardless of whether they were in direct communication with the individual initiating the error. Shared errors are likewise subdivided into independent or dependent according to the amount and accuracy of the information available (Sasou and Reason, 1999).

The error-recovery process includes three stages—detection, indication, and correction (Sasou and Reason, 1999). The initial stage, detection, is followed by the indication phase, in which an identified error is brought to the attention of the group. If this fails to occur, the error is not fully recovered, and actions taken to correct the error are not likely to work. The final stage involves actual correction of the error.

Sasou and Reason (1999) have applied this taxonomy to 21 error events occurring in the nuclear industry, 21 events in the aviation industry, and 25 events in the shipping industry. Human factors reports were used to identify 28 team errors in nuclear industry events, 8 in aviation industry events, and 9 in shipping industry events. The findings suggest that individual errors occur more frequently than shared errors and that failures to detect errors occur more often than failures to indicate or correct.

In this same study, the investigators identify internal and external factors that contribute to the errors made. They define these contributors as performance-shaping factors (PSFs), which include external factors such as darkness, temperature, and high work requirements that are shared by all team members working in the same environment. Internal PSFs include high stress, excessive fatigue, and deficiencies in knowledge and skill. According to Sasou and Reason (1999), internal PSFs are often influenced by external factors and may vary across individuals even under the same set of circumstances. Team PSFs are a third potential contributor to error. These include, for example, lack of communication, inappropriate task allocation, and excessive authority gradient (Sasou and Reason, 1999).

In their review of adverse events in the nuclear, aviation, and shipping industries, Sasou and Reason (1999) found the most common team PSF to be failure to communicate. Failure to communicate resulted in the inability to detect both individual and shared errors. Excessive professional courtesy, overtrusting, an air of confidence, and excessive belief were additional factors. Inadequate resources and deficient task management created errors and also led to detection failures. Excessive authority gradient was the most dominant factor in failures to indicate and correct errors, although excessive professional courtesy also led to team member reluctance to challenge error makers. Shared errors commonly occurred during the human–machine interface, where low task awareness, low situational awareness, and excessive adherence to overreliance on established practices contributed to mistakes. Failures to detect were influenced by deficiencies in communication and resource/task management, excessive authority gradient, and excessive belief. Failures to indicate/correct were influenced by excessive authority gradient, excessive professional courtesy, and deficiency in resource/task management. Based on these findings, the authors recommend that team error-reduction strategies focus on clarifying team member responsibility and accountability and on improving interpersonal skills performance. This includes efforts both to maximize communication success and to provide constructive feedback to established and well-respected team members.

A second theory of team behavior and safety processes proposes that four boundaries of safe or acceptable practice are evident in systems—physical, psychological, social, and economic (Bea, 1998). Individuals within systems function within a "safety space" created by these four boundaries and take action to withdraw when they perceive they are approaching one of the unsafe areas. In this model, the physical boundary reflects conditions in which the work or effort required is perceived to be excessive. When approaching this boundary, employees develop work shortcuts to reduce the perceived threat. The psychological boundary represents conditions in which mental effort, stress, or anguish is unacceptable. Safety protection behaviors when approaching this boundary include withdrawal and aggressive action. The social boundary clarifies the limits of acceptable group norms and behavior and may include legal or corporate expectations for performance. The economic boundary indicates where economic viability or security is threatened and when approached often leads to cost-cutting measures.

Strategies to keep teams and organizations functioning within the safety zone created by these boundaries involve designing robust structures that include attention to (1) redundancy, in which alternate paths are available to carry demands; (2) ductility, in which components are able to deform without failing and to shift demands to other paths when necessary; and (3) excess capacity, in which components are designed to carry demands beyond those normally expected. Full integration of these fail-safe measures requires the development of cohesive work teams that emphasize integrity, trust, and cooperation (Bea, 1998). Necessary also are sufficient training of members who have direct influence over the system's safety; the development of positive economic and psychological incentives that promote safety behaviors; the development of effective internal and external checking and verification procedures; and standards of performance, including procedures for disciplinary action when rules are breached and the introduction of methods to promote early identification of and response to emerging risks.

According to this model, three approaches can be used to maximize consistent practice within teams and return to safe systems. The first is a reactive approach, which results in analysis of the failure or failures of the system. This process focuses on understanding the reasons for failure and how to avoid it in the future. Most commonly, the process results in the development of safety guidelines, procedures, and rules for performance (Bea, 1998). The proactive approach works to analyze the system before it fails and to put into place measures that prevent the anticipated failure. One of the difficulties with this approach is its focus, which directs attention to what may go wrong rather than what is working right. For this reason, Bea adds a third approach, which he believes needs further development and exploration. This real-time approach stresses the responses that occur during a crisis when a buildup of danger signals requires immediate action to return the system to its normal state. The real-time approach recognizes those situations in which the sequence of events or the novelty of the situation is unpredictable and different from previous experiences. In this scenario, employees are provided with enhanced abilities to rescue themselves from the threatening event and to return the system to its usual safe state. Training, including the use of simulation techniques, is the most useful approach for developing these skills. Ideally, the training should address the three cognitive processes that govern how well people respond during a crisis: (1) overall knowledge of background information and related conditions; (2) attention dynamics, or the control and management of mental workload, maintenance of situation awareness, and avoidance of fixations; and (3) strategy development, which includes considering trade-offs between conflicting goals, dealing with uncertainty and ambiguity, setting effective priorities, and making good decisions (Bea, 1998).

A third team- and safety-related theory focuses on team effectiveness, including the ability to avoid or minimize the potential for error. In this model, team effectiveness is measured by the team's ability to solicit and value differences in team members' assumptions and world views (Korsgaard et al., 1995). Even in the best of circumstances, however, team members may become disengaged from the team if they believe the action taken by the team differs from their personal view. For this reason, reviews of effective team decision making should consider both the quality of the decision and the impact of the decision-making process on team members' commitment to the decision, their continued attachment to the team, and their trust in the team leader. These latter three dimensions serve as antecedents to cooperation among team members, which is essential to the ultimate support for and action on a decision made.

One approach to determining the potential level of team member support for a team decision is consideration of a team member's perceived level of procedural justice during the decision-making process. The tenets of procedural justice suggest that fair treatment is central to all humans and is a major determinant of their reaction to how decisions are made and executed (Korsgaard et al., 1995). The concept is focused in particular on the meaning of involvement in the decision-making process and less so on the individual's ultimate control over the decision outcome. Perceptions of fairness are influenced by the extent to which team members show consideration for the input of other team members and the extent to which individual members' input affects or is reflected in the final decision. In the case of health care teams designed according to hierarchical reporting determiners, procedural justice is influenced considerably by the senior members of the team. If the senior members routinely seek and incorporate junior members' opinions in decision making, junior members are more likely to perceive the team process as just and supportable. If, on the other hand, junior team members perceive the process as unjust, they are much less likely to cooperate with or support any decisions made. They also are far more likely to disengage from the group and to minimize the potential benefit of the group process for patient safety decisions.

This theory of team effectiveness and the impact of team leader consideration and responsiveness was tested in a study of intact teams of middle-

and upper-level managers of a Fortune 500 company (Korsgaard et al., 1995). In this study, decisions made in teams with high levels of consideration behavior by leaders were perceived by team members as much more fair than decisions in low-consideration groups. Members of high-consideration groups also were significantly more committed to the decisions made, especially when their level of influence was low. In addition, high-consideration group members increased their commitment to the team over time, while low-consideration group members disengaged. Member influence in decision making had the most dramatic effect, with the quality of decisions made in high-influence groups being significantly greater than that of decisions made in low-influence groups. A comparable effect on decision quality was not seen for level of leader consideration.

Organizational Behavior and Team Performance

More recent theories have been proposed concerning the ways in which organizations and work groups successfully reduce the potential for error. Some of these theories center on high-reliability organizations, defined as organizations that operate relatively free of error for long periods of time, frequently in hazardous environments (Bea, 1998; Gaba, 2000). High-reliability organizations view safety as the top functional objective for the organization (Gaba, 2000). They have extensive process auditing procedures to assist in the identification of safety problems and have well-established reward systems that reinforce error-reduction behaviors (Bea, 1998). High-reliability organizations focus their error-reduction activities at the systems level and incorporate rehearsals of familiar scenarios of failure. They also recognize the likelihood of human error and attempt to train their workforce to recognize and recover from such error (Reason, 2000).

According to Gaba (2000), health care institutions have viewed safety as a by-product of non-negligent care rather than a goal to be achieved. This world view differs from that of high-reliability organizations, in which safety is the focus of all actions. Altering this view has been difficult, especially in light of the problems associated with planning for and measuring the impact of accidents that do not occur (as a result of the focus on error-free outcomes). Gaba suggests that health care's decentralized system contributes to the proliferation of error. Individual practices and the reluctance to consolidate care delivery processes have led to highly variable performance patterns and the likelihood of negative events. Even in those cases in which health care organizations have joined larger health services systems, the focus on these collaborations has been on business operations and cost savings, not safe practices. Shifting this focus to coincide with the expectations of high-reliability organizations will be difficult.

An application of high-reliability theory has been described for and tested in organizations requiring nearly error-free operations to prevent the occurrence of catastrophes (Weick and Roberts, 1993). In this model, high-reliability organizations engage in aggregate mental processes that are more fully developed than those evident in organizations concerned with process efficiency. Weick and Roberts have tested this model with flight team members whose interactions with others are coordinated in explicit and visible ways and whose socialization is continual. In addition, when working alone, these workers have less of a grasp of the system than when working together. In this situation, the system is constructed of interdependent worker abilities and of individuals who react quickly to novel and rapidly occurring situations. Furthermore, the consequences of any lapse of team member attention are rapid and disastrous.

In this model, the collective mind of group members is a reflection of overlapping knowledge and actions that are taken with care, rather than any within-group similarity of attitudes (Weick and Roberts, 1993). Weick and Roberts define the actions taken with care as heedful actions—actions that are critical, consistent, purposeful, attentive, and vigilant. Heedful performance denotes continuous learning that is modified by previous performance. The more heedful the interactions among team members, the more developed is the team's collective mind and the greater is the team's ability to comprehend and respond to unexpected events that evolve quickly in unanticipated ways. When heedful actions are spread across more activities and more connections, group understanding is increased, and the potential for errors is reduced.

Weick and Roberts (1993) suggest that when heedful behaviors are visible, rewarded, modeled, and discussed, new team members learn this style of responding. The new team members subsequently incorporate these behaviors into the definitions of who they are in the system and reaffirm this style in their actions. Collective mind is renewed and reaffirmed during the socialization of new team members and is maximized when senior team members describe and review representative failures as well as successes. The style of senior member interactions also contributes to the development of heedful behaviors by new team members. If those interactions are poor, heedful behavior may suffer, resulting in errors in communication or action by new members. In addition, attention may be focused on individual actions or needs rather than group actions. If this process continues over time, small, individual errors can grow to large-scale group error. Weick and Roberts suggest that this process has important implications for team development strategies in which training may be focused exclusively on content rather than heedful behaviors. They also recommend that training programs include attention to the social processes and dynamics of the work group.

An additional theory of organizational behavior relevant to team inter-actions and patient safety is the microsystem concept described by Nelson and colleagues (2002). According to this model, the health system is com-posed of a front-line clinical microsystem, an overarching macrosystem, and patient subpopulations needing care. Two assumptions of this frame-work are that the microsystems produce the quality, safety, and cost out-comes associated with delivery of services and that the outcomes of the macrosystem can be no better than the microsystems of which it is com-posed. To bring about the changes needed to reduce errors in health care, fundamental changes need to occur at all levels of the system. In addition, efforts need to be made to optimize each individual microsystem and to establish seamless, timely, reliable, and efficient linkages among clinical microsystems. According to Nelson and colleagues, one of the benefits of this conceptual approach is its attention to the front-line component of service delivery.

Health care microsystems evolve over time and conduct the primary work associated with the core aims of the organization. They are composed of a small group of people who work together on a regular basis to provide care to a discrete subpopulation of patients (Nelson et al., 2002). In this framework, clinical microsystems are the essential building blocks of the health system and as such contribute significantly to the outcomes seen. They are tightly or loosely connected with one another and perform better or worse under different operating conditions.

This microsystem model was tested by Nelson and colleagues (2002) through the use of a qualitative design consisting of observation, interview, review of documents, and analysis of financial data. In this study, 20 high-performing clinical microsystems were identified through a review of lists of award winners, literature citations, previous research findings, expert opinion, and nominations from leaders of exemplary organizations. A struc-tured screening interview and questionnaire were used to select 20 micro-systems from an initial 75 sites. The investigators identified a set of nine success characteristics evident across all sites that led to highly favorable systemic outcomes: the leadership of the microsystem, the culture of the microsystem, the macro-organizational support of the microsystem, a focus on patients, a focus on staff, interdependence of care teams, the availability and use of information and information technology, a focus on process improvement, and an outstanding performance pattern (Nelson et al., 2002). An emphasis on patient safety, health professional education, and awareness of the impact of the external environment also were evident at these institutions.

Nelson and colleagues (2002) believe that the critical role of these natu-rally occurring microsystems has been ignored in previous efforts to reduce health system errors. They suggest that attention has been directed instead at clinicians, consumers, and others, thereby ignoring the essential building blocks of the health care system. They recommend pushing the decision making, process ownership, and accountability expectations out to the microsystems where the greatest potential for impact lies.

This micro- and macrosystem model can be linked to earlier work on "teams" and their role in health care delivery conducted by Schmitt (1991). Schmitt sorts the interdisciplinary health team literature into three different levels according to the extent of linkage between the microsystem and the macrosystem of the health care institution: (1) the functioning team as a small work group, which usually is defined as three or more members representing different disciplines who share responsibility for an integrated plan of care for a specific cohort of patients over time; (2) the unit-level microsystem, in which the mix of staff involved with patients varies from patient to patient; and (3) institutional policies and procedures that support either the small work group or unit-based care delivery process. The impact of team approaches on patient outcomes, including safety outcomes, potentially can be studied from any of these perspectives.

This shift in conceptualization is further described by Schmitt (2001), who introduces the ideas behind "team" as the second and third levels of relationship falling between microsystem and macrosystem. The basic shift in thinking in this approach is its focus on the concept of *collaboration* in the delivery of care among diverse health professions. Collaboration, which has been defined as "cooperatively working together, sharing responsibility for solving problems and making decisions to formulate and carry out plans for patient care" (Baggs and Schmitt, 1988:145), incorporates efforts to coordinate care. Interdisciplinary teams can be viewed as one specific form of collaboration that is relevant to certain situational circumstances of health care delivery. Questions can then be raised about other forms of collaboration between disciplines and the effects of that collaboration on care delivery outcome.

Examples of studies that fit into this refined framework include a study of differences in mortality outcomes in intensive care units (ICUs) in 13 U.S. hospitals. After performing risk adjustment for differences in patient severity of illness and ruling out several other potential explanations, Knaus and colleagues (1986) argue that the greater presence of interdisciplinary interaction and coordination of care among staff contributed to the differences seen. Included in their discussion of potential contributors to favorable care provider relationships is the availability of policies and procedures (e.g., joint care rounds) that support coordination and collaboration in care, which they suggest accounts for the lower mortality rates seen in some units. The identification of these differences in the care delivery process was retrospective, however, making the assurance of cause–effect relationships uncertain. In a second, prospective study of 42 randomly chosen ICUs

(Shortell et al., 1992, 1994), an ICU nurse–physician questionnaire was used to evaluate perceptions of the multiple dimensions of care delivery process, such as leadership, communication, coordination, and conflict management. Although not associated with risk-adjusted mortality, these caregiver performance variables were associated with better technical care, efforts to meet family needs, and decreased ICU length of stay.

In a second national study of 25 ICUs, Mitchell and colleagues (1996) found the flow of information that is characteristic of interdisciplinary collaboration to be associated with more-favorable staff perceptions of unit conflict management, collaboration, staff quality, and quality of care. It was not associated with any clinical outcomes, however. Moreover, many aspects of the care delivery process were examined in these studies, making it difficult to assess the actual contribution of interdisciplinary caregiver interaction to the outcomes seen.

Additional support for the interdisciplinary collaboration concept is provided by Baggs et al. (1992, 1999), who examined the relationship between collaborative discharge decision making between nurses and physicians and patient outcomes. In both studies, nurses' perceptions (but not physicians') of greater collaboration was found to be linked to a small but significant reduction in risk-adjusted mortality and readmission in the medical ICU. Higgins (1999) could not reproduce these findings, but there were significant differences in her study design compared with that of Baggs and colleagues. More recently Gittell et al. (2000:810) studied "relational coordination," defined as consisting of "four communication dimensions (frequent, timely, accurate, and problem-solving communication) as well as three relationship dimensions (shared goals, shared knowledge, and mutual respect)" among respondents representing five disciplines (physicians, nurses, social workers, physical therapists, and case managers) caring for hip and knee arthroscopy patients in nine hospitals. Greater perceived relational coordination was associated with patient perceptions of higher quality of care, less post-operative pain, greater post-operative functioning, and shorter length of stay.

Generally, the literature concerning collaboration in health care focuses primarily on nurse–physician interaction, whereas the literature on interdisciplinary teams focuses on a broader array of disciplines involved in care delivery. To develop a full appreciation of the impact of collaboration on safety outcomes, research must be expanded (as in Gittell et al.'s [2000] study) to include additional disciplinary groups.

Health Care Work Groups and Performance Outcomes

Much of the literature pertaining to interdisciplinary health teams has focused on the clinical microsystems level, particularly as it relates to multi-

or interdisciplinary care delivery teams. Following is a review of this research to date.

Six integrative reviews of research concerning interdisciplinary teams and care delivery outcomes were found in a search of medical, nursing, psychology, sociology, education, and business electronic databases. In the following summary of these integrative reviews, additional reports relevant to the content of the reviews are incorporated.

Integrative Review # 1

The earliest integrative review is that of Halstead (1976), focused on the literature pertaining to team delivery of care in the areas of chronic illness and rehabilitation. Halstead (1976:507) identifies three broad categories of literature in his review of 25 years of team-related reports: opinion articles, descriptions of programs, and "serious efforts to investigate the effectiveness of team care." The bulk of the literature falls into the first two categories.

Halstead (1976) identified only 10 studies published between 1951 and 1975 that met the criterion of requiring a comparison or control group as part of the design. Given the emphasis on chronic illness and rehabilitation, most of the outcomes focused on various types of patient functioning (e.g., social, intellectual, and activities of daily living). In about half of the studies, investigators focused on morbidity outcomes or measures of service utilization; few addressed employment, mortality, or costs of care. In judging the overall effectiveness of team interventions, six of the studies revealed an association between favorable outcomes and the team approach. In two studies, results were mixed, supporting greater effectiveness for only some of the outcomes seen. The results of the remaining two studies indicated that team approaches are as effective as usual care approaches (no difference). The results also were mixed in studies in which utilization of services and costs of care were assessed. In light of the meager evidence, Halstead (1976:507) concluded that team care is still "largely a matter of faith and the subject of many platitudes."

Integrative Review # 2

The second systematic review targeted research examining the effectiveness of interdisciplinary geriatric teams (Schmitt et al., 1988) and focused mainly on studies published in the early 1980s. Eleven studies were identified that met the criterion of having a comparison or control group, or other design features used to address the absence of such a group. The geriatric teams examined were almost all hospital-based. In a later review, Schmitt (2001) organized and summarized the outcome data from Schmitt et al. (1988) to allow for a clear comparison with Halstead's (1976) earlier results. Outcomes examined in these studies covered the same broad range represented in Halstead's review, with differences appropriate to the geriatric focus (i.e., the employment category is missing, but referrals to higher or lower levels of care are examined in about half the geriatric studies). Of the 11 studies included, the results from 7 demonstrated greater effectiveness with the team approach; results of 3 studies indicated that team care is similar to or more effective than (depending on the outcome studied) the care provided by the comparison group; and results for 1 study showed no differences in any of the outcomes compared.

In summarizing the similarities and differences between the reviews of Halstead (1976) and Schmitt et al. (1988), Schmitt (2001) notes that functional outcomes were the most frequently assessed in both cases. Functional status also demonstrated a positive change in response to the team approach. In the geriatric team studies, referral to reduced levels of care was a consistent finding with the team care approach. When mortality rates were examined, no difference is seen. Service utilization was investigated more often in recent studies, but with mixed results. Where investigators studied cost outcomes, no differences in costs or cost savings were found. In many of these studies, however, the financial impact of greater use of health services was not studied directly.

Integrative Review # 3

Schmitt (2001) provides a third summary of the outcomes of 24 studies of the effectiveness of geriatric (20 studies) and other team (4 studies) interventions, focusing on the mid-1980s to the mid-1990s. Of the 24 studies examined, 1 finds team intervention to be more effective, while 15 show the team approach to be similar to that of the comparison group for some outcomes and more effective for others. The more frequent pattern of mixed outcomes (i.e., some improved, others similar) may be related to the greater frequency with which multiple outcomes are examined in any given study, as compared with earlier studies in which the number of outcomes is limited to one or two. Results of 7 studies show no difference in outcomes. In 1 study results are mixed, with survivors in the experimental group having lower functioning than those in the comparison group, probably because team intervention reduces mortality by keeping sicker individuals alive. Results indicate that team consultation activities alone are not sufficient to produce improved outcomes. An impact was demonstrated, however, when expert teams provided both assessment and treatment interventions.

Looking across the above three reviews (Halstead, 1976; Schmitt, 2001; Schmitt et al., 1988), several things are apparent: (1) the study of team approaches to care delivery has focused primarily on the level of the functioning team as a small work group in which the same identified team members share responsibility for a specific cohort of patients over time; (2) there has been considerable growth in efforts to examine the impact of team approaches using more rigorous research designs; (3) a greater variety of outcomes is being examined in any given study; and (4) there is a slowly accumulating body of evidence, primarily in hospital settings and mainly with older populations, that conscious team approaches to care delivery can result in improvements in a range of outcomes. As a group, however, the studies have a number of serious limitations, identified in two of the reviews. Among the concerns mentioned by Schmitt (2001) and Schmitt et al. (1988) are the inability to rule out confounders, such as a "demonstration" effect; differences in skill mix between team and usual-care personnel; differences in treatment intensity; and a long-standing focus on the effects of a single team compared with the usual-care situation. From study to study, structural aspects of the teams, such as size, mix of disciplines, and communication frequency and pattern, also vary. In addition, only recently has an effort been made to determine the magnitude of the effectiveness of team interventions. As a result, the impact of the overall quality of such efforts on outcomes cannot be assessed. Moreover, little attention has been paid to the multifaceted dimensions of team relationships, with no attempt being made to assess the active elements of the team intervention (e.g., communication processes, joint care planning, improved coordination of care).

Very recently, researchers have attempted to define the minimum requirements for team structure and process and to assess the effectiveness of comprehensive team delivery of care on care delivery outcomes. In a national, multisite controlled trial of the impact of the Veterans Administration's (VA) inpatient unit and outpatient clinic geriatric evaluation and management (GEM) interdisciplinary teams on patient outcomes (Cohen et al., 2002), the core team members were clearly defined, and the elements of the intervention were well scripted. Process-of-care data assessing the perceptions of the effectiveness of team functioning were gathered at the initiation of the study and annually for three additional years. Team functioning and effectiveness data were compared with previously collected similar information from a representative sample of VA GEM teams (Schmitt et al., 2000).

No evidence was found that the GEM interventions reduced mortality as compared with usual care; however, the GEM inpatient unit treatment positively affected physical functioning and general health, pain, activities of daily living, and physical performance at discharge. Only the difference in pain levels was sustained at the 1-year follow-up point, regardless of type of follow-up care. Patients receiving outpatient GEM clinic treatment for a 1-year period posthospitalization improved only in mental health as compared with their hospital discharge score. No differences in costs of care among the alternative treatments were evident at 1 year. Ineffective team functioning was ruled out as an explanation for the lack of greater differences among the alternative treatments because team "functioning met the criteria generally accepted to characterize the best-functioning units, with team functions and processes of care that were equivalent to those of other highly effective programs" (Cohen et al., 2002:911).

Integrative Review # 4

A fourth integrative review is that of Schofield and Amodeo (1999), who searched education, psychology, medical, and sociology databases to identify work on interdisciplinary teams. Their review was designed to address a series of questions, two of which pertain to the relationships between interdisciplinary teams and treatment and cost of care. The reviewers identified 138 articles containing significant substantive content pertaining to interdisciplinary teams. Of these, 55 were labeled as descriptive because they addressed some aspect of interdisciplinary teams but did not include a specific description of team process or any empirical data on process or outcome. Fifty-one articles were identified as process-focused because they contained descriptions of interdisciplinary team processes but no formal data. Twenty-one articles were research-based, using either qualitative or quantitative methods to assess the effect of a variety of variables on the team itself. An additional 11 articles were defined as outcome-based because they used research methods to assess the impact of an interdisciplinary team on some outcome that was distinct from team functioning. Schofield and Amodeo noted that only 1 of the 11 investigations adhered to four study design elements they considered necessary for assessing whether a team had an effect. Unfortunately, the reviewers did not explicitly identify these criteria in their review, nor did they provide a table highlighting the studies reviewed. Based on the investigations mentioned in the article, however, and the reference list provided, there appears to be little overlap with the studies critiqued in other reviews.

Schofield and Amodeo's (1999) conclusions highlight the deficiencies associated with the existing research on interdisciplinary teams. They conclude that the available literature repeatedly endorses the team model, but contains little evidence of efforts to evaluate team effectiveness or assess team impact. The majority of the articles reviewed simply assume the value of interdisciplinary teams. Schofield and Amodeo also note the interchangeable use of the terms "interdisciplinary" and "multidisciplinary," which are rarely defined by investigators. They express concern about the absence of well-conceived conceptual models of interdisciplinary teamwork and the failure to assess the actual components of the interdisciplinary process. According to the authors, investigators routinely treat the team as a fixed entity rather than a multidimensional group consisting of diverse players, processes, and expectations for performance. Schofield and Amodeo suggest that the quality of the conceptualization of the teams is so poor that reliable conclusions cannot be drawn.

Integrative Review # 5

In a fifth review, Zwarenstein and Bryant (2002) include studies containing an explicit statement that the evaluated intervention was designed to improve collaboration between the nursing and medical professions. All randomized controlled trials, controlled pre- and postintervention studies, and interrupted time-series studies were eligible for inclusion. The authors searched the Cochrane Library and MEDLINE databases for evidence of research reports. Most of the articles identified in their search were descriptive reports of the problem, studies of professional substitution, and evaluations of undergraduate training programs and their impact on graduates' attitudes toward collaboration.

Two studies meet Zwarenstein and Bryant's (2002) inclusion criteria. The first study (Curley et al., 1998) was designed by an interdisciplinary continuous quality improvement team for the purposes of improving patient care on the inpatient medicine units of one hospital. This investigation was a randomized controlled firm trial of daily interdisciplinary rounds that included all disciplines involved in patient care, with order writing occurring during rounds. A "firm" was defined as a health care delivery "unit" that was part of the Firm System created in the study hospital. Three firm medical inpatient "units," consisting of two ward services in each firm unit, comprised similar groups of patients and physicians. Three medical inpatient wards implemented the new rounds, while three wards continued with traditional physician work rounds.

Because of the hospital's usual procedure of randomly assigning patients and physicians to firms, there were very few demographic or clinical differences among the 1,102 patients in the experimental and usual care groups. No differences between the experimental and usual care wards were seen for hospital mortality, type of hospital disposition, or readmission rates; after controlling for baseline differences in case mix, however, length of hospital stay for patients admitted to the experimental wards declined significantly following the intervention, as did total charges for care. A greater percentage of orders written for aerosol use were evaluated as appropriate on the experimental wards as compared with the control wards. In addition, a chart audit by nutritionists found dietary recommendations were implemented more frequently on the experimental wards. Staff on the experimental wards also reported more favorable perceptions of teamwork and communication patterns and a better understanding of patient care.

Control ward findings were unchanged during the same period. Subsequent to the study, interdisciplinary rounds were implemented on all six medical wards.

The second study reviewed by Zwarenstein and Bryant (2002) was conducted in Thailand (Jitapunkel et al., 1995) and involved the randomization of patients to a study or control ward, both of which were female wards, each in a separate hospital building. The new rounding process involving physicians and nurses occurred four times per week and consisted of joint decision making concerning treatment plans. A weekly team case conference of all disciplines involved in the care of these patients also was introduced. A historical comparison of current and past patient experience on the two wards was conducted as well. There were no differences in mean length of stay or mortality rate between the two study wards, during the trial or historically. However, reduced lengths of stay occurred on the experimental ward among those aged 60–74 who were discharged home. The benefits of collaboration were rated as "high" by team members.

Recent examples of reports evaluating the use of team-based, collaborative rounds that do not meet the rigorous design guidelines for a Cochrane systematic review include one focused on the care of cardiac surgery patients (Uhlig et al., 2002). This study was designed as a continuous quality improvement effort and nested conceptually in human factors science, the aviation safety literature, and high-reliability organization theory. A before–after single-case design was used to evaluate the introduction of daily interdisciplinary rounds that included the patient and family. In this process, a communication protocol was followed to maximize the consistency and completeness of the information exchanged and to facilitate effective decision making. During the rounding process, team members, patients, and families were encouraged to discuss anything they believed might have gone wrong in the care delivery process. The bedside round process was evaluated biweekly to ensure that the intended outcomes of the team process were achieved. According to the report's authors, mortality rates have declined significantly since the introduction of the team-based approach, and the levels of satisfaction with the care delivery process among both patients/families and team members have increased.

In a third randomized controlled trial identified by Zwarenstein and Bryant (2002), nonrecommended drug use was reduced in an experimental set of nursing homes that introduced pharmacist visits to an interdisciplinary team (Schmidt et al., 1998). This trial was excluded from the review because of the impossibility of separating the effects of the interdisciplinary team intervention from those of the additional pharmacist visits. Despite its exclusion, this study is only one of a few attempts to assess team interventions in long-term care settings. One other clinical trial of an interdisciplinary team intervention in a long-term care setting occurred much earlier

(Feiger and Schmitt 1979; Schmitt et al., 1982). In this study, team intervention was found to be associated with more positive changes in health and functioning and less decline at 1-year follow-up in a sample of ambulatory diabetics. Among the four experimental teams studied, degree of collegiality in the teams' interactions was correlated positively with patient outcomes. Unlike most studies in which collaboration is measured through self-report questionnaires, the degree of collegiality was assessed directly by means of coding interaction in videotaped team meetings.

More recently, Stone et al. (2002) examined a multidimensional interdisciplinary health care model introduced in 11 freestanding, not-for-profit long-term care facilities in eastern Wisconsin, which included interdisciplinary teams within and across sites. The investigators used both qualitative and quantitative means to measure program impact. The evaluation examined both the processes used to implement the model successfully and the outcomes associated with the model's adoption.

The model introduced into the nursing homes is called Wellspring Innovative Solutions. It consists of clinical consultation and education by a geriatric nurse practitioner, a shared program of staff training using modules developed by the nurse practitioner, the sharing of comparative data on resident outcomes, and interdisciplinary care resource teams that develop and implement interventions designed to improve resident care (Stone et al., 2002). The Wellspring model focuses on quality improvement activities and the creation of an environmental culture that supports decentralized decision making and the recognition and rewarding of staff directly involved in resident care. The cultural shift undertaken through Wellspring also has targeted interagency collaboration, with each of the nursing homes sharing outcome data and providing consultation and advice to member facilities.

Member facilities have formed a loosely coupled alliance that provides overall administrative support for the model. In addition, a program coordinator and interdisciplinary quality improvement teams assist the geriatric nurse practitioner with delivery of the model. The Wellspring coordinator serves as an educator and a facilitator of communication throughout the alliance. Membership on the care resource teams is voluntary and open to both nursing and non-nursing staff. Clinical training modules are used to ensure that facility staff are up to date on clinical practices that pertain to their patient populations (Stone et al., 2002).

The impact of the Wellspring program was assessed by comparing Wellspring and non-Wellspring facilities in Wisconsin. Outcomes were measured as "deficiencies," defined as being in noncompliance with various federal regulatory requirements. According to the investigators, Wellspring facilities had significantly fewer deficiencies postimplementation than did non-Wellspring facilities. A dramatic decline also was seen for the magnitude of deficiencies, with Wellspring facilities going from reporting three times as many severe deficiencies to having no severe deficiencies after implementation of the model. Findings also suggest that Wellspring staff became much more vigilant as a result of the model and took a more proactive approach to delivering resident care. This vigilance was perceived as having prevented several serious events, although these observational findings could not be substantiated by outcome data. Nurse retention rates also improved significantly following implementation of the model, as compared with reductions in nurse retention rates in non-Wellspring sites (Stone et al., 2002).

Integrative Review # 6

A sixth integrative review focused on innovative models of health care delivery, including the use of interdisciplinary teams (Wadhwa and Lavizzo-Mourey, 1999). The emphasis of this review was on the impact of innovative models on outcomes among two vulnerable populations—the terminally ill and the mentally ill. Reviewers searched medical literature databases, reviewed reference lists of published reports, and contacted known experts and authors to identify additional work. Twenty-four articles met the reviewers' criteria for inclusion, which required the presence of a control group.

Three studies included in the review evaluated the impact of interdisciplinary teams on outcomes among terminally ill patients, while seven examine their effect on the mentally ill (Wadhwa and Lavizzo-Mourey, 1999). Findings for the terminally ill population suggested the interdisciplinary team approach produced reductions in hospitalization rates and improvements in patient and family satisfaction. Few other differences were seen between control and experimental groups. The authors of the original studies and the integrative review suggest the absence of differences may be the result of the contamination of control groups, which frequently received interventions comparable to those of the experimental plan. Hospitalization rates and levels of patient and family satisfaction were found to be significantly improved for mentally ill patients overseen by interdisciplinary groups. Other outcome findings were comparable. In reviewing the evidence pertaining to the management of mentally ill populations, Wadhwa and Lavizzo-Mourey stressed the importance of including long-term support and outreach services with the use of interdisciplinary teams.

Teams and Patient Safety Outcomes

Reports of investigations of the impact of work teams on patient safety are limited. Most descriptions of work team success either are anecdotal or include only brief reviews of methods used to measure team effects. In many cases, the reports focus on the development and use of safety review committees and the structures used to support the work of these teams (Piotrowski et al., 2002; Sim and Joyner, 2002; Wong et al., 2002). Many describe continuous quality improvement efforts, including some that bring together representatives from multiple organizations within health care systems (Green and Plesk, 2002; Kosseff and Niemeier, 2001).

In the studies of interdisciplinary team outcomes described in previous sections, medical error reduction is not examined directly. It appears reasonable to assume, however, that some overlap exists in the outcomes studied and patient safety outcomes. Interdisciplinary assessment and treatment create multiple opportunities to improve diagnosis, reduce omissions in care, and reduce avoidable error. Conversely, a breakdown in interdisciplinary communication, the fundamental element in building effective collaboration, can result in serious medical error. In an exploratory study, Schmitt (1990) provides a content analysis of 13 appellate court malpractice cases from a variety of states, in which the interactions of medicine and nursing were relevant to the case. In these cases, multiple disciplines were sued, and the negligence was distributed across disciplines based on the nature of the communication that had or had not occurred between disciplines. Key problems in communication patterns included those in which nurses communicated information important to the diagnosis and management of the case that was ignored by the physician, as well as those in which nurses failed to communicate relevant information; both communication patterns resulted in errors in diagnosis and management. A set of related issues underpins these sorts of interdisciplinary error-producing communication problems. These issues include counterproductive hierarchical communication patterns that derive from status differences; disjunctions in the distribution of authority, responsibility, and accountability across disciplines; issues of respect (or its lack); and lack of clarity with regard to legal and ethical obligations across disciplines.

In the limited literature concerning the contribution of health teams to patient safety outcomes, some reports describe a beneficial effect (Leape et al., 1999; Sovie and Jawad, 2001), whereas others report none (Bates et al., 1998). These differences are likely the result of the variety of methods used to assess team impact, the size and makeup of the teams, the variable dimensions of the team intervention, and the frequency and magnitude of the outcomes assessed.

A recently completed 3-year national study of medical and surgical units in 29 university teaching hospitals provides some additional information pertaining to the effect of teams on positive and negative care delivery outcomes. In this study, the consequences of hospital restructuring were examined for their impact on nurse staffing and patient care (Sovie and Jawad,

2001). The study's investigators identified structure and process predictors of patient satisfaction and adverse patient outcomes, including falls, nosocomial pressure ulcers, and urinary tract infections. The Management Practices and Processes Questionnaire used to assess nurses' perceptions of process indicators was based on an instrument developed by Shortell and colleagues (1991) for use in ICUs. The structure variables of registered nurse (RN) hours and all nursing personnel hours worked per patient day were found to be significant predictors of patient satisfaction and adverse outcomes. On medical units, one of the predictors of urinary tract infections was found to be reported collaboration of nurses with physicians. Similarly, in combination with the structure variables, reduced falls were associated with increased communication, collaboration, and conflict resolution between nurses and physicians.

In an earlier study of potentially harmful drug-related errors, care delivery team characteristics and nurse manager behaviors were assessed for their impact on detected error rates (Edmondson, 1996). In this nonexperimental research design, eight hospital unit teams were randomly selected from two urban teaching hospitals affiliated with the same medical school. Potentially harmful drug-related errors were identified through daily chart reviews, informal visits to units to ask about unusual drug events, and incident reporting. Drug-related error data were collected for 6 months; team and nurse manager behaviors were assessed through nonparticipant observation and surveys distributed during the second month of the study.

Detected error rates were found to be strongly associated with high scores on nurse manager direction setting and coaching, perceived unit performance outcomes, and quality of unit relationships. Edmondson (1996) suggested that the unexpected association between more-favorable work environment and incidence of errors is actually a desirable outcome. She believed the increased numbers of detected errors were an indication of the influence of a safe reporting environment on error reporting. This perception is supported by comparable associations among nurse manager direction setting, quality of unit relations, and frequency of interceptions to prevent adverse drug events. Error interceptions also were found to be moderately correlated with unit tolerance for mistakes, suggesting that tolerant error-reporting environments facilitate both the detection of errors and the delivery of successful interventions to prevent harmful outcomes.

Team intervention in some studies is defined according to the products created by the team. For instance, Bates et al. (1998) measured team impact on the prevention of serious medication errors through the implementation of a recommended dilutions chart; a computerized drip-rate calculation program; the standardized labeling of intravenous bags, tubes, and pumps; and a pharmacy communication log for nursing and pharmacy staff. How the team devised these elements and how it influenced or oversaw each product's implementation is not clear. Whether all components were implemented equally also is unknown.

Methodological shortcomings have contributed to the difficulties inherent in determining the characteristics of effective teams and the processes used to reduce error. For example, in some cases team impact is assessed through the quality improvement performance of the attending physician (Posner and Freund, 1999). This approach is necessary when an institution assigns adverse events to the senior clinician overseeing the care delivery activities of the team. Although some justification can be made for using this reporting process, little useful information can be gleaned about what actually occurred within the team to produce the outcomes seen. In addition, the assignment of responsibility to the senior physician reinforces the hierarchical nature of the team, suggesting that regardless of what team members do, the overall product of the team is the result of the team director's actions.

Although findings concerning the relationship between the existence and performance of health care teams and patient outcomes are mixed, evidence suggests the relationship is present when measured carefully and with a clear indication of team process and interaction components. The concept of collaboration within and apart from prescribed teams appears to be an important dimension of what makes teams (and individuals, dyads, or small groups) successful. Clearly, interpersonal communication, regard for others, a strong focus on patient safety goals, and constant reassessment of the environment are important aspects of the relationship between team performance and care delivery outcomes.

Non–Health-Related Work Groups and Performance Outcomes

Studies of non–health-related work groups have focused primarily on productivity and workplace injury outcomes. Nonetheless, performance and outcomes among non–health worker teams have some similarities with those of health care work groups; in both, sphere of influence is expected to widen, and goal-focused actions are expected to result in safer production processes.

Findings concerning team formation and safe environment are informative, with some studies demonstrating significant reductions in on-site injury (Kaminski, 2001) and others identifying differences according to span of control and perceived level of empowerment among team members (Hechanova-Alampay and Beehr, 2001). Hechanova-Alampay and Beehr suggest that simply empowering employees with decision-making authority is insufficient to prevent product error. Attention to the team members' span of control also is necessary. If the span of control is too great, safety outcomes may suffer.

Industry-related safety studies have identified several organizational attributes that contribute to safe employee behaviors. Among these attributes are frequency of nonroutine work processes, level of work hazards, level of cooperativeness between employees and supervisors, level of work group cohesiveness, extent of supervisory management of safety actions, and supervisor experience (Simard and Marchand, 1995). Safety studies also suggest that the organization's climate of safety is detectable at the work group level and that the importance team members place on safety is influenced significantly by supervisor behavior rather than policies and procedures (Simard and Marchand, 1995; Zohar, 2000). In addition, when climates are perceived as less safe, work groups generate a greater number of safety errors.

The effect of work team performance on product quality and labor productivity has been tested in a few manufacturing (Banker et al., 1996; Shrednick et al., 1992) and service (Cohen and Ledford, 1994) industries. The makeup of the teams in these investigations has varied across organizations, and decision-making authority has ranged from limited to semiautonomous. In addition, the team makeup has been specified in some cases, while in others, employees have volunteered to participate.

In the investigation by Banker et al. (1996), the initial months of work team development focused primarily on establishing trust between production workers and management. This focus was particularly important in an institution in which the presence of a bargaining unit had created a history of poor cooperation between workers and administrators. Despite the difficulties of creating high-performance work teams and developing trusting relationships between employees and administration at the site, the introduction of work teams resulted in significantly reduced product defect rates. Productivity also increased.

In the Cohen and Ledford (1994) study, no differences were found in actual safety performance outcomes between self-managed and traditional teams. Significant differences in team members' perceptions of the quality of work and the desirability of work teams were seen, however, suggesting that the increased decision making and responsibility produced better work group relationships and assessment of group performance. These favorable perceptions did not extend to the organization as a whole.

Team members' perceptions of team desirability, organizational support, and organizational outcomes also have been assessed in industry (Bishop et al., 2000). The expectation of the investigators was that favorable employee perceptions would produce improved levels of organizational commitment and better production outcomes. In these studies, favorable perception of the work group was consistently found to be related to level of employee performance and intention to remain employed at the study institution. Similar findings have been reported in the nursing literature, where favorable perceptions of the work group result in intention to remain in the work setting and overall job satisfaction (Ingersoll, 1996; Ingersoll et al., 1996, 2000, 2002). These findings have the potential to influence patient safety performance through the retention of highly skilled and experienced employees.

Considerable interest has been expressed in the beneficial effects of a process defined as crew resource management (CRM), which is used primarily in the aerospace industry but increasingly is being applied to health services industries as well (Helmreich and Davies, 1997; Kosnik, 2002). CRM training in civilian aviation was developed in response to several investigations of airline accidents indicating that a considerable percentage of the accidents were crew-related (Aarons, 2002).

Discussions of CRM strategies for performance improvement and error reduction suggest it is particularly useful when newly trained individuals or persons unfamiliar with a complex process are placed in highly charged, specialized task performance conditions (George, 2002). In these cases, the new team member's attention is focused almost exclusively on mastering the complex demands of the task. Any additional unforeseen event or unexpected condition may be missed or misinterpreted because of the limited available cognitive processing ability of the novice team member.

Critical to the success of CRM strategies is the development of a culture in which all members of the team feel comfortable in verbalizing alternative opinions or in questioning the senior team member's view or planned action (George, 2002). Essential also is the availability of technology or task completion instruments that reduce the need for focused attention on the act of information gathering or the need for lengthy communications between team members. A third component of the CRM process is the routine use of standard operating procedures (SOPs), which define each team member's roles and responsibilities and describes the specific actions required for each phase of the process. These SOPs are designed to make the best use of each team member's time and to improve the situational awareness of the other team members (George, 2002). A concept alignment process is used to facilitate the expression of divergent opinions. In this case, an initial statement by a member of the team is either refuted or supported by another. If opinions differ, the team is responsible for seeking a third opinion. If one point of view can be validated with evidence and the other cannot, the validated view is accepted by the team. If both views can be validated, the senior member of the team chooses the action. If neither can be validated, the most conservative approach is taken (Kosnik, 2002).

CRM training generally includes several days of formal review of prior errors or accidents and in-depth self-assessments of communication style. These self-assessments are intended to facilitate team members' appreciation of the ways in which strengths and weaknesses in personal communication affect crew coordination (Aarons, 2002). Health-related training sessions in CRM have included sessions related to team culture, problem solving, team communication, team-building skills, and workload management strategies (Kosnik, 2002).

Formal investigations of these processes are limited at this point. Work to this end is under way, however, particularly at the University of Texas, where the CRM approach is being tested for its usefulness in a number of industries, including health care. The concepts associated with CRM make intuitive sense and support health researchers' and authors' suggestions concerning the structure, training, and goal-focused approach needed for successful team outcomes in high-risk settings.

CREATING EFFECTIVE TEAMS AND COLLABORATIVE WORK RELATIONSHIPS IN THE WORKPLACE

Barriers to Effective Team Development and Performance

One of the most difficult barriers to effective team performance in health care is the differences in world view that exist across participating health professionals (Baggs and Schmitt, 1997; Prescott and Bowen, 1985). As Shine (2002) notes, physicians of the twentieth century have prided themselves on their individual autonomy and their perceived decision-making infallibility. Eliminating or reframing this perception will be difficult for many physician members of interdisciplinary teams. As a result, the formation of teams will best be served by the careful selection of individuals who already demonstrate an awareness of the need to change and are amenable to different ways of planning for and providing care.

A number of factors have been identified that contribute to poor interdisciplinary working relationships. Larson (1999) suggests these barriers lead to unethical care delivery practices because of the likelihood of deficient care delivery outcomes and the potential for patient harm when disciplines fail to work together. Principal in Larson's summary of the literature is a divergence in perspective on the ability and authority of nurse members of interdisciplinary teams. In previous research concerning interprofessional relationships, physicians have routinely rated actual and ideal nurse authority significantly lower than have nurses (Larson, 1999). Physicians also have tended to focus on the need for nurses to provide more data when presenting information, whereas nurses have focused on the need to improve interpersonal relationships.

The creation of teams may increase the demands associated with the job and result in increased intraorganizational strain. In some cases, the benefits derived from using decision-making teams have not surpassed the costs associated with increased workforce stress (Landsbergis et al., 1999).

This problem may be a temporary one, however, with team members' stress declining significantly as their role expectations and participation demands evolve over time (Parker et al., 1997).

Historical communication patterns also may interfere with effective team performance. Previous research suggests these patterns are highly complex, with novice team members demonstrating undesirable modeling or withdrawal behaviors when tension among team members is high (Lingard et al., 2002). In some cases, these interactions have been outright abusive (Barnsteiner et al., 2001; Manderino and Berkey, 1997), while in others, poor communication patterns have resulted in major loss of life and diminished public faith in health care (Schmitt, 1990), private industry, and service agencies. Two particularly notable cases are cited as instances in which poor team decision making resulted in a disastrous outcome and the loss of public faith. In each of these cases—the Ford Pinto recall and Challenger shuttle disaster—the failure of team members to question other members' decision making and the fear of repercussions from senior management created an environment ripe for errors in decision making, as theorized within a groupthink framework.

In the Ford Pinto case, a reanalysis of internal and external documents, along with interviews of key informants, resulted in a reassessment of the factors contributing to the decision to market Pinto automobiles despite evidence of their poor crash test performance (Lee and Ermann, 1999). The investigators identified a number of such factors, including safety standards at the time; industry norms; the widespread assumption that smaller and cheaper cars were less crashworthy, resulting in a greater tolerance for poor performance; and the perception that the crash test procedures were inadequate and of limited usefulness.

The team errors that contributed to the undesirable outcome included the promotion of an inexperienced manager to a senior role in product safety recall and the manager's use of SOP scripts to determine which automobiles warranted recall. Decisions regarding recall were based solely on the frequency of documented problems and the evidence of causal links to design defects (Lee and Ermann, 1999). Group members' concerns over being ridiculed for recalling a car that did not meet recall specifications and fears of expressing their concerns to senior management also contributed in important ways. According to Lee and Ermann, team members stopped making requests for input because their recommendations were routinely rejected. Self-censorship also prevented senior administrators from hearing the growing concerns of employees working directly on cars. This combination of factors resulted in the continued production and sale of unsafe automobiles, which were recalled only after external pressure forced the action.

In the case of the Challenger launch decision, work group culture and restrictions on access to and dissemination of information silenced team members whose input into decision making might have prevented the space shuttle's takeoff (Roberts, 1997). Experts who might have provided alternative opinions about the safety of takeoff in adverse conditions were removed from the immediate decision-making process. In addition, the silence of key personnel was considered proof that the system was working rather than broken. Project team members also were pressured by political imperatives to adhere to cost estimates and liftoff schedule; bureaucratic expectations that stressed following procedural rules and relaying information according to hierarchical authority relations; and technical imperatives to use data, engineering analyses, and technical rationales to support opinion. Organizational rituals were common and their use widespread, contributing to the overall tendency for employees to behave in routine and nonspecific ways. The combination of these factors led to the shuttle disaster and the subsequent loss of public trust in the space program. According to Roberts, this case is particularly important to the study of team decision making and safe practice because poor decisions were made by a highly skilled team in an organization that would be described in today's terms as highly reliable and decentralized.

Facilitators of Effective Team Development and Performance

Favorable attitudes toward team performance and collaborative patient management approaches maximize team outcomes. These attitudes are particularly important for interdisciplinary groups composed of individuals with differing values and expectations for outside-discipline performance and scope of practice (Schaefer et al., 1994).

Accomplishing this blending of diverse opinions and world views requires a profound cultural shift within a health care organization or system (Shrednick et al., 1992). A 10-year experience at Corning International suggests this process is a constantly evolving one in which team members are vested with both the responsibility and the authority to deliver and manage customer service. The experience at Corning highlights eight key contributors to work team success: (1) a vision and clear goals that serve to communicate expectations at the outset and to guide the evolution of processes over time; (2) a clear commitment of senior management, including a willingness to take risks and to share power and authority for decision making; (3) a plan for focused attention on middle managers and others who may fear loss of control and power because of the shift to team-directed decision making; (4) the early and continuous inclusion of team members in all phases of project development; (5) the commitment to continuous, multi-format communication strategies; (6) a continuous focus on customer expectations and outcomes; (7) a program of education and training to support team member activities and those responsible for interacting with teams; and (8) the development of a reward system that promotes team success.

Corning's experiences are supported by reports of others in the literature. Overall findings concerning the effect of teams on error-free outcomes suggest the following factors contribute to team success or failure in error prevention, detection, and recovery:

Team-related

- Size and structure of team
- Tenure of team members
- Heterogeneity of team membership—cultural mix, functional expertise, professional groups represented
- Level of autonomy and decision-making authority
- Sphere of responsibility and authority
- Nature of member participation—voluntary versus assigned
- Relational properties (internal social structure)
  - Level of trust among team members
  - Knowledge of team members' experiences and expertise
- Team norms that support a focus on quality and safety
- Patterns of communication/information exchange
  - Processes for exchange and dissemination of information within and across teams
  - Amount and complexity of information exchanged
  - Information processing methods
- Knowledge and cognitive skills of team members
- Expected outcome or product
  - Goal or charge of group
  - Clarity of team expectations
  - Complexity of team expectations
- History of team members' experiences with team performance and outcome

Organization/systems-related

- Mission and philosophy—zero tolerance of risk and harm
- Level of specialization
- Technological complexity
- Organizational culture and climate
- Organizational structure
  - Centralized versus decentralized
  - Independent versus system-supported/derived

- History of organizational innovation, including the use of teams in decision-making and error reduction
  - Performance, staffing, workload, and other workforce standards
  - Error-reporting mechanisms and sanctioning processes
  - Amount and type of support provided to teams
    - Expert consultation for problem areas
    - Secretarial assistance for documentation of team activities and generation of reports
    - Educational programming
    - Support for process improvement activities
  - Level of senior management commitment
  - Level of midlevel management commitment and interpersonal style
  - Interdepartmental dependency

Strategies for Developing and Maintaining Effective Work Teams and Partnerships

According to Schaefer and colleagues (1994), simple adherence to standards and protocols is insufficient for reducing health system errors. As these authors note, the creation of environments in which ideas and concepts are actively sought, discussed, and evaluated without regard for the status of the person or the group providing the information is essential to ensure optimum care delivery outcomes.

A combination of strategies will be required to achieve the effective working relationships needed to reduce care delivery errors and optimize care delivery outcomes. Among these strategies are the development of clear position descriptions and explication of role expectations for all members of the team (Disch et al., 2001). Particular attention should be paid to those areas of responsibility that overlap, because these are often the least well understood by competing disciplines and are frequently sources of tension during the delivery of care (Trey, 1996).

Disch et al. (2001) further recommend discussing in detail the shared vision for the team. In this process, individual team members' expectations and concerns are explored to identify where misperceptions lie and what individuals expect from other members of the team. Essential also is the establishment of specific times and formats for evaluating the progress and performance of the team.

Attention also needs to be paid to team makeup, including the heterogeneity or homogeneity of team members in such areas as position within the organization or community, gender, socioeconomic status, ethnicity, age, and other characteristics that may increase the potential for restricted or open discussion and exchange of ideas. Ideal teams are those that represent the populations involved in both the delivery and the receipt of care. In reality, teams often reflect the dominant population or culture and therefore miss the opportunity to maximize team outcomes and reduce the potential for error.

The makeup of the team may result in different levels of perceived success depending on the stage of team development. One study suggests that homogeneous team members tend to report more favorable outcomes and working processes early in the team's development. Heterogeneous team members' perceptions change over time, with members reporting improved work relationships as the group evolves. Heterogeneous teams also report a greater range of perspectives and alternatives generated (Watson et al., 1993). In this study, task performance remained higher for the homogeneous group throughout the study period, although the overall quality of decision making and team performance was comparable by the study's end. In light of these findings, the investigators note the importance of allowing sufficient time for heterogeneous teams to develop the skills needed to work together effectively. The long-term impact, especially in the case of strategies for error identification and reduction, is worth the wait.

Team development strategies also need to include some attention to individual members' assessment of personal strengths and weaknesses and how these contribute to team performance. Also important is self-assessment of perceptions about how error occurs, and how stress and team performance contribute to errors and error identification. Evidence from a survey of ICU and operating room physicians and nurses suggests these individuals seriously underestimate the effect of stress on performance and the likelihood of error (Sexton et al., 2000). In this study, 60 percent of health care professionals rated their ability to perform when fatigued as comparable to their performance when not fatigued during critical conditions. This same percentage believed in the ability of professionals to leave their personal problems behind when working. In addition, a majority of respondents (70 percent) rated their ability to make decisions in emergency situations as comparable to that during routine conditions. The investigators expressed their concern about the clear indication that health care workers failed to recognize the impact of stress and fatigue on decision making. They also noted that the percentages seen in this study were significantly higher than those reported for a sample of airline pilots, who demonstrated a considerably greater level of awareness of the impact of stress, personal problems, and critical events on decision-making errors.

In this same study, physicians rated the presence of collaborative relationships significantly higher than did nurses. Surgeons rated the quality of teamwork with others highly, while others did not reciprocate. On the contrary, nurses and anesthesia staff described the level of teamwork with physicians as poor. Respondents also reported difficulty in discussing mistakes, citing damage to their personal reputation, the threat of malpractice suits, high expectations of family and society, possible disciplinary action, the threat to job security, and expectations of others as reasons for their reluctance to report. Recommendations for improving safety in the ICU focused on increasing staffing, while recommendations for the operating room centered on improved communication patterns (Sexton et al., 2000).

Mentioned frequently in discussions of strategies for error reduction and error recovery by teams is the use of simulations to create real-world conditions of uncertainty and decision-making response. A benefit of this approach is the ability to challenge team members concerning how to react in high-likelihood error situations without jeopardy to individual job security or risk to patients. According to experts, simulation training needs to be ongoing because of the potential for attitudes and skills to decay over time. Simulation procedures also need to be designed in accordance with conditions and experiences of the training organization (Helmreich, 2000).

Simulation methods help in assessing both technical skills and crisis management behaviors, including those associated with decision-making processes and team interaction (Gaba et al., 1998). Gaba and colleagues have successfully used simulations of perioperative crises to assess the technical and behavioral performance of team members and the overall team under high error situations. Included in their assessment of team performance is attention to orientation to case, inquiry/assertion, communication, feedback, leadership, group climate, anticipation/ planning, workload distribution, vigilance, and reevaluation behaviors. A limitation of their simulation process is the deliberate avoidance of combining nonphysicians and physicians on one team. Because most intraoperative crises are likely to include a variety of health care personnel, this restriction limits the application of the simulation procedure to actual practice.

At the University of Texas, an aviation model of threat and error has been adapted to the health care environment. According to the model developers, this approach fits with health care's input–process–outcomes concept of team performance. Included in the simulation model are individual, team, organizational, environmental, and patient characteristics that contribute to latent and immediate threats to safe care delivery. Immediate threats are those associated with the patient's condition or care provider's ability, while latent threats pertain to aspects of the system that predispose to threat or error, such as staffing mix and number of staff (Helmreich, 2000).

Because health care teams are often dissimilar in makeup from other groups that have used simulations successfully, some additional refinement and study are needed to ascertain the most effective use of this training technology. In keeping with the high levels of stress and uncertainty associated with decision making in health care, computer applications and other intelligent decision aids (IDAs) must be able to promote both high-level decision making under uncertainty and the ability to develop strategies for planning for and preventing stressful events (Kontogiannis and Kossiavelou, 1999). The most successful IDAs for team training purposes are those that mimic usual event escalation processes and contributors, including imagined action consequences, anticipation of rare events, and prioritization of tasks when time is limited. IDAs also can be used to provide information about an event or situation, to present multiple perspectives about potential contributors and possible outcomes, and to monitor task performance. In addition, they have potential relevance for facilitating contingency planning through the use of information displays concerning difficulties encountered in the past, critical errors associated with similar actions, and resources needed to activate the plan. Because the use of IDAs for assistance with decision making in highly stressful conditions is new, experiments and field evaluations of their effectiveness must be an integral part of their use (Kontogiannis and Kossiavelou, 1999).

Methods for Measuring the Safe Care Delivery Practices of Work Teams and Collaborative Groups

Reports on methods for monitoring team processes are few, with most evaluations of team performance focusing primarily on clinical outcomes rather than error or error avoidance. Although favorable outcomes are commonly interpreted as an indication of the absence of error, this assumption needs to be documented more clearly. Moreover, because the development and maintenance of effective teams are essential to safe care delivery processes and ideal outcomes, efforts need to be made to monitor and describe those collaborative groups and work teams that consistently produce safe care. Identifying teams and organizations as benchmarks for outcomes is insufficient; understanding and mimicking their processes also is required.

Strategies for evaluating team performance range from day-to-day quality assessment processes to formal investigations of team impact. Inherent in all discussions of the impact of interdisciplinary teams on patient safety and other care delivery outcomes, however, is the need for continuous assessment of team performance and impact. This continuous process is highlighted in a model of collaboration described by Sorine and colleagues (1996), who identify five essential components of the collaboration cycle, each requiring close monitoring of process and outcome. In Sorine et al.'s model, performance guidelines drive compliance agreements, which in turn influence preparedness training and implementation procedures. Once the procedures have been implemented, verification and improvement efforts are undertaken to ensure the quality and consistency of behaviors. These actions subsequently spur the refinement or revision of performance guidelines. This process is continuous, resulting in improvements in team performance and care delivery outcomes over time.

Using this model, the evaluation of performance guidelines might focus on whether they are evidence-based or reflective of documented best practices. Their scope, reasonableness, and usefulness for guiding the formulation of compliance agreements also might be assessed. Compliance agreements and subsequent preparedness components would require evaluation of the achievement of compliance expectations and the effectiveness of training. The implementation process aspects of the evaluation would focus on whether the collaborative model had been introduced as intended and how it evolved over time, while the verification and improvement practices would constitute the ongoing quality improvement monitoring associated with ensuring compliance and achieving safe practices.

One method for assessment of safe and unsafe practices recommended by a non–health-related (aviation) industry entails observational audits of pilots and flight crews (Croft, 2001). In this process, termed a line operations safety audit (LOSA), specially trained observers ride in the airplane's cockpit and observe the responses of the airplane's pilots to such inflight threats as severe weather or congested airports. The observers also interview the pilots during and after the observational period. Reports of the observations made and summaries of the pilot interviews are entered into a database where trends are identified and reported back to participating airlines. No identifying information is included with the data to ensure that individual pilots are not penalized for identified deficiencies as a result of the observational monitoring (Croft, 2001). The focus of the experience is on monitoring and managing the industry's overall training and safety program rather than on the individual pilot's performance.

Observers are trained to monitor for five types of error—procedural, communications, proficiency, decision, and intentional. Errors are categorized as consequential when the pilot's action puts the aircraft in an undesired state and inconsequential when safety is not adversely affected (Croft, 2001). In a review of observations conducted to date, observers have noted one threat to flight safety on 8 of every 10 flights and at least one error on every 6 of 10. These errors resulted in one undesired aircraft state in 3 of the 10 flights. Of importance in this observational process is the failure of pilots to detect over half of the errors made. In addition, when the pilots did catch an error, 1 of 20 (5 percent) was mismanaged. In the majority of cases, errors that compromised safety were caused by the pilot's lack of knowledge concerning the airplane's automation features.

The LOSA process is a lengthy and expensive one, incurring costs associated with observation of pilot performance, interview, and entry and analysis of data. Each audit requires approximately 3 months and is funded by the participating airline and grants from the Federal Aviation Administration (Croft, 2001). At the time of the report on the LOSA process, data from 13 airlines had been obtained, and audit developers were anticipating a 2-year time frame for determining program effects. Application of this approach to health care would require careful consideration of the costs involved and the possibility of obtaining comparable information through other methods.

NEEDS FOR FURTHER RESEARCH

Health professionals interact with others in multiple ways and often under the most challenging of situations. As a result, opportunities exist for promoting beneficial impacts on the delivery of health care through the partnering of professionals involved in care delivery. These partnerships may occur between two persons (e.g., patient and practitioner, nurse and physician, pharmacist and care provider) or through the linking of representatives from multiple disciplines. In all cases, a clear pattern of performance and supportive practices emerges as essential to the success of these relationships.

Nonetheless, the need for increased attention to and understanding of effective team processes is evident. Although some investigators have begun to explore the mechanics and makeup of teams and how these factors contribute to care delivery outcomes, additional work is needed. Team processes, as defined by Marks and colleagues (2001:356), consist of "members' interdependent acts that convert inputs into outputs through cognitive, verbal, and behavioral activities directed toward organizing taskwork to achieve collective goals." According to Marks et al., taskwork involves what the team is doing, whereas teamwork describes how they do it. Taskwork is dependent primarily on skill and member competence; teamwork requires higher-level behaviors, including the ability to direct, align, communicate, negotiate, and monitor taskwork.

Marks and colleagues (2001) stress the need to focus research and team development strategies on the interaction processes evident in teams. They suggest that previous research devoted to team cohesion and situational awareness, for example, has tapped qualities that reflect member attitudes, values, and motivation rather than interaction processes per se. They also describe these variables as emergent products of team experience. Using this framework, Marks and colleagues suggest these variables are indicators of team input that influence teamwork processes and taskwork. As a result, their use in the assessment of how team behavior influences care delivery outcomes and safety behaviors is limited. According to Marks and colleagues attention needs to be shifted to team performance episodes, where inputs, actions, and outcomes occur in a continuous, dynamic process. Inherent in this focus on performance episodes is attention to environmental and other influences that contribute to team processes at different points in time.

Team process dimensions include monitoring behaviors directed toward the assessment of goal achievement and feedback about that process. This monitoring activity identifies when goals have been achieved or abandoned and when new goals are needed for action. The monitoring activities undertaken by team members include the assessment of team resources and environmental conditions that contribute to goal achievement. Effective teams monitor internal and external factors that contribute to the team's ability to perform its task. The internal monitoring process may be devoted to the assessment of team members' performance errors and the development of strategies for eliminating or recovering from those errors. Team process behaviors also involve coordination activities, interpersonal processes, conflict management actions, motivating and confidence-building efforts, and regulation of team members' emotions (Marks et al., 2001).

Marks and colleagues (2001) framework of team processes and outcomes stresses the multidimensional and constantly changing nature of teamwork behavior. This constant movement of teams from periods of transition between existing and new goals makes the measurement of team performance difficult, especially if single one-shot assessments are performed. In cases in which an organization's safety outcomes are of interest, multiple measures and multiple assessment time frames are needed.

A variety of other explorations of team functioning and impacts on patient safety also are required. Among the areas of need identified in the literature are studies exploring the impact of stress (Sexton et al., 2000) and organizational culture on teamwork error and the role of the leader in facilitating or structuring team interaction. This aspect is particularly important in investigations of the relationships between team performance and error identification and reporting, where leader behavior may influence team members' beliefs about the consequences of and ability to discuss mistakes (Edmondson, 1996). When previous experiences with the reporting of errors are seen as nonthreatening, team members not only detect and report more errors, but also intervene more effectively to recover from errors and prevent serious adverse events.

The application and conduct of focused investigations concerning the use of CRM principles and other non–health-related strategies for error reduction are needed. Early reports of the effectiveness of these strategies are encouraging, but additional work is required. The environments in which health care is delivered are often more diverse and variable than those of other fields, and the makeup of the teams involved is clearly different as well. Moreover, applications to the health care environment should focus on team processes that incorporate the full range of individuals likely to be involved in clinical decision making and action.

Funding is needed to support these research initiatives and the education and training that will be required to build and sustain the teams and organizational environments necessary to achieve high-quality care delivery outcomes. Legislation and regulations alone will not affect the high-level processes required to promote and create safety cultures in health care organizations. The cognitive, decision-making, and behavioral skills required for successful team membership will need to be addressed during early educational experiences and continue throughout the team member's work life. Incentives also will be required to ensure that individuals and organizations move toward this new health care production framework. In general, the literature suggests the following areas are ripe for exploration and action in health care.

Theory-Testing Research

The literature to date suggests that the research concerning the relationships between work groups and safety outcomes would benefit from the testing of existing or evolving theories concerning work group relationships and work group safety. Several theories have been proposed, yet few have been tested in any sustained or evolutionary way. Although more recent studies demonstrate increased attention to theory-derived measures and hypothesized relationships, additional work is needed.

Collaboration, Communication, and Other Interpersonal Relationship Behaviors

Some evidence suggests and several authors recommend a broader focus on interpersonal interactions rather than team creation alone. These authors suggest that it is the interpersonal dynamics within team processes that contribute to favorable outcomes and reduced production error. They also stress the multiple ways in which health care workers interact in dyads, small groups, and unit-based teams. A focus on the characteristics of the interpersonal behaviors that facilitate effective interaction, decision making, and error-prevention performance may be more useful than a restricted focus on team behavior. Such a focus also may make the measurement aspects of assessing multidimensional team performance more manageable.

Patient Management and Oversight Responsibilities

Consistent with a focus on collaboration, communication, and interpersonal relationships is attention to the most effective patient management and care delivery approaches for reducing patient error. One of the difficulties apparent in the literature is the significant number of individuals involved directly or indirectly in decision making concerning patients' needs. Some limited evidence suggests that the use of case managers may be beneficial for facilitating desirable care delivery outcomes. Much of this beneficial impact is perceived to be related to the communication and collaboration skills of these individuals and the case manager's ability to overcome systems barriers. Additional information is needed to clarify the impact of models of care delivery on patient safety outcomes.

Application of Non–Health Care Industry Training Standards

The literature concerning the effectiveness of safety-focused work group strategies in non–health care industries suggests this may be a useful vehicle for health care. At present, the research concerning these processes (both outside and within health care) is limited, necessitating cautious movement to this field of training, decision making, and error-prevention behavior. Some efforts have been made to introduce these team development and training strategies in health care, although such efforts have not been widespread. Additional information is needed concerning how these methods work with diverse work groups and less intense environments.

CONCLUSION

The evidence to date reinforces the need to identify what interpersonal and group interaction processes contribute to the delivery of safe care. A number of theories exist concerning how teams perform and how their behaviors contribute to safe or unsafe practices. Clearly evident is the need for additional information about which of these theories is most applicable to the delivery of quality health care and which approaches in health care and other industries demonstrate the most potential for favorable effect. In this paper, the current evidence concerning work groups and patient safety has been reviewed, with recommendations made for future action.

REFERENCES

Aarons RN. 2002. Targeting failures: Human and structural new training recommendations from the Aspen tragedy, and an update on American Airlines Flight 587. *Business & Commercial Aviation*, 91(3), 154.

Baggs JG, Schmitt MH. 1988. Collaboration between nurses and physicians. *Image: Journal of Nursing Scholarship*, 20, 145–149.

Baggs JG, Schmitt MH. 1997. Nurses' and resident physicians' physicians' perceptions of the process of collaboration in a MICU. *Research in Nursing & Health*, 20, 71–80.

Baggs JG, Ryan SA, Phelps CE, Richeson, JF, Johnson JE. 1992. The association between interdisciplinary collaboration and patient outcomes in medical intensive care. *Heart & Lung*, 21, 18–24.

Baggs JG, Schmitt MJ, Mushlin AI, Mitchell PH, Eldredge DH, Oakes D, Hutson AD. 1999. Association between nurse–physician collaboration and patient outcomes in three intensive care units. *Critical Care Medicine*, 27, 1991–1998.

Banker RD, Field JM, Schroeder RG, Sinha KK. 1996. Impact of work teams on manufacturing performance: A longitudinal field study. *Academy of Management Journal*, 39, 867–890.

Barnsteiner JH, Madigan C, Spray TL. 2001. Instituting a disruptive conduct policy for medical staff. *AACN Clinical Issues*, 12, 378–382.

Bates DW, Leape LL, Cullen DJ, Laird N, Petersen LA, Teich JM, Burdick E, Hickey M, Kleefield S, Shea B, Vander Vilet M, Seger DL. 1998. Effect of computerized physician order entry and a team intervention on prevention of serious medical errors. *Journal of American Medical Association*, 280, 1311–1316.

Bea RG. 1998. Human and organization factors: Engineering operating safety into offshore structures. *Reliability Engineering and System Safety*, 61, 109–126.

Bishop JW, Scott KD, Burroughs SM. 2000. Support, commitment, and employee outcomes in a team environment. *Journal of Management*, 26, 1113–1132.

Chassin MR, Galvin RW, National Roundtable on Health Care Quality. 1998. The urgent need to improve health care quality. *Journal of American Medical Association*, 280, 1000–1005.

Cohen HJ, Feussner JR, Weinberger M, Carnes M, Hamdy RC, Hsieh F, Phibbs C, Courtney D, Lyles KW, May C, McMurtry C, Pennypacker L, Smith DM, Ainslie N, Hornick T, Brodkin K, Lavori P. 2002. A controlled trial of inpatient and outpatient geriatric evaluation and management. *The New England Journal of Medicine*, 346, 905–912.

Cohen SG, Ledford GE. 1994. The effectiveness of self-management teams: A quasi-experiment. *Human Relations*, 47, 13–43.

Croft J. 2001. Researchers perfect new ways to monitor pilot performance. *Aviation Week & Space Technology*, 155(3), 76–77.

Curley C, McEachern JE, Speroff T. 1998. A firm trial of interdisciplinary rounds on the inpatient medical wards: An intervention designed using continuous quality improvement. *Medical Care*, 36, AS4–AS12.

Disch J, Beilman G, Ingbar D. 2001. Medical directors as partners in creating healthy work environments. *AACN Clinical Issues*, 12, 366–377.

Edmondson AC. 1996. Learning from mistakes is easier said than done: Group and organizational influences on the detection and correction of human error. *Journal of Applied Behavioral Science*, 32, 5–28.

Farrell MP, Heinemann GD, Schmitt MH. 1986. Informal roles, rituals and humor in interdisciplinary health care teams: Their relation to stages of group development. *International Journal of Small Group Research*, 2(2), 143–162.

Farrell MP, Schmitt MH, Heinemann GD. 1988. Organizational environments of interdisciplinary health care teams: Impact on team development and implications for consultation. *International Journal of Small Group Research*, 4(1), 31–54.

Farrell M, Schmitt M, Heinemann GD. 2001. Informal roles and the stages of interdisciplinary team development. *Journal of Interprofessional Care*, 15, 281–293.

Feiger SM, Schmitt MH. 1979. Collegiality in interdisciplinary health teams: Its measurement and its effects. *Social Science & Medicine*, 13A, 217–229.

Gaba DM. 2000. Structural and organizational issues in patient safety: A comparison of health care to other high-hazard industries. *California Management Review*, 43, 83–102.

Gaba DM, Howard SK, Flanagan B, Smith BE, Fish KJ, Botney R. 1998. Assessment of clinical performance during simulated crises using both technical and behavioral ratings. *Anesthesiology*, 89, 8–18.

George F. 2002. Transitioning to a two-crew cockpit: Two heads are (almost) always better than one, but those new to shared responsibilities have to work for the benefits. *Business & Commercial Aviation*, 91(1), 64–70.

Gittell J, Fairfield K, Bierbaum B, Head W, Jackson R, Kelly M, Laskin R, Lipson S, Siliski J, Thornhill T, Zuckerman J. 2000. Impact of relational coordination on quality of care, postoperative pain and functioning, and length of stay. *Medical Care*, 38(8), 807–819.

Green PL, Plesk PE. 2002. Coaching and leadership for the diffusion of innovation in health care: A different type of multi-organization improvement collaborative. *Joint Commission Journal on Quality Improvement*, 28, 55–71.

Halstead LS. 1976. Team care in chronic illness: A critical review of the literature of the past 25 years. *Archives of Physical Medicine and Rehabilitation*, 57, 507–511.

Hambrick DC, D'Aveni RA. 1992. Top team deterioration as part of the downward spiral of large corporate bankruptcies. *Management Science*, 38, 1445–1466.

Headrick LA, Wilcock PM, Batalden PB. 1998. Continuing medical education: Interprofessional working and continuing medical education. *British Medical Journal*, 316, 771–774.

Hechanova-Alampay R, Beehr TA. 2001. Empowerment, span of control, and safety performance in work teams after workforce reduction. *Journal of Occupational Health Psychology*, 6, 275–282.

Heinemann GD, Farrell MP Schmitt MH. 1994a. Groupthink theory and research: Implications for decision-making in geriatric health care teams. *Educational Gerontology*, 20, 71–85.

Heinemann GD, Schmitt MH, Farrell MP. 1994b. The quality of geriatric team functioning: Model and methodology. Interdisciplinary Health Care Teams. *Proceedings of the Sixteenth Annual Conference*. Indianapolis, IN: Indiana University Medical Center. Pp. 77-91.

Helmreich RL. 2000. On error management: Lessons from aviation. *British Medical Journal*, 320, 781–785.

Helmreich RL, Davies JM. 1997. Editorial: Anaesthetic simulation and lessons to be learned from aviation. *Canadian Journal of Anaesthesia*, 44, 907–912.

Higgins LW. 1999. Nurses' perceptions of collaborative nurse–physician transfer decision making as a predictor of patient outcomes in a medical intensive care unit. *Journal of Advanced Nursing*, 29, 1434–1443.

Ingersoll GL. 1996. Organizational redesign: Effect on institutional and consumer outcomes. In: JJ Fitzpatrick & J. Norbeck (eds.) *Annual Review of Nursing Research* (Vol. 14). New York, NY: Springer Publishing Company. Pp. 121–143.

Ingersoll GL, Schultz AW, Hoffart N, Ryan SA. 1996. The effect of a professional practice model on staff nurse perception of work groups and nurse leaders. *Journal of Nursing Administration*, 26(5), 52–60.

Ingersoll GL, Kirsch JC, Merk SE, Lightfoot J. 2000. Relationship of organizational culture and readiness for change to employee commitment to the organization. *Journal of Nursing Administration*, 30(1), 11–20.

Ingersoll GL, Olsan T, Drew-Cates J, DeVinney BC, Davies J. 2002. Nurses' job satisfaction, organizational commitment, and career intent. *Journal of Nursing Administration*, 32, 250–263.

Janis IL. 1972. *Victims of Groupthink: A Psychological Study of Foreign-Policy Decisions and Fiascoes*. Boston, MA: Houghton Mifflin.

Janis IL. 1982. *Groupthink* (2nd Edition). Boston, MA: Houghton Mifflin.

Jitapunkul S, Nuchprayoon C, Aksaranugraha S, Chalwanichsiri D, Leenawat B, Kotepong W. 1995. A controlled trial of multidisciplinary team approach in the general medical wards of Culalongkorn Hospital. *Journal of Medical Association of Thailand*, 78, 618–623.

Kaminski M. 2001. Unintended consequences: Organizational practices and their impact on workplace safety and productivity. *Journal of Occupational Health Psychology*, 6, 127–138.

Knaus WA, Draper EA, Wagner DP, Zimmerman JE. 1986. An evaluation of outcome from intensive care in major medical centers. *Annals of Internal Medicine*, 104, 410–418.

Kontogiannis T, Kossiavelou Z. 1999. Stress and team performance: Principles and challenges for intelligent decision aids. *Safety Science*, 33, 103–128.

Korsgaard MA, Schweiger DM, Sapienza HJ. 1995. Building commitment, attachment, and trust in strategic decision-making teams: The role of procedural justice. *Academy of Management Journal*, 38, 60–84.

Kosnik LK. 2002. The new paradigm of crew resource management: Just what is needed to reengage the stalled collaborative movement? *Joint Commission Journal on Quality Improvement*, 28, 235–241.

Kosseff A L, Niemeier S. 2001. SSM health care clinical collaboratives: Improving the value of patient care in a health care system. *Joint Commission Journal on Quality Improvement*, 27, 5–19.

Landsbergis PA, Cahill J, Schnall P. 1999. The impact of lean production and related new systems of work organization on worker health. *Journal of Occupational Health Psychology*, 4, 108–130.

Larson EB. 1999. The impact of physician–nurse interaction on patient care. *Holistic Nursing Practice*, 13(2):38–46.

Leape LL, Cullen DJ, Clapp MD, Burdick E, Demonaco HJ, Erickson JI, Bates DW. 1999. Pharmacist participation on physician rounds and adverse drug events in the intensive care unit. *Journal of the American Medical Association*, 282, 267–270.

Lee MT, Ermann MD. 1999. Pinto "madness" as a flawed landmark narrative: An organization and network analysis. *Social Problems*, 46, 30–47.

Lingard L, Reznick R, Espin S, Regehr G, DeVito I. 2002. Team communications in the operating room: Talk patterns, sites of tension, and implications for novices. *Academic Medicine*, 77, 232–237.

Longley J, Pruitt DG. 1980. Groupthink: A critique of Janis' theory. In: L. Wheeler (ed.) *Review of Personality and Social Psychology*. Beverly Hills, CA: Sage Publications. Pp. 74–93.

Manderino MA, Berkey N. 1997. Verbal abuse of staff nurses by physicians. *Journal of Professional Nursing*, 13, 48–55.

Marks MA, Mathieu JE, Zaccaro SJ. 2001. A temporally based framework and taxonomy of team processes. *Academy of Management Review*, 26, 356–376.

Mitchell PH, Shannon SE, Cain KC, Hegyvary ST. 1996. Critical care outcomes: Linking structures, processes, and organizational and clinical outcomes. *American Journal of Critical Care*, 5, 353-363.

Nelson EC, Batalden PB, Huber TP, Mohr JJ, Godfrey MM, Headrick LA, Wasson J H. 2002. Microsystems in health care: Part 1. Learning from high-performing front-line clinical units. *Joint Commission Journal on Quality Improvement*, 28, 472–493.

Palmersheim TM. 1999. The 1999 ICSI/IHI colloquium on clinical quality improvement—"Quality: Settling the frontier." *Joint Commission Journal on Quality Improvement*, 25, 654–668.

Parker SK, Chmiel N, Wall T. 1997. Work characteristics and employee well-being within a context of strategic downsizing. *Journal of Occupational Health Psychology*, 2, 289–303.

Piotrowski MM, Saint S, Hinshaw DB. 2002. The safety case management committee: Expanding the avenues for addressing patient safety. *Joint Commission Journal on Quality Improvement*, 28, 296–305.

Posner KL, Freund PR. 1999. Trends in quality of anesthesia care associated with changing staffing patterns, productivity, and concurrency of case supervision in a teaching hospital. *Anesthesiology*, 91, 839–847.

Prescott PA, Bowen SA. 1985. Physician–nurse relationships. *Annals of Internal Medicine*, 103, 127–133.

Reason J. 1990. *Human Error*. Cambridge: UK: Cambridge University Press.

Reason J. 2000. Human error: Models and management. *British Medical Journal*, 320, 768–770.

Roberts KH. 1997. The Challenger launch decision: Risky technology, culture, and deviance at NASA. *Administrative Science Quarterly*, 42, 405–410.

Sasou K, Reason J. 1999. Team errors: Definition and taxonomy. *Reliability Engineering and System Safety*, 65, 1–9.

Schaefer HG, Helmreich RL, Scheideggar D. 1994. Human factors and safety in emergency medicine. *Resuscitation*, 28, 221–225.

Schmidt I, Claessen CB, Westerholm B, Nilsson LG, Svarstad BL. 1998. The impact of regular multidisciplinary team interventions on psychotropic prescribing in Swedish nursing homes. *Journal of American Geriatric Society*, 46, 77–82.

Schmitt MH. 1990. Medical malpractice and interdisciplinary team dynamics. *Proceedings of the 12th Annual Interdisciplinary Health Care Team Conference*. Indianapolis, IN: Indiana University. Pp. 53–66.

Schmitt MH. 1991. Alternative conceptualizations of "team" as the unit of analysis in examining outcomes of team health care delivery. *Proceedings of the 13th Annual Conference on Interdisciplinary Health Care Teams*. Indianapolis, IN: Indiana University. Pp. 9-16.

Schmitt MH. 2001. Collaboration improves the quality of care: Methodological challenges and evidence from U.S. health care research. *Journal of Interprofessional Care*, 15, 47–66.

Schmitt MH, Watson NM, Feiger SM, Williams TF. 1982. Conceptualizing and measuring outcomes of interdisciplinary team care for a group of long-term chronically ill, institutionalized patients. In: JE Bachman (ed.) *Interdisciplinary Health Care: Proceedings of the Third Annual Interdisciplinary Team Care Conference at Kalamazoo, Michigan*. Center for Human Services. Kalamazoo, MI: Western Michigan University. Pp. 169–182.

Schmitt MH, Farrell MP, Heinemann GD. 1988. Conceptual and methodological problems in studying the effects of interdisciplinary teams. *The Gerontologist*, 28, 753–764.

Schmitt MH, Heinemann GD, Farrell MP, Feussner JR, Cohen HJ. 2000. Evaluation of the process of care in the Cooperative Study of the Outcomes of Geriatric Evaluation and Management Inpatient and Outpatient Care. *Gerontologist*, 40, 343.

Schofield RF, Amodeo M. 1999. Interdisciplinary teams in health care and human services settings: Are they effective? *Health & Social Work*, 24, 210–219.

Sexton JB, Thomas EJ, Helmreich RL. 2000. Error, stress, and teamwork in medicine and aviation: Cross sectional surveys. *British Medical Journal*, 320, 745–749.

Shine KI. 2002. Health care quality and how to achieve it. *Academic Medicine*, 77, 91–99.

Shortell, SM, Rousseau DM, Gillies R, Devers K, Simons T. 1991. Organizational assessment in intensive care units (ICU): Construct development, reliability, and validity of the ICU nurse–physician questionnaire. *Medical Care*, 29, 709–726.

Shortell SM, Zimmerman JE, Gillies RR, Duffy J, Devers K, Rousseau DM, Knaus WA. 1992. Continuously improving patient care: Practical lessons and an assessment tool from the national ICU study. *Quality Review Bulletin*, 18(5), 150–155.

Shortell SM, Zimmerman JE, Rousseau DM, Gillies RR, Wagner DP, Draper EA, Knaus W, Duffy J. 1994. The performance of intensive care units: Does good management make a difference? *Medical Care*, 32, 508–525.

Shrednick HR, Shutt RJ, Weiss M. 1992. Empowerment: Key to IS world-class quality. *MIS Quarterly*, 16(1), 491–505.

Sim TA, Joyner J. 2002. A multidisciplinary team approach to reducing medication variance. *Joint Commission Journal on Quality Improvement*, 28, 403–407.

Simard M, Marchand A. 1995. A multilevel analysis of organisational factors related to the taking of safety initiatives by work groups. *Safety Science*, 21, 113–129.

Sorine AJ, Walls RT, Brantmayer MJ. 1996. Collaboration: A cornerstone of successful safety management. *Occupational Hazards*, 58, 149–152.

Sovie MD, Jawad AF. 2001. Hospital restructuring and its impact on outcomes: Nursing staff regulations are premature. *Journal of Nursing Administration*, 31, 588–600.

Stone RI, Reinhard SC, Bowers B, Zimmerman D, Phillips CD, Hawes C, Fielding J, Jacobson N. 2002 (August). *Evaluation of the Wellspring Model for Improving Nursing Home Quality*. Retrieved 01/13/03. The Commonwealth Fund.

Trey B. 1996. Managing interdependence on the unit. *Health Care Management Review*, 21(3), 72–82.

Uhlig PN, Brown J, Nason AK, Camelio A, Kendall E. 2002. System innovation: Concord Hospital. *Joint Commission Journal on Quality Improvement*, 28, 666–672.

Wadhwa S, Lavizzo-Mourey R. 1999. Do innovative models of health care delivery improve quality of care for selected vulnerable populations? A systematic review. *Joint Commission Journal on Quality Improvement*, 25, 408–421.

Watson WE, Kumar K, Michaelsen LK. 1993. Cultural diversity's diversity's impact on interaction process and performance: Comparing homogeneous and diverse task groups. *Academy of Management Journal*, 36, 590–602.

Weick KE, Roberts KH. 1993. Collective mind in organizations: Heedful interrelating on flight decks. *Administrative Science Quarterly*, 38, 357–381.

Wong P, Helsinger D, Petry J. 2002. Providing the right infrastructure to lead culture change for patient safety. *Joint Commission Journal on Quality Improvement*, 28, 363–372.

Zohar D. 2000. A group-level model of safety climate: Testing the effect of group climate on microaccidents in manufacturing jobs. *Journal of Applied Psychology*, 85, 587–596.

Zwarenstein M, Bryant W. 2002. Interventions to promote collaboration between nurses and doctors. *Cochrane Database of Systematic Reviews*, 4. Retrieved 01/12/03.

Appendix C

Work Hour Regulation in Safety-Sensitive Industries[1]

A substantive body of literature documents the effects of fatigue on worker performance, including the effects of shiftwork and sustained operations on employee alertness. The first section of this appendix reviews this evidence. The second section examines how various health care and non–health care industries have attempted to address consumer and public safety issues by restricting work hours through regulations or administrative guidelines. Since fatigue countermeasures programs are often recommended, a brief overview of these programs and their efficacy is included. Table C-1 at the end of the appendix summarizes hours-of-service regulations in various industries.

EFFECTS OF FATIGUE

Fatigue resulting from continuous physical or mental activity is characterized by a diminished capacity to do work and is accompanied by a subjective feeling of tiredness. Fatigue may also result from inadequate rest, sleep loss, or nonstandard work schedules (e.g., working at night). Whatever its origin, fatigue has predictable effects, such as slowed reaction time, lapses of attention to critical details, errors of omission, compromised problem solving (Van-Griever and Meijman, 1987), reduced motivation, and decreased vigor for successful completion of required tasks (Gravenstein et

---

[1]This appendix was prepared for the committee to inform its deliberations by Ann E. Rogers, Ph.D., R.N., F.A.A.N., of the University of Pennsylvania School of Nursing.

al., 1990). Thus, fatigue causes decreased productivity; tired workers accomplish less, especially if their tasks demand accuracy (Krueger, 1994; Rosa and Colligan, 1988).

Since almost all physiological and behavioral functions are affected by circadian rhythms, the time of day when work occurs is important. Overall capacity for physical work is reduced at night (Cabri et al., 1988; Cohen and Muehl, 1977; Rosa, 2001; Wojtczak-Jaroszowa and Banaszkiewicz, 1974). Reaction times, visual search, perceptual–motor tracking, and short term memory are worse at night than during the daytime (Folkard, 1996; Monk, 1990). On-the-job performance also deteriorates; for example, railroad signal and meter reading errors increase at night, minor errors occur more often in hospitals, and switchboard operators take longer to respond to phone calls (Monk et al., 1996).

The human circadian rhythm strongly favors sleeping during the nighttime hours. Although one study notes that nurses working a permanent night shift or rotating shifts obtained more sleep on average than nurses working day or evening shifts, almost one-fifth of the nurses reported having struggled to stay awake while taking care of a patient at least once during the previous month (Lee, 1992). Another study found that falling asleep during the night shift occurred at least once a week among 35.3 percent of nurses who rotated shifts, 32.4 percent of nurses who worked nights, and 20.7 percent of day/evening shift nurses who worked occasional nights (Gold et al., 1992). It was also found that nurses working night or rotating shifts made more on-the-job procedural errors and medication errors because of sleepiness than nurses working other shifts. Sleepiness appeared to be confined to the night shift, as none of the shift rotaters or day/evening nurses who worked occasional nights reported significant difficulties remaining alert on other shifts.

These subjective reports of sleeping on duty were recently verified by both activity (wrist actigraphy) and sleep (polysomnographic) recordings of 15 French nurses who worked at night (Delafosse et al., 2000). Only 4 of the 15 nurses were able to remain awake all night at work; the others averaged 86.5 (standard deviation [SD] ± 77.6) minutes of sleep while on duty.

Moreover, difficulties maintaining alertness at night are not confined to nurses; episodes of both subjective (or self-reported) and objective sleep were recorded while U.S. Air Force traffic controllers were on duty at night (Luna et al., 1997), and episodes of drowsiness at the wheel were observed in the majority of 80 commercial truck drivers (Wylie et al., 1996).

A person who is not sleep deprived performs tasks more efficiently after prolonged wakefulness and can cope better with nonstandard work hours (nights or rotating shifts) than someone with a sleep deficit (Dinges et al., 1996). Individuals working nights and rotating shifts rarely obtain optimal amounts of quality sleep. Their sleep is shorter, lighter, more fragmented, and less restorative than sleep at night (Knauth et al., 1980; Lavie et al., 1989; Walsh et al., 1981).

Workers are more likely to report greater fatigue at the end of 12-hour work shifts than at the end of 8-hour workshifts (Mills et al., 1983; Rosa 1995; Ugrovics and Wright, 1990). There are exceptions, however: mineworkers reported no differences in fatigue after 8- and 12-hour shifts despite high physical workloads (Duchon et al., 1994), and computer operators reported reduced tiredness throughout the shift after switching from 8-hour to 12-hour shifts (Williamson et al., 1994). Although the timing and duration of meal breaks and "coffee" breaks were not described in these studies, in the case of unionized mineworkers, it is likely they were allowed to stop working for brief periods during their work shift.

Sustained operations (shifts of 12 or more hours with limited opportunity for rest and no opportunity for sleep) (Krueger, 1989) often occur among health care providers who staff busy emergency rooms and intensive care units (ICUs), work overtime shifts on nursing units, or work as members of surgical teams that perform lengthy or consecutive procedures (Krueger, 1989). The majority of anesthesiologists and anesthesia residents report having made errors in the administration of anesthesia when fatigued (Gravenstein et al., 1990). The California Nurses Association (CNA) website (CNA, 2001a) reports several serious errors committed by nurses mandated to work 16-hour shifts, in addition to cases in which nurses did not make errors but were at high risk for doing so. For example, a nurse who worked on average one mandatory double shift (16 hours) every 2 weeks for a 2-month period reported that "by 4 a.m. I was so exhausted that I would stop between going from one baby to the next and completely forget why I was going to the other bedside. Another time, again about 4 a.m., I would sometimes stop in the middle of the floor and forget what I was doing."

Studies have shown that accident rates increase during overtime hours (Kogi, 1991; Schuster, 1985), with rates rising after 9 hours, doubling after 12 consecutive hours (Hanecke et al., 1998), and tripling by 16 consecutive hours of work (Akerstedt, 1994). Data from aircraft accident investigations of the National Transportation Safety Board (NTSB) also show higher rates of error after 12 hours (NTSB, 1994a). Finally, night shifts longer than 12 hours and day shifts longer than 16 hours have consistently been found to be associated with reduced productivity and more accidents (Rosa, 1995).

Laboratory studies have shown that moderate levels of prolonged wakefulness can produce performance impairments equivalent to or greater than levels of intoxication deemed unacceptable for driving, working, and/or operating dangerous equipment (Dawson and Reid, 1997; Lamond and Dawson, 1998). In one study, performance on neurobehavioral tests remained relatively stable during the first 17 hours of testing, a period the researchers called the normal working day, then decreased linearly, with the poorest performance occurring after 25–27 hours of wakefulness (Lamond and Dawson, 1998). Performance on the most complex task—grammatical reasoning—was impaired several hours before performance on vigilance accuracy and response latency (20.3 versus 22.3 and 24.9 hours, respectively). Although Dawson and colleagues (Dawson and Reid, 1997; Lamond and Dawson, 1998) were the first to report that prolonged periods of wakefulness (i.e., 20–25 hours without sleep) can produce performance decrements equivalent to a blood alcohol concentration (BAC) of 0.10 percent, numerous other studies have shown that prolonged wakefulness significantly impairs speed and accuracy, hand–eye coordination, decision making, and memory (Babkoff et al., 1988; Florica et al., 1968; Gillberg et al., 1994; Linde and Bergstrom, 1992; Mullaney et al., 1983).

The combination of sustained wakefulness and working at night is particularly hazardous (Gold et al., 1992; Smith et al., 1994). When the *Exxon Valdez* ran aground around midnight on March 23, 1989, the third mate had been awake 18 hours and anticipated working several more hours (Alaska Oil Spill Commission, 2001). Although the explosion of the Challenger space shuttle occurred during the daytime, the decisions made the night before the launch by mission control staff have been cited as a major factor contributing to the explosion (Mitler et al., 1988).

The lack of adequate rest periods between workshifts can also exacerbate fatigue. Sleep loss is likely to occur when there are only short durations between work shifts. Most adults require at least 6–8 hours sleep to function adequately at work (Krueger, 1994). The loss of even 2 hours of sleep affects waking performance and alertness the next day (Dinges et al., 1996). After 5 to 10 days of shortened sleep periods, the sleep debt (sleep loss) is significant enough to impair decision making, initiative, information integration, planning, and plan execution (Krueger, 1994). The effects of sleep loss are insidious and until severe, usually are not recognized by the sleep-deprived individual (Dinges et al., 1996; Rosekind et al., 1999).

Very short off-duty periods (i.e., 8 hours or less) do not allow for commuting time, recovery sleep, or time to take care of domestic responsibilities (Dinges et al., 1996; Rosa, 1995, 2001). Off-duty intervals ranging from 10 to 16 hours are either suggested or already mandated for many transportation workers (Dinges et al., 1996; Gander et al., 1991b; Mitler et al., 1997). No amount of training, motivation, or professionalism will allow a person to overcome the performance deficits associated with fatigue, sleep loss, and the sleepiness associated with circadian variations in alertness (Dinges et al., 1996; Rosekind et al., 1995). Nor will training, motivation, or professionalism reduce the greater crash risk and increased drowsiness or sleepiness reported by commercial truckers after fewer than 9 hours off duty (McCartt et al., 2000). Recovery from extended work periods requires several days; schedules that require workers to return to work after an 8-hour rest period or to transition from night to day or evening shifts without at least 24 hours off are considered particularly dangerous (Olson and Ambrogetti, 1998; Rosa and Colligan, 1988).

Fatigue is also exacerbated by increased numbers of shifts worked without a day off (Dirkx, 1993; Knauth, 1993), and working more than four consecutive 12-hour shifts is associated with excessive fatigue and longer recovery times (Wallace and Greenwood, 1995). However, two consecutive nights of recovery sleep can return performance and alertness to normal levels, even following two or three 12-hour shifts (Dinges et al., 1996; Tucker et al., 1996), and longer intervals between works days are even more beneficial. Workers obtain more sleep and start their next shifts with less fatigue. The first or second night in a new series of night shifts, however, may be the most fatiguing because of circadian desynchrony (Rosa, 2001).

Predictability of work schedules assists in planning ahead for rest periods. Gold and colleagues (1992) found that nurses who worked rotating shifts reported more accidents than those who were day/evening rotaters. Unscheduled overtime, especially when added to a scheduled work shift, may require 16–20 hours of consecutive work for health care providers and those working in other professions (Rosa, 2001).

WORK SCHEDULES OF SELECTED HEALTH CARE PROVIDERS

The work schedules of both physicians and nurses, as outlined later in this appendix, are often quite demanding. Although the work hours of truck drivers, locomotive engineers, and pilots are regulated to protect the public from fatigue-related errors, hospitalized patients lack similar protections. At present, there are no restrictions on the number of hours a nurse may voluntarily work in a 24-hour or a 7-day period in the United States. Nor are there restrictions on the number of hours that may be worked by other hospital employees, such as pharmacists (another profession with a developing shortage), and only minimal restrictions exist on hours worked by physicians.

Nurses

The hours worked by registered nurses (RNs) are of particular concern since they provide the bulk of direct inpatient hospital care; moreover, studies have demonstrated that the care provided by RNs is vital for maintaining the well-being of hospitalized patients (Aiken et al., 2002; Kovner and Jones, 2002; Needleman et al., 2001). RNs must be alert enough to provide safe care for their patients and to recognize potentially dangerous errors in medication orders. Most previous studies evaluating medical errors took place in environments where nurses had obtained adequate amounts of sleep and were not unduly stressed by workloads, subjected to understaffing, or fatigued from working overtime (Cullen et al., 1997). Today, however, hospital nurses report extremely stressful working conditions, increased numbers of acutely ill patients, inadequate staffing, and working long hours without breaks (Murray and Smith, 1988; Schrader, 2000; Seccombe and Smith, 1996). The effects of these working conditions on patient safety are unknown, but may be significant since a large number of medication errors reported in one study were attributed to poor staffing and onerous work schedules (Leape et al., 1995).

Scheduled shifts may be 8, 10, or 12 hours, and may not follow the traditional pattern of day, evening, or night shifts. Although 12-hour shifts usually start at 7 p.m. and end at 7 a.m., some start at 3 a.m. and end at 3 p.m. Nurses working on specialized units, such as the operating room, dialysis units, and some ICUs may be required to be "on call" in addition to their regularly scheduled shifts. Shifts lasting 24 hours are becoming more common, particularly in emergency rooms (ERs) and on units where the nurses self-schedule (personal communications, ER nurse, June 2002, and ICU nurse, September 2002, University of Pennsylvania Hospital).

Maintaining adequate staffing levels is a difficult problem, especially during nursing shortages. Hospitals can hire contract staff for specific periods to cover vacant positions or to cope with seasonal fluctuations in demand. Agency nurses, who are not employees of the hospital, can also be used. The use of agency nurses, however, is very expensive, and the quality of care provided by these nurses has been questioned (Brusco et al., 1993). Asking regular nursing staff to work extra hours is often attractive to administrators since it costs less than hiring agency nurses, and the nurses are already familiar with the hospital (Brusco et al., 1993). Furthermore, unless specified in collective bargaining agreements, there are no federal (and only a few state) regulations restricting the number of hours a nurse can work in a 24-hour period or over a period of 7 days.

To maintain adequate staffing levels, hospitals frequently offer nurses significant incentives to work extra hours. For example, nurses at the University of Pennsylvania Hospitals are paid time and a half plus an extra $25.00 per hour for working overtime (personal communication, October 2002), while nurses in the University of California system are paid double time (CNA, 2001b). Likewise, nurses at the University of Michigan Medical Center recently approved a contract that requires the hospital to pay 2.5 times their normal wage when they volunteer for overtime in advance (CNA, 2001b). Everyone appears to benefit. When the incentives are high enough, hospital administrators can cover open shifts without hiring additional staff, agency nurses, or traveling nurses, and nurses can significantly increase their salaries by working extra hours or shifts. The effects on patient care, however, are unknown.

The use of overtime, whether mandatory or voluntary, to cope with staffing shortages is quite common in hospital and nursing home settings. Interviews with staff members who worked at 17 nursing homes studied by Louwe and Kramer (2001) revealed that in 13 of the 17 facilities, at least one nursing staff member, and usually more, had worked between one and three double (16-hour) shifts during the previous 7 days. In 5 of the facilities, at least one staff member had worked four to seven double shifts in the last seven days. And in one facility, more than one-third of the nursing staff had worked between eight and eleven double shifts in the past 14 days. Although all direct-care nursing staff (RNs, licensed practical nurses [LPNs]/ licensed vocational nurses [LVNs] and nursing assistants) worked extra hours, the majority of double shifts were worked by nursing assistants.

Anecdotal evidence suggests that hospital nurses are also working large amounts of overtime because of short staffing. Nurses continue to report working over 13 hours with only a 20-minute break (Northcott, 1995), and working "four eight hour shifts in two days—32 hours during a 40-hour stretch, leaving the hospital only once for an eight-hour break" (CNA, 2001a). A recent poll conducted by the American Association of Critical Care Nurses (AACCN) indicated that the use of mandatory overtime is also quite common in the United States (AACCN, 2001). Only 40 percent of 2,125 respondents had never been required to work mandatory overtime. Approximately one-third (31 percent) reported working mandatory overtime at least once a month, another 22 percent at least once every 2 weeks, and 7 percent (n = 149) at least once a week. Another poll conducted by the American Nurses Association showed similar results: approximately 60 percent of respondents (n = 4,258) reported being forced to work voluntary overtime (ANA, 2001).

Decisions about mandatory overtime are usually made at the last minute, and nurses may receive less than 60 minutes' notice that they will not be allowed to go home at the end of their scheduled shift (author's unpublished data). No special accommodations are made for nurses working an extra shift; they are simply assigned a group of patients and expected to provide high-quality care with no additional breaks or a chance to take a short nap between shifts (author's unpublished data). This practice is particularly dangerous when nurses are required to work extra hours at night. Under such conditions, the nurse may have been awake up to 24 hours, working 16 of those hours and often having only a 30- or 60-minute break.

The potential dangers posed by such overtime hours have been clearly documented. For example, the extensive use of overtime has been identified as a contributor to two separate outbreaks of *Staphylococcus aureus* (Arnow et al., 1982; Russell, et al., 1983). At the time, both hospitals were contending with an unexpected increase in patient census, coupled with understaffing. Investigations showed that the nurses, who were fatigued and stressed, compromised the usual standards of care by skipping steps or rushing through aseptic procedures.

Legislation has been introduced at both the federal and state levels to ban mandatory overtime. Two bills were introduced during the 107th U.S. Congress that would prohibit mandatory overtime for nurses and other licensed health care providers (Golden and Jorgensen, 2002). The first bill[2] would amend Title XVIII of the Social Security Act (Medicare Act), while the second bill[3] would amend the Fair Labor Standards Act. The Safe Nursing and Patient Care Act of 2001 also contained provisions that would have required the Agency for Healthcare Research and Quality to conduct a study to determine the numbers of hours a nurse can work without compromising the safety of patients. Similar legislation has been introduced in the 108th Congress.

State legislatures in approximately 19 states have considered bans on mandatory overtime for nurses and other health care professionals. Most proposed measures prohibit hospitals from requiring nurses to work more than their regularly scheduled 8- or 12-hour shifts. Some bills specify that nurses cannot be required to work more than 40 hours a week, while others prohibit hospitals from requiring employees to work more than 80 hours of overtime in any consecutive 2-week period (Golden and Jorgensen, 2002). Maine's law (Ch. 401) also mandates that if nurses work longer than 12 hours, they must be given at least 10 hours off before their next shift (Golden and Jorgensen, 2002). To date, bills prohibiting mandatory overtime for nurses have passed in only four states—California, Maine, New Jersey, and Oregon. No measure, either proposed or enacted, addresses how long nurses may work on a voluntary basis.

Physicians

The hours physicians work, particularly during their residency training, are often quite demanding. Although the Association of American Medical Colleges (AAMC) and the Accreditation Council for Graduate Medical Education (ACGME) have recommended that house staff work no more than 80–84 hours per week, it is still common for medical residents to work over 100 hours per week for prolonged periods (Patton et al., 2001). Work days are typically 12–14 hours (Czeisler et al., 2002), and workloads vary by specialty (Patton et al., 2001), with surgical residents typically working

---

[2]Safe Nursing and Patient Care Act of 2001. S. 1686, H.R. 3238 (2001).
[3]Registered Nurses and Patient Protection Act. H.R. 1289 (2001).

the longest hours (Committee of Interns and Residents, 2002a; Owens et al., 2001; Silberger et al., 1988). Despite recommendations that work shifts not exceed 24 consecutive hours, many interns and residents remain subject to call schedules requiring duty periods of up to 36 consecutive hours or longer on weekends (Czeisler et al., 2002; Leonard et al., 1998; Owens et al., 2001). Other residents opt to work 60–84 consecutive hours (Friday or Saturday morning through Monday afternoon) in a single "power week-end" each month (Czeisler et al., 2002).

The work hours of resident physicians have been the subject of research and frequent debate over the past 20–25 years. Although errors made by a sleep-deprived resident in a New York City hospital are believed to have caused a patient's death, few studies have shown a direct link between fatigue and patient safety (Asken and Raham, 1983; Friedman et al., 1971; Parker, 1987; Poulton et al., 1978). The findings of Smith-Coggins and colleagues are typical. Emergency room physicians working at night reported feeling significantly more sluggish, less motivated, and less clear-thinking than when working days. Although, they were able to maintain their accuracy in interpreting 12-lead electrocardiograms (ECGs) and rhythm strips, their reactions times were slower and they took longer to intubate a mannequin when working the night shift (Smith-Coggins et al., 1997).

Only a few studies have demonstrated that clinical performance is adversely affected by sleep deprivation. Unlike earlier studies, recent studies have been tightly controlled. Earlier methodological flaws (e.g., tests that were too short or tested factual knowledge, which is relatively insensitive to sleep deprivation; included performance incentives; or, most significantly, failed to control for the residents' actual sleep schedules prior to and during the studies) (Weigner and Ancoli-Israel, 2002) have been corrected. Researchers no longer expect to find differences between "rested" residents— e.g., those who had more than 4 hours of sleep (Bartle et al., 1988; Deaconson et al., 1988; Light et al., 1989), more than 5 hours of sleep, (Hawkins et al., 1985; Reznick and Folse, 1985), or "regular" sleep (Denisco et al., 1987; Storer et al., 1989), or were not on call (Orton and Gruzelier, 1989)—and "fatigued" residents. They assume all residents have a significant sleep deficit, even those tested when not on call (Weigner and Ancoli-Israel, 2002).

Several studies have shown impaired performance on measures of alertness and concentration, standardized tests of creative thought processes, and cognitive performance on a standardized computerized test battery after on-call periods ranging from 24 hours to an entire weekend (Leonard et al., 1998; Nelson et al., 1995; Wesnes et al., 1997). In studies using virtual-reality simulations, surgical residents made more errors and were slower to complete electrocoagulation of bleeding tissue as sleep loss increased

(Taffinder et al., 1998). Moreover, error rates were higher among residents after a night on call than during normal daytime hours (Grantcharov et al., 2001). Realistic patient simulators have also been used to evaluate the performance of anesthesiologists at night when fatigued and during regular workdays (Ou et al., 2001), as well as under conditions of acute sleep deprivation (e.g., awake for 25 hours) or being well rested (2 hours of extra sleep on average for four consecutive nights before the study) (Gaba, 1998; Weigner et al., 1998). Videotapes from the latter study showed sleep-deprived residents actually falling asleep while administering anesthesia.

Despite evidence that patient care may be compromised if a fatigued, sleep-deprived clinician is allowed to operate, administer anesthesia, manage a medical crisis, or deal with an unusual or cognitively demanding clinical presentation (Weigner and Ancoli-Israel, 2002), there is significant resistance to limiting the hours worked by resident physicians. Concerns have been expressed about reduced learning opportunities if resident work hours are curtailed (Greenfield, 2001; Holzman and Barnett, 2000; Suk, 2001), as well as decreased professionalism and commitment to patients (Holzman and Barnett, 2000). Current resident work hours have also been defended on economic grounds (Green, 1995; Patton et al., 2001; Thorpe 1990).

Only the state of New York limits the hours worked by resident physicians. The "Bell Regulations"[4] were enacted following the death of Libby Zion, the 18-year old daughter of Sidney Zion, an attorney and writer for the *New York Times*, in 1984. Her death triggered an aggressive media campaign questioning the quality of care in teaching hospitals, as well as a grand jury investigation into her death (Asch and Parker, 1988; Kwan and Levy, 2002). Although neither the hospital nor physicians were faulted, the grand jury did find fault with the residency training system and physician staffing patterns that allowed Libby Zion's death to occur. Five specific factors were identified as contributing to her death: (1) she was not examined by an attending physician with experience in emergency medicine when admitted to the ER in an agitated condition, complaining of fever; (2) after transfer to a medical unit, she was cared for by first- and second-year residents who were largely unsupervised; (3) she was admitted at 2:00 a.m., when both residents caring for her had been at work for 18 straight hours; (4) the first-year resident ordered that she be placed in physical restraints without reevaluating her condition; and (5) she was given meperidine (Demerol) despite the resident's knowledge that she was also taking phenalzine.[5]

---

[4]New York State Health Code. The Bell Regulations. N.Y.C.R.R. § 405.4 (1989).
[5]Meperidine is contraindicated for a patient taking phanelzine.

In March 1987, the New York State Commissioner of Health appointed an Ad Hoc Advisory Committee on Emergency Services to analyze the grand jury's findings. The committee, chaired by Dr. Bertand Bell, reviewed the grand jury's report and issued several recommendations to the New York State Department of Health, including that residents should not work more than 80 hours per week, more than 24 consecutive hours, or more than 6 days without at least one 24-hour period off duty (Holzman and Barnett, 2000; Kwan and Levy, 2002). Rest periods of at least 8 hours between shifts were also mandated (Holzman and Barnett, 2000). ER residents and attending physicians were limited to 12-hour shifts (Kwan and Levy, 2002). The committee's recommendations were then incorporated into the New York State Code in 1989. Although the New York Hospital Association immediately filed suit contending that the regulations were arbitrary, had been improperly adopted, and failed to provide adequate reimbursement for the increased costs of their implementation,[6] its appeal to the State Supreme Court failed (Patton et al., 2001).

Also in 1989, the ACGME amended its regulations to require accredited internal medicine residency programs to limit the hours worked by residents. Internal medicine residents could spend no more than 80 hours per week providing patient care, could be on call no more than every third night, and on average would have to have the opportunity to spend at least 1 of every 7 days free of patient care duties (Green, 1995). Today there are 26 sets of different guidelines, each developed by a different Residency Review Committee. Weekly work hour limitations range from "whatever is considered 'appropriate' by residency directors" (general surgery) to 72 hours (emergency medicine) (Gurjala et al., 2001; Kwan and Levy, 2002). Not only are the guidelines inconsistent across the various specialties, but they are also voluntary, not mandatory.

Neither the Bell Regulations in New York nor the ACGME guidelines have been effective in curtailing the hours worked by resident physicians (Gurjala et al., 2001; Kwan and Levy, 2002). Fully 92 percent of New York hospitals were not complying with the Bell Regulations during 1991–1992, a fact known by the New York State Department of Health (Patton et al., 2001). In a survey conducted almost 10 years after the Bell Regulations were enacted, residents in all New York teaching hospitals reported working an average of 95 hours per week (Anonymous, 1998). In 1998, a surprise investigation conducted by the New York State Department of Health found all 12 hospitals visited to be violating resident work hour limits. Over one-third of the residents (38 percent) had worked in excess of 24 consecutive hours, 37 percent were working more than 85 hours per week,

---

[6]Hospital Association v. Axelrod, 546 N.Y.S.2d 531. 1989.

and 20 percent had exceeded 95 hours per week, while 60 percent of surgical residents had exceeded 95 hours per week (Kennedy, 1998). Despite increased fines and stepped-up enforcement efforts, some residency programs in New York continue to violate daily and weekly work hour limitations (Committee of Interns and Residents, 2002b).

All residency programs in the United States undergo periodic accreditation reviews by the ACGME. Although none have lost their accreditation solely for overworking residents (Kwan and Levy, 2002), 20 percent of the residency programs reviewed in 1999 were cited for noncompliance with work hour standards (Kwan and Levy, 2002). In 2000, only 8 percent of the programs reviewed that year were cited (Lamberg, 2002).

During the past year, increasing attention has been paid to hours worked by resident physicians. The ACGME has recommended that all residency programs limit resident work hours to 80 hours/week and have a maximum shift length of 24 hours (although a resident could be required to put in an additional 6 hours for transfer of patient care responsibilities, educational debriefing, didactic activities, and seeing patients in a post-call continuity clinic), and that night call be limited to every third night. Recommendations from the American Medical Association (AMA) and the AAMC are quite similar, and stress a voluntary approach (AMA, 2002; AAMC, 2002). A petition submitted in spring 2002 to the Occupational Health and Safety Administration (OSHA) by Public Citizen and the American Medical Student Association called for federal regulation, civil penalties, and public disclosure of violating hospitals (Gurjala et al., 2001). OSHA denied the petition on October 10, 2002, citing the voluntary standards being adopted by the ACGME (Public Citizen, 2002).

As discussed earlier, legislation to amend title XVIII of the Social Security Act (Medicare Act) was introduced in both houses of the U.S. Congress during the 107th session. The Patient and Physician Safety Act of 2001[7] would have required any hospital receiving Medicare funding to limit the hours worked by postgraduate trainees to no more than 80 hours per week and 24 hours per shift. H.R. 3236 was introduced on November 6, 2001, and referred from the House Energy and Commerce Committee to the House Subcommittee on Health on March 5, 2002.[8] The Senate version of the bill (S. 2614) was introduced June 12, 2002, and immediately referred to the Senate Committee on Finance.[9] No further action was taken.

In June 2001, legislation was introduced and passed by the New Jersey State Assembly limiting the work hours of resident physicians in that state

---

[7]The Patient and Physician Safety Act of 2001. S. 2614, H.R. 3236 (2001).
[8]Bill Summary and Status for the 107th Congress (2002).
[9]Bill Summary and Status for the 107th Congress (2002).

to an average of 80 hours/week over a 4-week period and 24 consecutive hours of duty (A. No. 1852) (Committee of Interns and Residents, 2002b). If the bill is passed by the state senate and approved by the governor, on-call duties during night shifts will also be limited to no more than every third night, and hospitals will not be able to require residents to work more than 6 days per week.

OTHER PUBLIC SERVICE PROVIDERS

Police and Firefighters

Although the services of police officers and firefighters are required 24 hours a day, 7 days a week, their typical work schedules are quite different. Firefighters in many jurisdictions work for 24-hour periods followed by 48 hours off, whereas police officers are often subjected to rotating shifts, must put in extra hours to appear in court and/or complete paperwork, and may moonlight to supplement their income. Only limited research is available about the effects of fatigue in these two occupational groups.

Although overwhelming fatigue was described by police officers testifying at hearings conducted by the National Commission on Sleep Disorders Research in 1991 (DHHS, 1993), it was not known whether the witnesses' experiences were representative of the larger population of police officers. Over the past 10 years, newspaper reports of automobile accidents due to police officers falling asleep and running red lights, running off the road and hitting trees or joggers, or crashing while chasing fleeing motorists have provided anecdotal evidence that at least some police officers have significant problems with fatigue (Vila and Kenney, 2002). Results of a recent study of four medium-sized metropolitan police departments suggest that 6 percent of officers on duty at any one time are severely impaired by fatigue, and that nearly half have clinical sleep pathologies (Vila, 1996). Fewer than 26 percent of the participating officers reported averaging 7 hours of sleep a day, and nearly 12 percent obtained less than 5 hours per day. Nearly 16 percent reported trouble staying awake during normal activities such as driving, eating meals, or engaging in social activities.

There are no regulations limiting the number of hours worked by police officers. Surveys have shown that at least a few officers in most departments work substantial overtime, and that more than half of the officers in many departments moonlight (Vila and Kenney, 2002). Mean overtime hours range from 17.5 to 100 per month.

Several studies suggest that lengthening work shifts and decreasing the number of days worked per week may reduce fatigue among police officers. Officers working 10- and 12-hour days reported that the longer shifts were less fatiguing. They also reported fewer sleep problems and significantly less fatigue at the beginning of their shifts (Vila and Kenney, 2002). Switching to a compressed work week (three 13.5-hour shifts followed by four days off) also improved productivity in Bexar County, Texas, and did not lead to greater fatigue or increased moonlighting (Vega and Gilbert, 1997). Finally, changing the direction of shift rotation (from backward to forward), speeding up the rate of shift rotation, lengthening the shift to 8.5 hours, and reducing the number of consecutive shifts to four resulted in a four-fold decrease in the numbers of Philadelphia police officers reporting poor sleep, twice as many reporting no daytime fatigue, a decrease in sleep episodes on duty, a decline in the number of on-the-job motor vehicle accidents per mile driven, an increase in alertness on night shifts, and a reduction in the use of sleeping pills and alcohol (Center for Design of Industrial Schedules, 1988).

Agencies are being encouraged to review their policies and procedures related to shift scheduling, moonlighting, and number of consecutive days worked and to provide in-service training on the importance of adequate sleep, the hazards associated with shift work, and strategies for managing those hazards (Vila, 1996, 2000). Information is scarce on whether these recommendations are being adopted and if so, how effective they are.

Firefighters typically work approximately 9 to 10 days per month and average 52–56 hours on duty per week (Anonymous 2002 a,b). Although they are on duty for longer periods than most people, not all hours spent at the firehouse are devoted to working; part of the time is devoted to meal preparation, housekeeping chores, recreational activities, and sleep.

Military Personnel

Although the U.S. military has few regulations or guidelines regarding hours of service or duty restrictions, all branches are acutely aware of the adverse effects of fatigue on performance. During normal conditions at post, camp, and duty stations where personnel can go home at night, work hours are quite similar to those of civilians. When personnel are deployed in the field or at sea, they tend to work about 70 hours per week (U.S. Congress Office of Technology Assessment, 1991c).

Combat operations impose unique demands. Work demands are often continuous, requiring individuals to maintain performance for 12 hours or more. Sleep may be difficult or impossible. Nighttime operations, jet lag due to rapid aerial deployments, extra tasks associated with the first day or two at sea, and a faster-than-usual tempo of operations can further limit endurance (U.S. Congress Office of Technology Assessment, 1991c).

Tasks requiring physical activity and effort (e.g., infantry marches, handling supplies, and preparing fortifications) are affected less than other tasks by time of day, moderate sleep loss, or other circadian disruptions (Belenky et al., 1987; Haslam, 1982; Ryman et al., 1987). Several days of sustained operations will degrade the vigilance, memory, and cognitive task performance of infantry soldiers, tank crews, and artillery fire direction teams (Krueger, 1989), while performance on tasks requiring constant vigilance (e.g., sonar operations) can degrade within less than an hour (Krueger, 1989; Poulton, 1972).

Long flights and sustained operations involving aircraft can be quite hazardous. Fighter pilots can maintain physical coordination despite extreme sleepiness (Krueger et al., 1985), but judgment and planning abilities are extremely sensitive to the onset of fatigue (Graeber et al., 1986; Kopstein et al., 1985; Word, 1987). Although not studied, the performance of other tasks, such as maintenance, preparation, and operation of equipment (e.g., weapon systems, communication systems, and construction equipment), is also likely to be affected by fatigue and time of day (U.S. Congress Office of Technology Assessment, 1991c).

The Army, Air Force, and Navy have regulations governing flight times and duty periods for pilots. The Army specifies both the maximum amount of time pilots are allowed to fly and their maximum duty periods. Flight times are adjusted for such factors as time of day (flying 1.0 hour at night is considered the same as flying 1.4 hours during the day), instrument conditions, and whether the pilot is required to wear night vision devices or protective gear (U.S. Congress Office of Technology Assessment, 1991c). Flight times for Air Force pilots are longer (up to 12 hours in duration for a single crew). Total flying time is limited to 75 hours per 30-day period and 200 hours per 90 consecutive days. A minimum rest period of 12 hours is mandated between flights and must include 8 hours of uninterrupted, continuous rest. If a crew member is interrupted and cannot get 8 hours of rest, he or she must be given 8 more hours of uninterrupted time for rest, plus additional time for other activities. Flight surgeons and aviation safety officers are usually involved in scheduling missions. However, the commanding officer can waive the regulations for high-priority missions and in combat situations.

Naval regulations are quite similar, but specify that pilots cannot be assigned to flight duty on more than 6 consecutive days or assigned continuous alert or flight duty for more than 18 hours. If the 18-hour rule is exceeded, 15 hours of continuous off duty time must be given to the crewmember. Any deviation from this protocol requires that the individual be closely monitored and cleared for each flight by the commanding officer in consultation with the flight surgeon (U.S. Congress Office of Technology Assessment, 1991c).

Flight surgeons also have the authority to issue stimulants and hypnotic medications to pilots to facilitate sleep and maintain alertness during combat conditions. Crewmembers are encouraged to defer non–flying-related duties in the days before a mission, take short frequent naps, consume nutritious meals, and use caffeine judiciously (Naval Strike and Air Warfare Center, 2000). If a long flight or compromised alertness during a flight is anticipated, pilots may be issued several tablets of amphetamine (5 mg) at the beginning of the flight. No one is required to take amphetamines, and any leftover doses are collected at the end of the flight. Hypnotics are never issued prior to a flight to prevent their inadvertent use in place of a stimulant.

The use of medications to promote sleep and/or alertness among pilots is not new. According to *Performance Maintenance during Continuous Flight: A Guide for Flight Surgeons* (Naval Strike and Air Warfare Center, 2000), both British and German pilots used amphetamines during World War II. British pilots used sedatives during the Falklands conflict, and both Air Force and Navy pilots were given amphetamines in Viet Nam and most recently during Desert Storm. Flights during Desert Storm often exceeded the legal durations, sometimes lasting up to 15–18 hours. Amphetamine use was most common in the early morning hours or just after dawn during extended combat air patrol missions.

Although there are no specific guidelines for work and duty schedules for most Army activities and operations, commanding officers are responsible for ensuring that personnel under their command are rested and fit for duty. Commanders are encouraged to plan for at least 6 hours of rest for combat personnel (those doing the fighting) (U.S. Congress Office of Technology Assessment, 1991c). However, actual conditions dictate the nature and scheduling of rest periods during combat conditions, reinforcement operations, and special operations.

The Air Force has maximum duty limits for all personnel (e.g., flight and nonflight) that apply even during combat. Staff can work 10 hours a day, 6 days a week, for a total of 247 hours a month during continuous operations, and up to 12 hours a day, 6 days a week, for a maximum of 30 days during sustained operations (U.S. Congress Office of Technology Assessment, 1991c). Crews manning intercontinental ballistic missile silos are on alert duty for 24-hour periods. Regulations require that all crewmembers have at least 6 hours for rest or sleep during their duty period. Crews are rotated and tend to be on duty every third day (U.S. Congress Office of Technology Assessment, 1991c).

At-sea schedules for nonflight naval personnel can be quite rigorous. Workweeks of 70–80 hours are not uncommon. Even under noncombat conditions, rotating watch schedules can cause significant circadian disruption (U.S. Congress Office of Technology Assessment, 1991c). Submarine crews typically use 18-hour watch schedules involving three sections of personnel rotating 6 hours on and 12 hours off. Because of maintenance tasks and administrative and training requirements, crewmembers sleep on average only 4 hours out of every 18-hour period (U.S. Congress Office of Technology Assessment, 1991c). Although 12-hour watch schedules are typical, this does not imply that personnel on surface ships have 12 consecutive hours off duty. Instead, crewmembers usually work for 6 hours, then have 6 hours off for other tasks, including sleeping and eating. During normal conditions, crewmembers average about 6 hours of sleep in 24 hours (U.S. Congress Office of Technology Assessment, 1991c). Although crews manning aircraft carriers usually do not follow a rotating watch schedule as do crews on other surface ships, they usually work for somewhat longer periods (14–16 hours). Combat conditions, which require the entire crew of a ship to remain on duty without relief or rest periods, can induce significant acute fatigue, especially after 1 or 2 days.

Many Marine Corps missions are planned to begin before dawn, when the enemy is believed to be less vigilant and effective. There is generally a very intense period of sustained operations, usually the first 36–48 hours, after an amphibious assault, when personnel are almost continuously active (U.S. Congress Office of Technology Assessment, 1991c). Marine air forces, which provide air support for amphibious assaults and other ground operations, are normally governed by the same flight regulations as other Navy flight crews, although these regulations may be waived during the first 36–48 hours of an amphibious assault (U.S. Congress Office of Technology Assessment, 1991c).

Nuclear Power Plant Workers

Although the dangers of a nuclear power plant accident have been recognized from the industry's inception in the 1950s, regulations have focused exclusively on reactor design, training programs, and licensing requirements. The dangers of operator fatigue were not acknowledged until 1980 (U.S. Nuclear Regulatory Commission, 1980), when the Nuclear Regulatory Commission (NRC) reported that "inspections of personnel performance and training since the accident at Three Mile Island, have shown that in certain situations facility personnel are either required or allowed to remain on duty for extended periods of time." The NRC recommended that (1) workers not be permitted to work more than 12 hours straight, (2) there be at least a 12-hour break between all work periods, (3) individuals not work more than 72 hours in any 7-day period, and (4) that workers not work more than 14 consecutive days without having 2 days off.

A second generic letter sent 6 months later to all licensees of operating power plants and applicants for operating licenses (Eisenhut, 1980) recommended that enough plant operating personnel be employed to provide adequate coverage without the routine heavy use of overtime, but stated that when unforeseen problems occurred and/or the reactor was shut down for refueling, major maintenance, or major plant modifications, workers could work up to 16 consecutive hours as long as they had a break of at least 8 hours between shifts. In addition, workers could not work more than 24 hours in any 48-hour period or more than 72 hours in a 7-day period. If there were extenuating circumstances, however, the plant manager or his/ her designee could authorize additional hours. Although further clarifications were issued in 1982 (Eisenhut, 1982), no substantive changes were made to these guidelines.

It is important to note that these are guidelines or recommended policies, not regulations. Although the Director of the Division of Licensing, Office of Nuclear Reactor Regulation, can suggest in a generic letter to all licensees of operating plants, applicants for an operating license, and holders of construction permits that they "take action as necessary to revise the administrative section of [their] technical specifications to assure [their] plant administrative procedures follow the revised work hour guidelines" (Eisenhut, 1982), plant owners cannot be compelled to follow those recommendations. Nuclear power plant operators can choose to incorporate the recommendations into their technical specifications and administrative procedures, but are not required to do so (U.S. Congress Office of Technology Assessment, 1991b). Once incorporated into a plant's technical specifications and administrative procedures, however, these policies can be, although rarely are, enforced by the NRC.

Most nuclear power plant employees work 8-hour shifts, although a growing number of power plants have sought permission to implement 12-hour shift schedules (U.S. Congress Office of Technology Assessment, 1991b). Workers usually rotate shifts and have every other weekend off. Overtime is common, especially in outage situations, when every day off line (not functioning) costs the utility revenue (U.S. Congress Office of Technology Assessment, 1991b). Staff shortages, usually associated with an employee failing to show up for a scheduled shift, often result in employees being required to work a double shift (if on 8-hour shifts) or split a second shift with another worker.

Plant workers' claims that they often work more than 70 hours a week when the reactor is operating and 80 or 90 hours a week when the plant is shut down for refueling or other tasks (TiredNukes.Org, 2002) have been substantiated. For example, data collected by the Nuclear Energy Institute showed that one-third of nuclear power plants were authorizing more than 1,000 and as many as 7,500 approvals[10] a year to exceed the guidelines

---

[10]An approval by the plant manager is required every time a worker is asked to work more than 12 hours/day, more than 72 hours/week, or more than 14 consecutive days. Therefore, one-third of the plants studied were authorizing between 3 and 21 workers/day to exceed work hour guidelines.

(Travers, 2001). In addition, over one-quarter of the sites surveyed reported that more than 20 percent of their personnel covered by the guidelines were working more than 600 hours (per person) of overtime per year (U.S. Nuclear Regulatory Commission, 2000a). This number is more than two to three times the level allowed for operators at some foreign nuclear power plants and more than twice the level recommended by an expert panel in 1985 (NUREG/CR-4248) (U.S. Nuclear Regulatory Commission, 2000a).

Although fatigue was not identified as a causal factor in the Three Mile Island accident, NRC inspectors ruled that fatigue from excessive overtime was the main contributor to an accident at Braidwood Unit 1 in Illinois, where three workers were accidentally sprayed with 180°F water (U.S. Nuclear Regulatory Commission, 1991). Other plants were also criticized in Information Notice No. 91-36 (sent to all holders of operating licenses or construction permits for nuclear power reactors) for using excessive overtime, preparing overtime authorizations after the fact, and maintaining poor documentation of overtime (Union of Concerned Scientists, 2000).

Although concerns about operator fatigue and excessive overtime have been voiced in numerous generic letters and information notices and during the 1990 Fitness for Duty Rulemaking Process, no action was taken until 2001, when the NRC concluded that earlier guidelines had not been "wholly effective" in addressing worker fatigue. Four events occurring within an 8-month period apparently stimulated NRC staff members to begin investigating the impact of worker fatigue in nuclear power plants. In February 1999, the Chairman of the NRC received a letter from three congressmen expressing their concerns about staffing levels and excessive overtime in nuclear power plants (Markey et al., 1999; Travers, 2001). A month later, similar issues were raised by the Union of Concerned Scientists in a report entitled *Overtime and Staffing Problems in the Commercial Nuclear Power Industry* (Travers, 2001; Union of Concerned Scientists, 2000). Finally, in September 1999, the NRC received a petition for rulemaking (PRM-26-2) (Quigley, 1999).

After reviewing several options, the NRC recommended expanding Part 26 of the Fitness for Duty Program to include a broad range of possible impairments, including fatigue. Rather than imposing absolute limits on the number of hours an individual could work in any 48-hour period, specific restrictions on 16-hour shifts, or annual limits on work hours, the NRC opted to "establish thresholds for work hour controls." However, no specific thresholds were set or recommended in the NRC's rulemaking plan (U.S. Nuclear Regulatory Commission, 2000b), even though NRC staff considered "the limit of no more than 16 hours in any 24-hour period [was] too high to ensure that personnel [were] not impaired by fatigue," and that a limit of 72 hours in a 7-day period did not appear adequate to prevent cumulative fatigue. Proposed work hour limits would apply regardless of the plants' operating state (e.g., operating or in outage). Some deviations would be allowed if the plant could demonstrate that the extra hours of work would cause no undue risk.

A final rule is not anticipated until at least December 2003 (U.S. Nuclear Regulatory Commission, 2002). Significant opposition to any efforts to regulate work hours is expected.

TRANSPORTATION INDUSTRY

Operator fatigue was recognized as a danger over 100 years ago, long before scientists were able to demonstrate the adverse effects of fatigue on performance. Traditional modes of passenger transportation, such as railroads and ships, were the first to be regulated. Aviation and trucking were added to the list of industries with work hour restrictions during the 1930s. The aerospace industry, which developed during the latter half of the twentieth century, has no statutes or regulations limiting work hours.

Despite the Department of Transportation's acknowledgment that current work hour rules are outdated and that fatigue remains a significant factor, none of the regulations or statutes limiting hours of service have been modified since 1989. Attempts to incorporate the findings of recent research on fatigue into hours-of-service regulations have not been successful.

Railroad Employees

Although railroads were the predominant mode of intercity travel at the beginning of the twentieth century, rail travel was dangerous for employees and passengers alike. Between 1902 and 1907, over 19,000 employees and passengers were killed in railroad accidents, and another 276,722 were injured (U.S. Congress Office of Technology Assessment, 1978). Four years later, the number of fatalities had risen to 37,907 and the number of injuries to 516,669. Deaths and injuries did not decline until the early 1920s, when the last of the early safety laws,[11] the Signal Inspection Law, was enacted (U.S. Congress Office of Technology Assessment, 1978).

The contribution of fatigue to these early accidents is unknown. Although various sources mention the extended or excessive hours worked by railroad employees of that era (Adams, 1879), the actual hours worked by

---

[11]Other measures included the Hours of Service Act of 1907; the Ash Pan Act, designed to prevent injury to workers cleaning ashes from engines not equipped with ash pans; the Safety Appliances Act, requiring standardized equipment for breaking, couplers, and handholds; the Block Signal Act, which provided incentives for the testing and installation of automatic signaling devices; and the Locomotive Boiler Inspection Act.

employees is not known. The 1907 Hours of Service Act limited those who were "engaged in or connected to the movement of trains" to 16 hours of consecutive work and mandated a 10-hour rest break between work shifts (Friends of the Railroad Museum of Pennsylvania, 2002; U.S. Congress Office of Technology Assessment, 1978). Employees connected with "train dispatching and train ordering" were restricted to working no more than 9–13 hours in a 24-hour period (U.S. Congress Office of Technology Assessment, 1978). Employees could not be required or volunteer to either go on duty or remain on duty if these limits would be exceeded.

It is not known how Congress arrived at these limits on railroad employee work hours; there were no studies of fatigue and railroad safety to guide their decision-making process. Perhaps they had read some of the accounts referred to by Munsterberg (1913—as cited in Intermodal Transportation Institute, 2000a): "We have in the literature concerned with accidents in transportation numerous popular discussions about the destructive influence of loss of sleep on the attention of the locomotive engineer." Or as text from a 1917 U.S. Court Decision[12] explains, "It is common knowledge that the enactment of this legislation was induced by reason of the many casualties in railroad transportation which resulted from requiring the discharge of arduous duties by tired and exhausted men whose power of service and energy had been so weakened by overwork as to render them inattentive to duty, or incapable of discharging the responsible labors of their positions." Even without evidence from research studies, the U.S. Congress and other writers at the beginning of the twentieth century were aware that working for long hours without adequate rest periods had an adverse effect on public safety.

Although some modifications have been made to the Hours of Service Act over the past 95 years,[13] the basic provisions remain the same. Railroad employees are entitled to 8 consecutive hours off duty in the preceding 24 hours, or 10 consecutive hours off duty after working 12 consecutive hours (49 U.S.C. 21101(a)). Although compliance with the Hours of Service Act has been quite high (the U.S. General Accounting Office [GAO, 1992] found that 99.4 percent of the time, engineers had been given at least 10 hours off duty following a work shift of 12 or more hours), fatigue-related accidents continue to occur.

Over 30 studies (U.S. DOT, 2002) and numerous reports on fatigue among railway employees have been published since Grant's (1971) initial

---

[12]Atchison Topeka and Santa Fe Railroad Co. v. United States No. 267. U.S. Supreme Court (1917).

[13]Hours of Service Act. C.F.R. Title 49, Volume 4, Parts 200–399, Chapter 211 (1994; Revised October 1, 1996), and Rail Safety Enforcement and Review Act. 106 S. 972 (1992).

study. Irregular start times, uncertainty about the time of the next assignment, excessive working hours, long commutes and waiting times before beginning work, unsatisfactory conditions for sleeping at some terminals, and work/rest schedules less than 24 hours in length have been cited as factors contributing to the fatigue experienced by railroad crews (Moore-Ede, 2002; Pilcher and Coplen, 1999; Pollard 1991; Sussman and Coplen, 2002). Even though studies and accident investigations have shown that current hours-of-service regulations are not sufficient to prevent fatigue-related accidents, additional modifications of the Hours of Service Act are not planned.

Barriers to legislative change include labor contracts that maximize employee earnings by placing members on 24-hour call, employee resistance to any measure that would reduce the number of trips made and/or lengthen the intervals between trips since their pay is dependant on the number of trips made, and a culture that promotes "working when you want" (Intermodal Transportation Institute, 2000a; Sussman and Coplen, 2002). The development of new, scientifically based standards is also hampered by a lack of scientific consensus on the best way to manage shiftwork schedules, difficulties in translating research findings into operational environments, and recognition that the wide variety of settings (commuter rail, long-haul freight, and short-haul lines) makes it impossible to develop a single set of standards. Educating employees about fatigue management is considered more acceptable to all stakeholders (e.g., employees, railroad management) than prescriptive hours of service (Sussman and Coplen, 2002). As a result, most railroads now offer training modules in fatigue countermeasures for all employees, scheduled days off, confidential screening for sleep apnea, and improved sleeping facilities at railroad terminals (Intermodal Transportation Institute, 2000a,b). Although the programs are varied in the material presented, scheduling approaches, management of emergencies, and outcomes measured, several best practices have emerged. These include (1) assigned days off, particularly after an extended period of work; (2) allowing napping on duty under predetermined and controlled circumstances; and (3) educational interventions tailored to the needs of employees at a specific location (Intermodal Transportation Institute, 2000a).

Marine Employees

U.S. Coast Guard studies indicate that fatigue is a contributing factor in 16 percent of critical vessel casualties[14] and 33 percent of personal injuries

---

[14]Defined as severe damage to the vessel, capable of causing crew fatalities.

(McCallum et al., 1996). Sleep is often severely restricted by traditional watch schedules, particularly the 1-in-4 schedule[15] (Comperatore et al., 2001). The 1-in-5 schedule, while allowing for longer periods off duty, still requires crewmembers to start work 4 hours earlier every day. Advancing sleep and wake-up times by 4 hours each day is difficult if not impossible for most people. Long workdays, reduced time between watches, sleep disruptions, and fragmented sleep are also common (Comperatore et al., 1999; U.S. Coast Guard Research and Development Center, 1996). All-hands drills and other conditions further fragment sleep.

Manning requirements for Great Lakes vessels, ocean-going vessels, coastwise vessels (vessels that travel only along the coast), offshore supply vessels, towing vessels, and tankers are spelled out in Title 46 of the United States Code, Part F, Manning of Vessels, Section 8104.[16] Until 1990, the regulations, which date back to the early part of the twentieth century, focused more on the numbers and types of crewmembers required (e.g., licensed master, three mates, three or four licensed engineers) than on how long crewmembers could work (Maquire, 1984; NTSB, 2002a). The grounding of the *Exxon Valdez* on March 24, 1989, dramatically changed 46 U.S.C. 8101–8105. The Oil Pollution Act of 1990, which amended 46 U.S.C. 8101–8104, added specific hours-of-service limitations for licensed individuals and seamen; provisions forbidding deck officers to combine both navigation and cargo watch duties using a 6 hours on, 6 hours off schedule; and a requirement that officers on watch during departures from port be sufficiently rested.

Work hours in port as well as at sea are spelled out in the regulations. Seamen cannot be required to work more than 9 out of 24 hours while in port or more than 12 out of 24 hours at sea (on oceangoing or coastwise vessels of not more than 100 gross tons). Crewmembers on vessels operating in the Great Lakes can work up to 15 out of 24 hours, but cannot work more than 36 out of any 72 hours (Clifton, 2002). Work while anchored in a safe harbor is limited to 8 hours per day.[17] Licensed individuals or seamen on oil tankers are not permitted to work more than 15 hours in any 24-hour period or more than 36 hours in any 72-hour period. Administrative

---

[15]A 1-in-4 watch schedule requires crew members to work two 4-hour periods the first day (e.g., 2400–0400 and 1600–2000), and one 4-hour period the next (0800–1200). A 1-in-5 schedule requires crew members to stand watch from 2400 to 0400 and from 2000 to 2400 on the first day, from 1600 to 2000 the second day, from 1200 to 1600 the third day, from 0800 to 1200 on the fourth day, and from 0400 to 0800 on the fifth day.

[16]1990 Amendment, Manning of Vessels. United States Federal Regulations 46, 8101–8104 (1990).

[17]1990 Amendment, Manning of Vessels. United States Federal Regulations 46, 8101–8104 (1990).

duties, whether performed on board or on shore, are to be counted as work by vessel operators.[18] Crewmembers on the largest type of ocean-going vessels—those over 200 gross tons—traveling over 600 nautical miles from their home port have the shortest workday of all—8 hours (Clifton, 2002). Workers on other types of vessels are limited to working 12 hours in a 24-hour period. The number of watches per day (e.g., two or three) is also prescribed for vessels of various sizes, and unnecessary work is forbidden if the vessel is in port on Sundays and/or certain holidays. Restrictions, however, can be waived in emergencies, such as if work is necessary for the safety of the vessel or to save a life on board another vessel[19] (U.S. Congress Office of Technology Assessment, 1991d). Finally, an officer in charge of a deck watch when a vessel leaves port must have been off duty at least 6 of the 12 hours prior to the ship's departure (U.S. Congress Office of Technology Assessment, 1991d).

These regulations apply to all vessels registered in the United States, as well as those from other countries using U.S. ports. Owners, charterers, or managing operators can face civil penalties if the U.S Coast Guard discovers that work hour limits have been exceeded (Clifton, 2002). Individual mariners are expected to obey work hour limitations and to report suspected watchkeeping and work hour violations to the Coast Guard. Tips are kept confidential, and those who report code violations are protected from discrimination, including discharge, by 46 U.S.C. 2114 (Clifton, 2002).

The Oil Pollution Act of 1990 also directed that the U.S. Coast Guard undertake the development of a research program to establish safe manning levels (U.S. Congress Office of Technology Assessment, 1991a), and that results of research on the effects and reduction of fatigue be disseminated to industry personnel (National Transportation Safety Board, 1990). Although safe manning levels have not been established, research over the past 10 years has confirmed that fatigue among mariners is quite common (e.g., up to 70 percent of Coast Guard personnel showed evidence of compromised alertness [Comperatore, et al., 2001]); very complex; and influenced by a wide variety of environmental, operational, and individual factors (NTSB, 2002a). Specialized programs for fatigue countermeasures have been developed and tested by the U.S. Coast Guard, the Crew Endurance Management System (for members of the U.S. Coast Guard [Comperatore et al., 2001], and the Commercial Mariner Endurance Management System (Comperatore and Kingsley, undated).

---

[18]1990 Amendment, Manning of Vessels. United States Federal Regulations 46, 8101–8104 (1990).

[19]1990 Amendment, Manning of Vessels. United States Federal Regulations 46, 8101–8104 (1990).

The U.S. Coast Guard has also begun working closely with the International Maritime Organization to highlight the issue of fatigue and collaborated in the development of the 1995 Amendments to the International Convention on Standards of Training, Certification, and Watchkeeping for Seafarers (NTSB, 2002a). These regulations, which apply to all employees sailing on ocean-going vessels, specify that an officer in charge of a watch or a rating forming part of a watch be provided with a minimum of 10 hours of rest in a 24-hour period and that two rest periods be given, one of these being at least 6 hours in length (International Maritime Organization, 1995). Section B-VIII/1 of the 1995 Amendments also cautions that "the minimum rest periods specified in Section A-VIII/1 should not be interpreted as implying that all other hours may be devoted to watchkeeping or other duties" (International Maritime Organization, 1995).

Despite efforts to publicize their recommendations and work with industry personnel to implement effective programs for fatigue countermeasures, vessels are still running aground because crewmembers are asleep at the helm. Unfortunately, falling asleep at the helm is not a rare or isolated event. Within a 1-week period in 1999, three fishing vessels out of Southeastern New England ran aground after a crewmember fell asleep at the helm (Harrington, 1999). One of the boats was broken apart by the action of the waves; the other two were severely damaged but salvageable, and two of the three crews had to be rescued by the U.S. Coast Guard.

Long-Haul Truck Drivers

Work hours of long-haul truckers have been regulated since the 1930s, when Congress passed the Motor Carrier Act of 1935. This act authorized economic regulation of the trucking industry and directed the Interstate Commerce Commission (ICC) to establish qualifications and maximum hours of service for drivers working for private and for-hire interstate property carriers and for-hire interstate passenger carriers (Federal Motor Carrier Safety Administration, 1999; United Transportation Union, 2001). Although safety was included in the mission of the ICC, the major focus of the agency in 1935 was on the financial plight of the trucking industry (United Transportation Union, 2001).

By December 1937, the ICC had published its final version of the Hours of Service regulations (Federal Motor Carrier Safety Administration, 1999). Drivers could not be permitted or required to be on duty more than 15 out of 24 hours, only 12 hours of which could be spent working (e.g., loading, unloading, driving, handling freight, preparing reports, preparing vehicles for service, or performing any other duties pertaining to the transportation of passengers or property). The extra 3 hours was intended for meals and rest breaks. The need for off-duty time was also recognized:

It is obvious that a man cannot work efficiently or be a safe driver if he does not have an opportunity for approximately 8 hours sleep in 24. It is a matter of simple arithmetic that if a man works 16 hours a day he does not have the opportunity to secure 8 hours sleep. Allowance must be made for eating, dressing, getting to and from work, and the enjoyment of ordinary recreations.

A 48-hour rest period was mandated once a driver reached the maximum weekly work limit. Weekly on-duty limits were set at 60 hours in any 7 consecutive days or 70 hours in 8 consecutive days, depending on whether the carrier operated 7 days a week or less[20] (Federal Motor Carrier Safety Administration, 1999).

Within a year, organized labor and trucking companies had successfully petitioned the ICC to revise the Hours of Service regulations (Federal Motor Carrier Safety Administration, 1999). Revisions to the regulations allowed drivers to work up to 16 hours a day as long as they drove only for 10 of those 16 hours. The mandated rest period was also decreased from 9 to 8 consecutive hours. Total work hours per week remained capped at 60 and 70 hours (3 FR 1875). In 1938, the Hours of Service regulations were modified again, this time allowing an extra 2 hours of driving if drivers encountered "unfavorable weather conditions." Other exceptions—such as emergency conditions, driver-salespeople, oilfield operations, 100 air-mile radius drivers, retail store deliveries, sleeper berths, operations in Alaska and Hawaii, and nondriving travel time—were later granted (Federal Motor Carrier Safety Administration, 1999). However, no substantive changes were made in the regulations until 1962, when the ICC dropped the 24-hour limit.[21] The revised rules retained the 10-hour driving limit and the requirement for an 8-hour rest period. By alternating 10-hour driving periods and 8-hour rest periods, drivers were now legally permitted to drive 16 out of 24 hours (Federal Motor Carrier Safety Administration, 1999). Drivers were to maintain logbooks documenting driving periods and mileage.

Neither the original regulations nor the amendments were based on scientific evidence. Although the ICC expressed hope in 1938 that changes in the Hours of Service regulations would not be used to lengthen drivers' hours, truckers engaged in interstate commerce generally work longer hours than any other group of employees in the United States. Typically paid by the mile and exempt from overtime pay by the Fair Labor Act of 1945 (Federal Motor Carrier Safety Administration, 1999), up to 73 percent of tractor trailer drivers exceed the daily and/or weekly driving limits (Beilock

---

[20]If a carrier operates 7 days a week, a driver may work 70 hours in 8 consecutive days. If a carrier operates less than 7 days a week, a driver may work only 60 hours in 7 consecutive days.

[21]"Hours of service" 49 C.F.R. Part 395 (1962).

and Capelle, 1987). Not only are hours-of-service violators more likely to speed or drive longer hours when given unrealistic driving times, but they are also more likely to report having fallen asleep at the wheel (Braver et al., 1992). Higher crash rates have also been reported by hours-of-service violators (Braver et al., 1992; Jones and Stein, 1987).

A notice of proposed rulemaking to update the Hours of Service regulations was issued in May 2000, generating over 50,000 comments and significant controversy (NTSB, 2002b). To date, none of the following changes have been adopted: (1) increase the on-duty/off-duty cycle to a normal 24-hour work cycle; (2) increase time off to allow sufficient time for 7 to 8 hours of sleep; (3) require mandatory "weekend" recovery periods consisting of at least 2 nights of recovery sleep to enable drivers to resume baseline levels of sleep structure and waking performance and alertness; (4) address the effects of operations between midnight and 6:00 a.m., requiring off-duty periods that enable restorative sleep by including two consecutive periods between these hours; (5) allow "weekends" of sufficient length to ensure safety and provide adequate protection for driver health and safety; and (6) increase operational flexibility by offering a menu of hours-of-service options customized to different major or distinct operational segments while maintaining an appropriate level of safety (Federal Motor Carrier Safety Administration, 1999).

Aviation Industry

Although Charles Lindbergh was not the first pilot to experience the effects of fatigue, his description of fighting fatigue during his 1927 transatlantic flight graphically illustrates the dangers of tired pilots:

> My mind clicks on and off. I try letting one eyelid close at a time while I prop the other with my will. But the effort is too much, sleep is winning, my whole body argues dully that nothing, nothing life can attain is quite so desirable as sleep. My mind is loosing resolution and control. (Printup, 2000)

Lindbergh landed safely near Paris after flying for 33.5 hours. Others have not been so lucky, either flying across the Atlantic or within the borders of the United States. The U.S. Air Mail Service was founded in 1918, 15 years after the Wright brothers' initial flight. Accident rates were extremely high: 31 of the original 40 Air Service pilots died in work-related airplane crashes between 1918 and 1921 (Leape, 1994). Lack of attention to safety and "efforts to meet delivery schedules in all kinds of weather" were believed to be the cause of this extraordinarily high accident rate (Leape, 1994). By 1926, the aviation industry, worried that the airplane would not reach its full commercial value without federal action to improve and maintain safety standards, convinced Congress to pass the Air Commerce Act. This act established the Aeronautics Branch of the Department of Commerce, and charged the Secretary of Commerce with fostering air commerce, issuing and enforcing air traffic rules, licensing pilots, certificating aircraft, establishing airways, and operating and maintaining aids to air navigation (Federal Aviation Administration [FAA], 2002). Lighted airways became more common, and aeronautical radio communications were improved through the use of radio beacons. Hours-of-service limitations were not established by the FAA until 1964 (Patton et al., 2001).

The duty schedules for pilots, air traffic controllers, engineers, flight attendants, airline mechanics, and various other types of crew members are regulated by the FAA under statute 11 C.F.R. 121 (P-S). Rules on duty hours for pilots vary by the size of the flight crew (e.g., one pilot versus a crew consisting of two or more pilots). Pilots working during both scheduled and unscheduled operations (e.g., corporate/executive operations), cannot work more than 8 hours in a 24-hour period if there is only one pilot. When larger flight crews are used, pilots are allowed to work an additional 2 hours (Patton et al., 2001; U.S. Congress Office of Technology Assessment, 1991d). Domestic air carriers are not permitted to issue, and pilots are not permitted to accept, an assignment for a flight if the crew member's total flight time will exceed 100 hours in a calendar month, 30 hours in 7 consecutive days, or 8 hours between required rest periods (U.S. Congress Office of Technology Assessment, 1991a). Rest periods are also mandated and vary according to the length of the scheduled flight time. If the scheduled flight is less than 8 hours in duration, 9 consecutive hours of rest are mandated between flights; if the scheduled flight is 8–9 hours in duration, 10 consecutive hours of rest are mandated; and if the scheduled flight is 9 hours or more in duration, 11 consecutive hours of rest are mandated (U.S. Congress Office of Technology Assessment, 1991a). Longer rest periods are also mandated if pilots exceed the daily flight time limitations because of circumstances beyond their control (e.g., adverse weather conditions). If flight time limitations are exceeded by less than 30 minutes, a pilot cannot be assigned or accept an assignment that does not allow for 11 consecutive hours of rest. If the flight time limitations are exceeded by more than 30 minutes, but less than 60 minutes, 12 consecutive hours of rest are mandated. And when flight time limitations are exceeded by 60 minutes or more, 16 consecutive hours of rest are mandated before the next flight (Patton et al., 2001).

Although commercial airline pilots typically work only 13–15 days a month (Meenan, 1999), there is ample evidence that fatigue remains a significant problem. Surveys, observational data, and anecdotal reports have documented that flight crews frequently experience unintentional sleep episodes while flying (Co et al., 1999; Gander et al., 1991a; Rosekind et al.,

2000). Maintenance of vigilance, particularly at night, is quite difficult. Pilots are expected to remain alert despite high levels of automation, low light levels on the flight deck, and regulations that require the pilots to remain in their seats for the duration of the flight unless their absence is necessary for the performance of duties in connection with the operation of the aircraft or biological needs, or if the crew member is taking a rest break and relief is provided. Getting up just to stretch or walk around is not allowed (Circadian Information, 2000; Neri et al., 2002). Non–24-hour duty/rest cycles, circadian desynchronization associated with transmeridian flights, and even time zone changes of only a few hours further compromise the pilot's ability to remain alert (Mann, 1999).

Approximately 21 percent of the incidents reported to the National Aeronautics and Space Administration's (NASA) Aviation Safety Reporting System (ASRS), a confidential self-reporting system for flight crews and others to report difficulties and incidents, are fatigue related (NTSB, 2002a). Data sets for both air carriers (Federal Aviation Regulations [FAR] 121) and commuter and corporate operations (FAR 91/135) contain numerous references to fatigue and difficulties maintaining vigilance (Aviation Safety Reporting System, 1998a,b). Fortunately, only one crash has been attributed to fatigue—that of American International Airways flight 808, which missed the runway at the U.S. Naval Air Station in Guantanamo Bay, Cuba, on August 18, 1993. According to the NTSB's investigation, the probable causes of that accident included the following factors: impairment of the judgment, decision-making, and flying abilities of the captain and flight crew because of fatigue; the captain's failure to properly assess the conditions for landing and maintaining vigilant situational awareness of the airplane while maneuvering onto final approach; his failure to prevent the loss of airspeed and avoid a stall; and his failure to execute immediate action to recover from a stall. Also mentioned in the report were the "inadequacy of the flight and duty time regulations applied to 14 C.F.R., Part 121, Supplemental Air Carrier, international operations and the circumstances that resulted in the extended flight/duty hours and the fatigue of the flight crew members" (NTSB, 1994b; Ranter and Luian, 2002).

John Meenan, Senior Vice President of the Air Transport Association of America, was technically correct when he told a House subcommittee that "there has never been a scheduled commercial airline accident attributed to pilot fatigue"(Meenan, 1999). However, several NTSB reports have played down or omitted the role of pilot fatigue even when the agency's own investigators have considered it a significant factor (Circadian Information, 2000). For example, even though the NTSB report on a China Airlines Boeing 707 flight in February 1985 omitted any mention of crew fatigue, a later analysis of the accident by the Aviation Human Factors Team at NASA concluded that inattention caused by crew fatigue was a key factor in the near disaster. Other accidents in which pilot fatigue played a significant but officially unacknowledged role include the KLM–Pan American collision in the Canary Islands in March 1977; the Eastern Airlines DC-9 crash in Charlotte, North Carolina, in 1974; and the Pacific Southwest–Cessna collision over San Diego in 1978 (Circadian Information, 2000).

Air traffic controllers obviously have an essential role in maintaining airline safety. Almost all air traffic controllers rotate shifts, and are limited to working 10 consecutive hours or 10 hours during a 24-hour period unless they have been allowed a rest period of at least 8 hours before or at the end of the first 10 hours of duty.[22] Air traffic controllers, like pilots, must be given at least 1 day off during each consecutive 7-day period (U.S. Congress Office of Technology Assessment, 1991d).

Many air traffic controllers appear to have a significant sleep deficit (Marcil and Vincent, 2000). The air traffic controllers studied by Rhodes and colleagues (1996) obtained only about 6–6.5 hours sleep on day shifts and only about 5 hours sleep when working on night shifts. And controllers may get even less sleep if their mandated rest period of 8 hours falls at a time when it is difficult to sleep. The accident investigation following the crash of a United Airlines DC-8 freighter into the side of a mountain in Utah at 1:38 a.m. in December 1977 revealed that the air traffic controller, who had omitted a critical radial number when giving holding instructions to the pilot, had had approximately 2 hours of sleep prior to starting his second shift that day at 11 p.m. (he had also worked the 7 a.m. to 3 p.m. shift that day) (Circadian Information, 2000).

Aerospace Industry

No regulations or guidelines limit work hour durations in the aerospace industry. Most employees work a traditional 40-hour week, then dramatically increase their hours in the weeks before a launch or during the mission. Early missions were short, lasting only a few hours or days. Today's missions, by contrast, may last weeks or even months, placing more demands on mission control staff and astronauts.

Shuttle launches frequently occur at night, requiring flight controllers at Kennedy Space Center to switch from day to night shifts (Kelly et al., 1993). After launch, responsibility for flight operations switches to the Missions Operations Directorate at Johnson Space Center in Houston, Texas, where three flight control teams (FCTs) are used to staff the Missions Operations Directorate for flights of less than 10 days. When flights of 10 days or longer are planned, a fourth FCT is added to allow team members time

---

[22]Certification: Airmen Other than Flight Crewmembers. 14 C.F.R. 65.47.

off. Although shift lengths vary, 10-hour shifts are not uncommon. Flight controllers average less than one break per shift (range 0.1 to 0.9) (Kelly et al., 1993).

Although the explosion of the Challenger space shuttle occurred during the daytime, the decisions made the night before the launch by mission control staff have been cited as a major factor contributing to the explosion (Mitler et al., 1988). Flight controllers are responsible for a wide range of cognitive tasks, including sustained trend analysis, monitoring of multiple voice channels, and rapid responses to emergency situations. Cognitive processing and vigilance must remain high because even small mistakes can be operationally significant (Kelly et al., 1993).

Although the aerospace industry has a history that includes several accidents and near accidents associated with fatigue, there are no regulations on how long workers employed by NASA and/or manufacturers supplying spacecraft components may work in the days prior to or during a mission. In contrast, the sleep patterns of astronauts have been monitored since the early days of the space program (Aschoff, 1965; Pittendrigh, 1967). Several passages from *Apollo 13* (Lovell and Kluger, 1994) illustrate the attention paid to the sleep/wake patterns of astronauts during a mission:

> After just a day or so in translunar drift, the astronauts got accustomed to the constant flickering and went about their sleep-wake, work-rest schedules as if the sun were rising and setting outside their craft just as it did outside their homes in Houston. As long as the crew maintained that schedule, NASA's flight surgeons had learned, their circadian rhythms would remain largely undisturbed.
>
> Even on a routine flight, no one expected the pilots to sleep a full eight hours. The almost total lack of physical exertion in space and the almost constant output of adrenaline that accompanied the business of flying to the moon made five or six hours of sack time the most the medics could hope for. Those five or six hours, however, were absolutely essential if a crew that was flying even a nominal mission was going to make it through their day without making some serious, and perhaps disastrous, mistake. A crew that was flying a less than nominal mission would need even more rest. (Lovell and Kluger, 1994:202)
>
> In the second row of Mission Control, the flight surgeon had been copying down the answers the men gave, and the totals had begun to alarm him. Since Monday night, the crew had been averaging about three hours of sleep apiece per day. It was 2:30 Friday morning. . . . (Lovell and Kluger, 1994:313)

These anecdotal reports of shortened sleep times have been confirmed by both subjective and objective studies (Dijk et al., 2001; Frost et al., 1976, 1977; Grundel et al., 1993, 1996, 1997; Monk et al., 1998; Santy et al., 1998). Despite preflight circadian adaptation measures and in-flight schedules to optimize circadian adaptation and minimize sleep loss, astronauts typically sleep only 6 to 6.5 hours. Polysomnography (sleep studies using electroencephalogram [EEG], electro-occulogram [EOG], and electromyogram [EMG] recordings) have shown more wakefulness and less slow-wave (deep) sleep in the final third of sleep episodes while in space and marked increases in rapid eye movement (REM or dreaming) sleep after return to earth (Dijk et al., 2001).

Astronauts frequently use hypnotics during flights (Putcha et al., 1999), and stimulants are available to ensure alertness during critical phases of the mission. Like Air Force pilots, as discussed earlier, astronauts are allowed to decide whether to take stimulants (usually dextroamphetamine). A final selection from *Apollo 13* illustrates one astronaut's decision-making process regarding the use of stimulants:

> In the spacecraft, Lovell, Haise, and Swigert were in their accustomed places, all awake and all feeling reasonably alert. Lovell had decided against the Dexedrine tablets Slayton had prescribed for his crew last night, knowing that the lift from the stimulants would be only fleeting, and the subsequent letdown would leave them feeling even worse than they did now. For the time being, the commander had decided, the astronauts would get by on adrenaline alone. (Lovell and Kluger, 1994:318)

FATIGUE COUNTERMEASURES PROGRAMS

Fatigue countermeasures programs usually consist of an educational component (Comperatore and Kingsley, undated; Comperatore et al., 2001; Intermodal Transportation Institute, 2000a; NASA Ames Research Center, 1997; Smith-Coggins et al., 1997) and sometimes include schedule alterations (Intermodal Transportation Institute, 2000a; Sussman and Coplen, 2002). Employees are generally given information about circadian rhythms, sleep hygiene measures, shiftwork and its adverse affects, and a variety of strategies that can be used to counter fatigue (e.g., judicious use of caffeine, napping during night shifts) (NASA Ames Research Center, 2001; Rosekind et al., 1997). Some industries have also added information about sleep disorders to their presentations (Intermodal Transportation Institute, 2000a). Managers are urged to consider altering the starting times of shifts whenever possible to make schedules more compatible with circadian rhythms; to avoid scheduling employees to work more than two or three consecutive night shifts; and to provide adequate recovery times between shifts, especially when an employee is rotating off night shift. By 1997, 497 people from 230 organizations in 17 countries had participated in a 2-day trainers' workshop run by the NASA Ames Fatigue Countermeasures Group (NASA Ames Research Center, 1997). Attendees have included representatives from all areas of aviation; other modes of transportation, including the rail, trucking, and maritime industries; health care; the petrochemical industry;

nuclear energy; and law enforcement. Follow-up data gathered from workshop attendees suggest that over 125,000 flight crews and other employees, including some physicians, have received educational materials on combating fatigue.

Although over 170,000 employees have been exposed to fatigue countermeasures programs, there is very limited information about their efficacy. Typical reports indicate that some aspects of a particular program were successful (e.g., employees slept longer at night [Pollard, 1991], napping improved alertness on duty [Neri et al., 2002])], and that participants used most of the suggested strategies (Smith-Coggins et al., 1997), but rarely assess the overall efficacy of programs in improving alertness on the job and/or reducing errors.

Smith-Coggins and colleagues (1997) found that, although resident physicians (n = 6) reported increased subjective alertness after using the suggested strategies for 1 month, there were no improvements in their performance, mood, or amount of sleep obtained when working night shifts. To date, no one has tested the efficacy of this type of intervention in a population of hospital staff nurses. A fatigue countermeasures program for nurses is currently being developed at the University of Pennsylvania, and will soon be tested using nurses from four ICUs (two control and two intervention). Subjective and objective measures of alertness and vigilance will be obtained before the program is implemented and 4 weeks following implementation. Although errors and near errors will also be recorded during the baseline and later data collection periods, this pilot study may not have sufficient power to detect changes in error rates.

CONCLUSIONS

Hours-of-service regulations have not always emerged from the results of rigorous scientific research. Many of the original regulations were written in response to a disaster, such the grounding of an oil tanker or the death of young woman (Libby Zion) in a New York City hospital, or to protect a particular industry or group of employees (e.g., trucking and manning rules for seagoing vessels). Amending existing hours-of-service regulations has often been a difficult if not impossible undertaking, even when the proposed changes are supported by scientific evidence. Employees, unions, owners, and professional associations often oppose any regulation that is perceived to reduce the earning power of employees, involve hiring more employees, or cost more money.

Guidelines, which are more flexible than regulations, are not enforceable and do not prohibit employees from working for long periods each day and/or accruing large amounts of overtime. Other regulations, such as driving-time limits for truckers, although enforceable, are easily circumvented.

Fatigue countermeasures programs, which require employees to take responsibility for acquiring sufficient sleep and remaining alert on the job, are often used in place of and along with hours-of-service regulations.

Although no particular approach, whether work hour regulation, guidelines, fatigue countermeasures programs, or some combination of these, can be applied to all industries or all settings within a particular industry, there appears to be some agreement that working longer than 12 consecutive hours without at least 8 hours off duty can be hazardous. Accident rates rise exponentially after 12 hours of work, particularly when employees work at night. Some work environments limit nighttime workers to shorter shifts (e.g., 8 hours) or consider 1 hour of nighttime flying to be equal to 1.4 hours of flight time during the day (U.S. Army). Many industries in which fatigued employees could compromise public safety do not allow employees to work more than 8–12 consecutive hours.

More research is needed to understand the effects of fatigue on patient safety. Controlled trials are needed to determine optimal work schedules in hospital settings and to test fatigue countermeasures. According to Olson and Ambrogetti (1998): "We do know enough to end the worse abuses of the human sleep-wake cycle, and we need to see a shift by both hospital employers and the medical [nursing] profession towards addressing this issue." The authors of the early hours-of-service regulations understood that people cannot work for long periods of time each day without adequate time to sleep. It is perhaps time to acknowledge that nurses cannot provide safe care when they are fatigued, have worked for more than 12 hours, and/or have not had at least 12–16 hours off between shifts.

TABLE C-1 A Comparison of Work Hour Limitations in Selected Safety-Sensitive Industries

Occupational Group	Regulatory Body and Type of Regulation	Maximum Work Hours in 24-Hour Period and/or 7-Day Period	Minimum Rest Period	Other Provisions
Health Care Professionals				
Registered nurses	No federal regulations	May not work more than 16 hours in any 24-hour period, with some exceptions for emergencies and rural hospitals (Oregon)	If a nurse works more than 12 hours, must be given at least 10 hours off before the next shift assignment (Maine)	• Mandatory overtime beyond 8 hours/day or 40 hours/week prohibited unless declaration of emergency or natural disaster (California) • 12-hour shifts allowed for hospital employees; employee may be required to stay 13th hour if someone fails to show up for work, but cannot be mandated to work more than 16 hours per shift (California) • Employees cannot be mandated to work more than 80 hours of overtime in any consecutive 2-week period (Maine) • Nurses cannot be required to work more than 12 consecutive hours (Maine) • Nurses cannot be required to work more than 2 hours beyond their regularly scheduled shift (Oregon)
Physicians	No federal regulations	May not work more than 80 hours/week or 24 consecutive hours (New York)	Must have at least 8 nonworking hours between shifts (New York)	• Guidelines of the Association of American Medical Colleges suggest that residents work no more than 80 hours/week. • No prohibitions on working extra hours (moonlighting)

*Non–Health Care
Public Service
Industries*

U.S. Military
Air Force

Guidelines

- Pilots limited to flying 12 hours in a 24-hour period, 75 hours in a 30-day period, and 200 hours in a 90-day period
- Even in combat, all personnel (flight and nonflight) are limited to working 10 hours/day, 6 days a week, for a total of 247 hours a month during continuous operations, and up to 12 hours a day, 6 days a week, during sustained operations
- Crews manning intercontinental ballistic missile silos work 24-hour shifts with 2 days off

- After 12 hours of flying, pilot must have 12 hours off duty, 8 hours of which must be consecutive and without interruptions
- Crews manning intercontinental ballistic missile silos must have at least 6 hours for sleep during their duty period

- Pilots have the option of taking small doses of stimulants during prolonged missions (e.g., flights of 15–18 hours)
- Hypnotics may be prescribed to ensure that pilots obtain adequate amounts of sleep
- Any deviations from flight limits must be approved by the flight surgeon

continued

TABLE C-1 Continued

Occupational Group	Regulatory Body and Type of Regulation	Maximum Work Hours in 24-Hour Period and/or 7-Day Period	Minimum Rest Period	Other Provisions
Army	Guidelines	• Pilots limited to 16-hour duty period and 8 hours of flying time in 24 hours, working 27 hours and flying no more than 15 hours in a 48-hour period, and working 36 hours and flying no more than 22 hours in a 72-hour period • Caps on flying time and maximum duty period in 30 days differentiate between peacetime and combat conditions	Encouraged to plan for at least 6 hours of rest for all combat personnel	• Flight times are based on daytime flying conditions; if flights require instruments, occur at night, require night vision devices, etc., maximum allowed flight times are reduced • Commanding officers are responsible for ensuring that personnel are rested and fit for duty • Guidelines can be ignored if commanding officers deem necessary (e.g., combat and other special missions)
Navy	Guidelines	• Pilots limited to flying 6.5 hours/day for single-seat aircraft and 12	• Eight hours must be made available for sleep every 24 hours for pilots	• In situations in which jet lag might occur, flight crews are not grounded, but are monitored closely by the flight surgeon • Any deviations from flight limits must be

continued

	hours/day for other types of aircraft • Pilots cannot be assigned to flight duty for more than 6 consecutive days	• If scheduled for continuous alert or continuous flight duty (which requires being continuously awake) for more than 18 hours, pilots must be given 15 hrs of continuous off-duty time	approved by the commanding officer in consultation with a flight surgeon • Guidelines can be ignored if commanding officers deem necessary (e.g., combat and other special missions)
Nuclear power plant workers	U.S. Nuclear Regulatory Commission guidelines	Individuals should not work more 14 consecutive days without 2 days off, more than 72 hours in any 7-day period, or more than 12 hours straight	Workers should have at least a 12-hour break between all work periods	Guidelines regarding overtime can be waived by plant managers or designees in "very unusual situations"
Police officers	No federal or state regulations	May not work more than 60 hours/week (Albuquerque, New Mexico)	None	No prohibitions on moonlighting
Transportation Industries				
Aerospace employees in manufacturing plants, mission control staff	No federal or state regulations	None	None	

TABLE C-1 Continued

Occupational Group	Regulatory Body and Type of Regulation	Maximum Work Hours in 24-Hour Period and/or 7-Day Period	Minimum Rest Period	Other Provisions
Astronauts	No federal or state regulations	None	None	Sleep and waking periods prior to and during missions are closely monitored by NASA
Aviation				
Air traffic controllers	Department of Transportation, FAA Regulations	Individuals limited to working 10 consecutive hours or a total of 10 hours in a 24-hour period, and no more than 6 days in each 7-day period	Individuals must have at least 8 hours off duty between shifts	
Pilots	Department of Transportation, FAA regulations	• Pilots cannot work more than 8 hours in a 24-hour period; if two or more pilots, then may work for 10 hours in a 24-hour period • Pilots cannot be assigned to fly more than 100	A 9-hour rest period is mandated for flights of 8 hours or less; 10 hours of consecutive rest is required for flights of 8–9 hours; and 11 hours of consecutive rest is required for flights of 9 hours or more	Longer rest periods are mandated if pilots exceed the daily flight time limitations because of circumstances beyond their control

		hours in a calendar month or 30 hours in 7 days	
Maritime employees	Department of Transportation, U.S. Coast Guard regulations and 1995 Amendments to the International Convention on Standards of Training, Watchkeeping for Seafarers	• May not work more than 8 hours in 24 (oceangoing vessels over 200 gross tons), 12 hours in a 24-hour period, and 15 hours in 24 hours (oil tankers and vessels operating in the Great Lakes) • If allowed to work 15 consecutive hours, cannot work more than 36 hours in a 72-hour period	• While in port, seamen cannot work more than 9 hours out of 24, and unnecessary duties are forbidden on Sundays • The officer in charge of a deck watch when a vessel leaves port must have been off duty at least 6 of the 12 hours prior to departure • Work hour restrictions can be waived if work is necessary to ensure the safety of the vessel or to save a life on board another vessel • Regulations do not apply to fishing, fish processing, and fish tender vessels
Railroad employees Dispatching and other operations	Department of Transportation, Federal Railroad Administration	Individuals may not work more than 9–13 hours in a 24-hour period	

continued

TABLE C-1 Continued

Occupational Group	Regulatory Body and Type of Regulation	Maximum Work Hours in 24-Hour Period and/or 7-Day Period	Minimum Rest Period	Other Provisions
Engineers	Department of Transportation, Federal Railroad Administration	Individuals can work up to 16 hours in a 24-hour period	If individuals work 12 hours or more, must be given a 10-hour rest break between work periods; otherwise must be given at least an 8-hour rest period every 24 hours	
Trucking industry	Department of Transportation, Federal Motor Carrier Safety Administration	Individuals may drive 10 hours out of every 18-hour period, with a weekly limit of 60 hours in 7 consecutive days or 70 hours in 8 consecutive days	Individuals must have 8 consecutive hours between trips and 48 hours off-duty after reaching the maximum	• Drivers allowed 2 hours of extra driving if they encounter "unfavorable weather conditions" • Driver-salespeople, those involved in oilfield operations or operations in Alaska and Hawaii, and 100-mile-radius drivers are also exempted from limits on driving time • Drivers are required to keep a logbook detailing their hours driven each day

REFERENCES

(AACCN) American Association of Critical Care Nurses. 2001. *AACN Online; Quick Poll Results.* [Online]. Available: http://www.aacn.org/AACN/Surveys.nsf/prarchivelist? OpenForm [accessed April 24, 2001].

AAMC (American Association of Medical Colleges). 2002. *AAMC Policy Guidance on Graduate Medical Education.* [Online]. Available: http://www.aamc.org/hlthcare/gmepolicy/start.htm [accessed November 1, 2002].

Adams CF. 1879. *Railroad Accidents.* New York, NY: G.P. Putnam's Sons. P. vi.

Aiken LH, Clarke SP, Sloan DM, Sochalski J, Silber JH. 2002. Hospital nursing staffing and patient mortality, nurse burnout, and job dissatisfaction. *Journal of the American Medical Association* 288(16):1987–1993.

Akerstedt T. 1994. Work injuries and time of day-national data. *Proceedings of a Consensus Development Symposium Entitled "Work Hours, Sleepiness, and Accidents."* Stockholm, Sweden: Karolinska Institute. P. 106.

Alaska Oil Spill Commission. 1990. *Spill: The Wreck of the Exxon Valdez.* [Online]. Available: http://www.oilspill.state.ak.us/facts/details.html [accessed July 29, 2003].

AMA (American Medical Association). 2002. *AMA (RFS) AMA Resident Work Hour Policies.* [Online]. Available: http://www.ama-assn.org/ama/pub/category/7094.html/#H310-979 AMA. [accessed November 1, 2002].

ANA (American Nurses Association). 2001. *Analysis of the American Nurses Association Staffing Survey.* Warwick, RI: Cornerstone Communications Group.

Anonymous. 1998. Work rules pose conflict. *MS Journal of the American Medical Association* 41(44). November 23/30, 1998. [Online]. Available: http://www.ama-assn.org/sci-pubs/msjama/articles/vol_280/no_21/medicare.htm [accessed October 26, 2002].

Anonymous. 2002a (September 14). *2001 Firefighter Work Schedule.* [Online]. Available: ladder54.com [accessed at http://www.ladder54.com/schedule.htm on November 1, 2002].

Anonymous. 2002b. Alexandria Fire Department Shift Schedules. City of Alexandria. [Online]. Available: http://ci.alexandria.va.us/fire/shift_schedule.htm [accessed November 1, 2002].

Arnow PM, Allyn PA, Nichols EM, Hill DL, Pezzio M, Barlett RH. 1982. Control of methicillin-resistant *Staphlococcus aureus* in a burn unit: Role of nurse staffing. *The Journal of Trauma* 22(11):954–959.

Asch DA, Parker RM. 1988. The Libby Zion case: One step forward or two steps backward? *The New England Journal of Medicine* 318(12):771–775.

Aschoff J. 1965. Significance of circadian rythms for spaceflight. In: Bedwell TC, Strughhold H, eds. *Proceedings of the Third International Symposium on Bioastronautics and the Exploration of Space.* U.S. Air Force. Pp. 465–484.

Asken MJ, Raham DC. 1983. Resident performance and sleep deprivation. *Journal of Medical Education* 58(5):382–388.

Aviation Safety Reporting System. 1998a. *Air Carrier (FAR 121) Flight Crew Fatigue Reports: ASRS Database Report Set (Update 1.0).* Mountain View, CA: Battelle Memorial Laboratories.

Aviation Safety Reporting System. 1998b. *Commuter and Corporate Flight Crew Fatigue Report: ASRS Database Report Set (Update 3.0).* Mountain View, CA: Battelle Memorial Laboratories.

Babkoff H, Mikulincer M, Caspy T, Kempinski D, Sing H. 1988. The topology of performance curves during 72 hours of sleep loss. *The Quarterly Journal of Experimental Psychology* 324(4):737–756.

Bartle EJ, Sun JH, Thompson L, Light AI, McCool C, Heaton S. 1988. The effects of acute sleep deprivation during residency training. *Surgery* 104(2):311–316.

Beilock R, Capelle RB. 1987. Economic pressure, long distance trucking and safety. *Journal of Transportation Research Forum* 28(1):177–185.

Belenky GI, Krueger GP, Balkin RJ, et al. 1987. *Effects of Continuous Operations (CONOPS) on Soldier and Unit Performance. Review of the Literature and Strategies for Sustaining the Solder in the CONOPS.* Report No. WRAIR BB-87-1. Washington, DC: U.S. Department of the Army, Medical Research and Development Command, Walter Reed Army Institute of Research.

Braver ER, Preusser CW, Preusser HM, Baum HM, Beilock R, Ulmer R. 1992. Long hours and fatigue: A survey of tractor-trailer drivers. *Journal of Public Health Policy* 13(3):341–366.

Brusco MJ, Futch J, Showalter MJ. 1993. Nurse staff planning under conditions of a nursing shortage. *Journal of Nursing Administration* 23(7–8):58–64.

Cabri J, De Witte B, Clarys J. 1988. Circadian variation in blood pressure responses to muscular exercise. *Ergonomics* 31(11):1559–1566.

Center for Design of Industrial Schedules. 1988. *Final Report on the Philadelphia Police Department Shift Rescheduling Program.* Boston, MA: Center for Design of Industrial Schedules.

Circadian Information. 2000. Aviation Safety and Pilot Error. In: *24 x 7 Operations: Optimizing Human Performance.* Cambridge, MA: Circadian Information. Pp. 6.1–6.14.

Clifton, J. 2002. Watchkeeping and work hour limitations. *Marine Safety Bulletin* II(I):9–10.

CNA (California Nurses Association). 2001a. *Mandatory Overtime Is Detrimental to Patient Care and the Health of Nurses.* [Online]. Available: http://www.Calnurse.org/CNA/patient/nursespeak.html [accessed April 20, 2001].

CNA. 2001b. *Supervisor's Update: Nurses Ratify Agreement.* [Online]. Available: http://for.healthcare.UCLA.edu/JuneCNAUpdate.htmn [accessed on October 4, 2002].

Co EL, Gregory KB, Johnson JM, Rosekind MR. 1999. *Crew Factors in Flight Operations XI: A Survey of Fatigue Factors in Regional Airline Operations.* Technical Memorandum No. 1999-208799. Moffett Field, CA: NASA Ames Research Center.

Cohen C, Muehl G. 1977. Human circadian rhythms in resting and exercise pulse rates. *Ergonomics* 20(5):475–479.

Committee of Interns and Residents. 2002a. *NY State Hours Regs Get Enforcement Boost.* [Online]. Available: http:// www.cirseiu.org/BNew/226breakingnewspage.htm [accessed October 24, 2002].

Committee of Interns and Residents. 2002b. NJ Assembly passes bill to limit resident work hours. [Online]. Available: http://www.cirseiu.org/news/271/breakingnewspage.htm [accessed October 24, 2002].

Comperatore CA, Kingsley LC. Undated. The commercial mariner endurance management system. Groton, CT: Crew Endurance Management Team, United States Coast Guard, Research and Development Center.

Comperatore CA, Bloch C, Ferry C. 1999. *Incidence of Sleep Loss and Wakefulness Degradation on a U.S. Coast Guard Cutter Under Exemplar Crewing Limits.* CG-D-14-99. Groton, CT: U.S. Coast Guard Research and Development Center.

Comperatore CA, Rothblum AM, Riveria PK, Kingsley LC, Beene D, Carvalhais AB. 2001. *U.S. Coast Guard Guide for the Management of Crew Endurance Risk Factors.* CG-D-13-01. Groton, CT: U.S. Coast Guard Research and Development Center.

Cullen DJ, Sweitzer BJ, Bates DW, Burdick E, Edmondson A, Leape LL. 1997. Preventable adverse drug events in hospitalized patients: A comparative study of intensive care and general care units. *Critical Care Medicine* 1289(8):1297.

Czeisler C, Lockley SW, Landrigan NT, Rothschild JM, Kaushal R. 2002. Current resident work hours: Too many or not enough? *Journal of the American Medical Association* 287(14):1802–1803.

Dawson D, Reid K. 1997. Fatigue, alcohol, and performance impairment. *Nature* 388(6639): 235.

Deaconson TF, O'Hair DP, Levy MF, Lee MBF, Schueneman AL, Condon RE. 1988. Sleep deprivation and resident performance. *Journal of the American Medical Association* 260(12):1721–1727.

Delafosse J, Leger D, Quera-Salva M, Samson O, Adrein J. 2000. Comparative study of actigraphy and ambulatory polysomnographic in the assessment of adaptation to night shift work in nurses. *Revue Neurologique* (Paris) 156(6–7):641–645.

Denisco RA, Drummond JN, Gravenstein JS. 1987. The effect of fatigue on the performance of a simulated anesthetic monitoring task. *J Clin Monit* 3(1):22–24.

DHHS (Department of Health and Human Services). 1993. *Report of the National Commission on Sleep Disorders Research*. Washington, DC: U.S. Government Printing Office.

Dijk DJ, Neri DF, Wyatt JK, Ronda JM, Riel E, Ritz-De Cecco A, Hughes RJ, Elliott AR, Prisk GK, West JB, Czeisler CA. 2001. Sleep, performance, circadian rhythms, and light-dark cycles during two space shuttle flights. *Am J Physiol Regulatory Integrative Comp Physiol.* 281(5):R1647–R1664.

Dinges D, Graeber R, Rosekind M, Samel A, Wegmann H. 1996. *Principles and Guidelines for Duty and Rest Scheduling in Commercial Aviation*. NASA Technical Memorandum 110404. Moffett Field, CA: NASA, Ames Research Center.

Dirkx J. 1993. Adaptation to permanent night work: The number of consecutive work nights and motivated choice. *Ergonomics* 36(1–3):29–36.

Duchon JC, Keran C, Smith T. 1994. Extended workdays in an underground mine: A work performance analysis. *Human Factors* 36(2):258–269.

Eisenhut DG. 1980 (July 31). *Letter to All Licensees of Operating Plants and Applicants for Operating Licenses and Holders of Construction Permits—Interim Criteria for Shift Staffing*. Washington, DC: U.S. Nuclear Regulatory Commission.

Eisenhut DG. 1982 (June 12). *Generic Letter No. 82-12, Letter to All Licensees of Operating Plants and Holders of Construction Permits: Nuclear Power Plant Staff Working Hours*. Washington, DC: U.S. Nuclear Regulatory Commission.

FAA (Federal Aviation Administration). 2002. *FAA History, Information and Resources*. [Online]. Available: http://www.faa.gov/apa/history/briefhistory.htm [accessed October 9, 2002].

Federal Motor Carrier Safety Administration. 1999. *Proposed Hours of Service, Hours of Service NPRM Background and Synopsis*. U.S. DOT. [Online]. Available: http://www.mesa.dot.gov/hos/backgrounjd.htm [accessed August 21, 2002].

Florica V, Higgins EA, Iampietro PF, Lategola MT, Davis AW. 1968. Physiological responses of men during sleep deprivation. *Journal of Applied Physiology* 24(2):169–175.

Folkard S. Effects on performance efficiency. 1996. In: Colquhoun W, Costa G, Folkard S, Knauth P, eds. *Shiftwork: Problems and Solutions*. Franfort am Main, Germany: Peter Lang. Pp. 65–87.

Friedman RC, Bigger JT, Kornfeld DS. 1971. The intern and sleep loss. *The New England Journal of Medicine* 285(4):201–203.

Friends of the Railroad Museum of Pennsylvania. 2002. *Railroad History Timeline*. [Online]. Available: http://www.rrmuseumpa.org/education/historytimeline3.htm [accessed August 29, 2002].

Frost JD, Shumate WH, Salamy JG, Booher CR. 1976. Sleep monitoring: The second manned Skylab mission. *Aviat Space Environ Med* 47(4):372–382.

Frost JD, Shumate WH, Salamy JG, Booher CR. 1977. *Experiment M133: Sleep Monitoring on Skylab*. Johnson RS, Dietlein LF, eds. Washington, DC: NASA. Pp. 113–126.

Gaba DM. 1998. *Physician Work Hours: The "Sour Thumb" or Organizational Safety in Tertiary Health Care.* Scheffler AL, Zipperer LA, eds. Chicago, IL: National Patient Safety Foundation. Pp. 302–305.

Gander PH, Graeber RC, Connell LJ, Gregory KB. 1991a. *Crew Factors in Flight Operations VIII: Factors Influencing Sleep Timing and Subjective Sleep Quality in Commercial Long-Haul Flight Crews.* Technical Memorandum No. 103852. Moffett Field, CA: NASA, Ames Research Center.

Gander PH, McDonald JA, Montgomery JC, Paulin MG. 1991b. Adaptation of sleep and circadian rhythms to the Antarctic summer: A question of zeitgeber strength. *Aviation, Space and Environmental Medicine* 62(11):1019–1025.

GAO (General Accounting Office). 1992 (August 21). [Online]. Available: http://www.du.edu/transporation/fatigue/fatigue_chap1.html.

Gillberg M, Kecklund G, Akerstedt T. 1994. Relations between performance and subjective ratings of sleepiness during a night awake. *Sleep* 17(3):236–241.

Gold D, Rogocz S, Bock N, Tosteson T, Baum M, Speizer F. 1992. Rotating shift-work, sleep and accidents related to sleepiness in hospital nurses. *American Journal of Public Health* 82(7):1011–1014.

Golden L, Jorgensen H. 2002. *Time After Time: Mandatory Overtime in the U.S. Economy* [Briefing Paper]. Washington, DC: Economic Policy Institute.

Graeber JG, Rollier RI, Salter JA. 1986. *Continuous Operations SOP for BIFV Units.* USARI Research Note 86-60. Fort Benning, GA: U.S. Department of the Army, Research Institute for the Behavioral and Social Sciences, Field Unit.

Grant JS. 1971. Concepts of fatigue and vigilance in relation to railway operations. *Ergonomics* 14(1):111–118.

Grantcharov TP, Bardram L, Funch-Jenson P, Rosenberg J. 2001. Laparoscopic performance after one night on call in a surgical department: Prospective study. *British Medical Journal* 323(7323):1222–1223.

Gravenstein J, Cooper J, Orkin F. 1990. Work and rest cycles in anesthesia practice. *Anesthesiology* 72(4):737–742.

Green MJ. 1995. What (if anything) is wrong with residency overwork? *Annals of Internal Medicine* 123(7):512–517.

Greenfield L. 2001. *Surgical Residency Review Committee Perspective.* Alexandria, VA: Conference on Sleep, Fatigue and Medical Training. October 28-29, 2001.

Grundel A, Nalishiti V, Reucher E, Vejvoda M, Zulley J. 1993. Sleep and circadian rhythm during a short space mission. *Clin Investig* 71(9):718–724.

Grundel A, Polyahov VV, Zulley J. 1996. Circadian rhythms and sleep structure in space. *Soc Res Biol Rhythms* 5:9.

Grundel A, Polyahov VV, Zulley J. 1997. The alteration of human sleep and circadian rhythms during spaceflight. *Journal of Sleep Research* 6(1):1–8.

Gurjala A, Lurie P, Haroona L, Rising JP, Bell B, Strohl KP, Wolfe SM. 2001 (April 30). Petition requesting a limit on medical resident work hours through a standard issued under the authority of the Occupational Safety and Health Administration.

Hanecke K, Tiedemann S, Nachreiner F, Grzech-Sukalo H. 1998. Accident risk as a function of hour at work and time of day as determined from accident data and exposure models for the German working population. *Scandinavian Journal of Work Environment Health* 24(Supplement 3):43–48.

Harrington T. 1999. *Fatigue Lessons Learned from the Coast Guard; Coast Guard Responds to 3 Incidents Caused by Fishermen Asleep at the Helm in One Week.* U.S. Coast Guard. [Online]. Available: http:// www.uscg.mil/hq/mne/ptp/lessons/cgfatigue.htm [accessed August 29, 2002].

Haslam DR. 1982. Sleep loss, recovery sleep and military performance. *Ergonomics* 25(2):163–178.

Hawkins MR, Vichick DA, Silsby HD, Kruzick DJ, Butler R. 1985. Sleep and nutritional deprivation and performance of house officers. *Journal of Medical Education* 60(7):530–535.

Holzman IR, Barnett SH. 2000. The Bell Commission: Ethical implications for the training of physicians. *The Mount Sinai Journal of Medicine* 67(2):136–139.

Intermodal Transportation Institute. 2000a. *Fatigue Countermeasures in the Railroad Industry, Past and Current Developments. Chapter 1 Introduction.* [Online]. Available: http://www.du.edu/transportation/fatigue/fatigue-chapterone.html [accessed September 9, 2002]. Intermodal Transportation Institute.

Intermodal Transportation Institute. 2000b. *Fatigue Countermeasures in the Railroad Industry, Past and Current Developments. Chapter 3 Early Industry Projects.* [Online]. Available: http://www.du.edu/transportation/fatigue/fatigue-chapterthree.html [accessed September 9, 2002]. Intermodal Transportation Institute.

Intermodal Transportation Institute. 2000c. *Fatigue Countermeasures in the Railroad Industry, Past and Current Developments. Chapter 5 Conclusions.* [Online]. Available: http://www.du.edu/transportation/fatigue/fatigue-chapterfivee.html [accessed September 9, 2002]. Intermodal Transportation Institute.

International Maritime Organization, U.S. Coast Guard. 1995. 1995 Amendments to Standards of Training, Certification, and Watchkeeping for Seafarers. Chapter VIII, Guidance regarding watchkeeping, Section B-VIII/1. [Online]. Available: http://www.USCG.mil.stcw/95 amendments/5-chj8B.htm.

Jones IS, Stein HS. 1987. *Effect of Driver Hours on Service on Tractor-Trailer Crash Involvement.* Arlington, VA: Insurance Institute for Highway Safety.

Kelly SM, Rosekind MR, Dinges DF, Miller DL, Gillen KA, Gregory KB, Aguiler RD, Smith RM. 1993. *Flight Controller Alertness and Performance during MOD Shiftwork Operations.* Houston, TX: Space Technology Interdependency Group. Pp. 405–416.

Kennedy R. 1998 (May 1). Residents' work hours termed excessive in hospital study. *The New York Times.* Section A, Page 1.

Knauth P. 1993. The design of shift systems. *Ergonomics* 36(1–3):15–28.

Knauth P, Landau K, Droge C, Schwitteck M, Widynski M, Rutenfranz J. 1980. Duration of sleep depending on the type of shift work. *International Archives of Occupational and Environmental Health* 46(2):167–177.

Kogi K. 1991. Job content and working time: The scope for joint change. *Ergonomics* 34(6):757–773.

Kopstein G, Siegal A, Corm J, et al. 1985. Soldier performance in continuous operations. USARI Research Note 85-68. Wayne, PA: U.S. Army Research Institute for the Behavioral and Social Sciences; Applied Psychological Services, Inc.

Kovner C, Jones C. 2002. Nurse staffing and postsurgical adverse events: An analysis of administrative data from a sample of U.S. hospitals, 1990–1996. *Health Services Research* 37(3):611–629.

Krueger GP. 1989. Sustained work, fatigue, sleep loss and performance: A review of the issues. *Work and Stress* 3(2):129–141.

Krueger GP. 1994. Fatigue, performance, and medical error. In: Bogner M, ed. *Human Error in Medicine.* Hinsdale, NJ: Lawrence Erlbaum Associates, Publishers. Pp. 311–326.

Krueger GP, Armstrong RN, Cisco RR. 1985. Aviator performance in week-long extended flight operations in a helicopter simulator. *Behavior Research Methods Instruments and Computers* 17(1):68–74.

Kwan R, Levy R. 2002. *A Primer on Resident Work Hours: Everything You Always Wanted to Know but Were Afraid to Ask!* Reston, VA: American Medical Student Association.

Lamberg L. 2002. Long hours, little sleep: Bad medicine for physicians-in-training. *Journal of the American Medical Association* 287(3):303–306.

Lamond N, Dawson D. 1998. *Quantifying the Performance Impairment Associated with Sustained Wakefulness* (March/April Edition). South Australia: The Centre for Sleep Research, The Queen Elizabeth Hospital.

Lavie P, Chillag N, Epstein R, Tzischinsky O, Givon R, Fuschs S, Shahal B. 1989. Sleep disturbances in shift-workers: A marker for maladaptation syndrome. *Work and Stress* 3(1):33–40.

Leape LL. 1994. Error in medicine. *Journal of the American Medical Association* 272(23): 1851–1857.

Leape LL, Bates D, Cullen D, Cooper J, Demonaco H, Gallivan T, Hallisey R, Ives J, Laird N, Laffel G, Nemeskal R, Petersen L, Porter K, Servi D, Shea B, Small S, Sweitzer B, Thompson B, Vander Vleit M. 1995. Systems analysis of adverse drug events. *Journal of the American Medical Association* 274(1):35–43.

Lee K. 1992. Self-reported sleep disturbances in employed women. *Sleep* 15(6):493–498.

Leonard C, Fanning N, Attwood J, Buckley M. 1998. The effect of fatigue, sleep deprivation, and onerous working hours on the physical and mental wellbeing of pre-registration house officers. *I.J.M.S.* 167(1):22–25.

Light AI, Sun JH, McCool C, Thompson L, Heaton S, Bartle EJ. 1989. The effects of acute sleep deprivation on level of resident training. *Curr Surg* 46(1):29–30.

Linde L, Bergstrom M. 1992. The effect of one night without sleep on problem-solving and immediate recall. *Psychological Research* 54(2):127–136.

Louwe H, Kramer A. 2001. *Case Studies of Nursing Care Facility Staffing Issues and Quality of Care.* In Baltimore, MD: CMS. 2001. *Report to Congress: Appropriateness of Minimum Nurse Staffing Ratios in Nursing Homes—Phase II Final Report.* [Online]. Available: www.cms.gov/medicaid/reports/rp1201home.asp [accessed June 25, 2002]. Site stated, "last modified on Wednesday June 12, 2002." Pp. 6-1–6-30

Lovell J, Kluger J. 1994. *Apollo 13.* New York, NY: Houghton Mifflin Co. P. 378.

Luna T, French J, Mitcha J. 1997. A study of USAF air traffic controller shiftwork: Sleep, fatigue, activity, and mood analyses. *Aviation, Space & Environmental Medicine* 68(1): 18–23.

Mann, M. 1999. Deputy Associate Administrator, Office of Aero-Space Technology, National Aeronautics and Space Administration. Testimony to the Aviation Subcommittee of the House Subcommittee on Transportation and Infrastructure of the U.S. Congress on August 3, 1999. [Online]. Available: http:// legislative.nasa/hearings.Mann.h-3.html.

Maquire CJ. 1984. *Appendix C: Laws and Regulations of the United States Concerning Vessel Manning.* Committee on Effective Manning; Marine Board; Commission on Engineering and Technical Systems, and National Research Council. Washington, DC: National Academy of Sciences. Pp. 99–114.

Marcil I, Vincent A. 2000. *Fatigue in Air Traffic Controllers: Literature Review.* Final Report TP 13457. Canada: Transport Canada, Air Navigation Services and Airspace.

Markey EJ, Dingell JD, Klink R. 1999 (February 25). *Letter to Shirley Ann Jackson, Chairman, Nuclear Regulatory Commission.* Washington, DC: U.S. Nuclear Regulatory Commission.

McCallum MC, Raby M, Rothblum AM. 1996. *Procedures for Investigating and Reporting Human Factors and Fatigue Contributions to Marine Casualties.* U.S. Coast Guard Report No. CG-D-09-97. Groton, CT: U.S. Coast Guard Research and Development Center.

McCartt A, Rohrbaugh J, Hammer M. 2000. Factors associated with falling asleep at the wheel among long-distance truck drivers. *Accident Analysis & Prevention* 32(4):493–504.

Meenan JM. 1999. Senior Vice President, Industry Policy Air Transport Association of America. Testimony to the House Transportation and Infrastructure Committee of the U.S. Congress on August 3, 1999. [Online]. Available: http:// www.air-transport.org/ publictestimony/pda.asp?pid=861.

Mills ME, Arnold B, Wood CM. 1983. Core 12: A controlled study of the impact of 12-hour scheduling. *Nursing Research* 32(6):356–361.

Mitler MM, Carskadon M, Czeisler C, Dement W, Dinges D, Graeber R. 1988. Catastrophes, sleep, and public policy: Consensus report. *Sleep* 11(1):100–109.

Mitler MM, Miller JC, Lipsitz, J, Walsh JK, Wylie CD. 1997. The sleep of long-haul truckers. [comment]. *The New England Journal of Medicine* 337(11):755–761.

Monk TH. 1990. *Shiftworker Performance.* Scott A, ed. Philadelphia, PA: Hanley and Belfus, Inc. Pp. 183–198.

Monk TH, Folkard S, Wedderburn A. 1996. Maintaining safety and high performance on shiftwork. *Applied Ergonomics* 27(1):17–23.

Monk TH, Buysse DJ, Billy BD, Kennedy KS. 1998. Sleep in circadian rhythms in four orbiting astronauts. *J Biological Rythms* 13:188–201.

Moore-Ede M. 2002. Prepared statement to Railroads Subcommittee of the Transportation and Infrastructure Committee. Washington, DC.

Mullaney DJ, Kripke DF, Fleck PA, Johnson LC. 1983. Sleep loss and nap effects on sustained continuous performance. *Psychophysiology* 20(6):643–651.

Murray M, Smith S. 1988. Nurses resigning their hospital jobs in Toronto: Who are they, why are they resigning, and what are they going to do? Report for the Nursing Manpower Taskforce of the Hospital Council of Metropolitan Toronto. Toronto, Ontario: Health Care Research Unit, University of Toronto.

NASA Ames Research Center. 1997. Crew fatigue research focusing on development and use of effective countermeasures. *ICAO Journal* 52:20–22, 28.

NASA Ames Research Center. 2001. *NASA Fatigue Countermeasures Education and Training Module Workshops.* [Online]. Available: http://human-factors.arc.nasa.gov/zteam/fcp/ etm.html [accessed April 18, 2001].

Naval Strike and Air Warfare Center. 2000. *Performance Maintenance during Continuous Flight Operations: A Guide for Flight Surgeons.* NAVMED P-6410. U.S. Navy. [Online]. Available: http://www.safetycenter.navy.mil/aviation/aeromedical/downloads/ performancemanual.pdf [accessed July 18, 2003].

Needleman J, Buerhaus P, Mattke S, Stewart M, Zelevinsky K. 1928. *Nurse Staffing and Patient Outcomes in Hospitals.* Contract No. 230-99-0021. Washington, DC: DHHS, HRSA.

Nelson, C, Dell'Angela K, Jellish W, Brown IE, Skaredoff M. 1995. Residents' performance before and after night call as evaluated by an indicator of creative thought. *Journal of the American Osteopathic Association* 95(10):600-603.

Neri DF, Oyung RL, Colletti LM, Mallis MM, Tam PY, Dinges D. 2002. Controlled breaks as a fatigue countermeasure on the flight deck. *Aviation, Space, and Environmental Medicine* 3(7):654–664.

Northcott N. 1995. Twelve-hour shifts: Helpful or hazardous to patients? *Nursing Times* 91(7):29–31.

NTSB (National Transportation Safety Board). 1990. *Marine Accident Report: The Grounding of the Exxon Valdez on Bligh Reef, Prince William Sound, AK March 24, 1989.* NTSB/Mar-90/94. Springfield, VA: National Technical Information Service.

NTSB. 1994a. *A Review of Flightcrew-Involved Major Accidents of U.S. Air Carriers, 1978 though 1990.* NTSB #SS-94-01/PB94-917001. Washington, DC: NTSB.

NTSB. 1994b. Uncontrolled collision with terrain. American International Airways Flight 808. Douglas DC-8-61. N814CK. NTIS No. PB-910406. U.S. Naval Air Station, Guantanamo Bay, Cuba: NTSB.

NTSB. 2002a. *Safety Issue: Human Fatigue in Transportation Operations.* [Online]. Available: http://www.ntsb.gov/recs/mostwanted.fatigue.htm [accessed August 29, 2002].

NTSB. 2002b. Fatigue in Transportation. [Online]. Available: http://www.ntsb.gov.ITSA.fatigue.htm [accessed October 17, 2002].

Olson LG, Ambrogetti A. 1998. Working harder-working dangerously? Fatigue and performance in hospitals. *Medical Journal of Australia* 168(12):614–616.

Orton DI, Gruzelier JH. 1989. Adverse changes in mood and cognitive performance of house officers after night duty. *British Medical Journal* 298(6665):21–23.

Ou JC, Weigner MB, Mazzei WG, Al E. 2001. Further evaluation of the effects of nighttime work on mood, task patterns, and workload during anesthesia care [abstract]. *Anesthesiology* 95:A1196.

Owens JA, Veasey SC, Rosen RC. 2001. Physician, heal thyself: Sleep, fatigue, and medical education. *Sleep* 24(5):493–495.

Parker JB. 1987. The effects of fatigue on physician performance: An underestimated cause of physician impairment and increased patient risk. *Can J Anaesth* 34(5):489–495.

Patton DV, Landers DR, Agarwal IT. 2001. Legal considerations of sleep deprivation among resident physicians. *Journal of Health Law* 34(3):377–417.

Pilcher JJ, Coplen MK. 1999. Predictive models of on-duty alertness in irregular work/rest cycles. *Sleep Research Online* 2(Supplement 1):264.

Pittendrigh CS. 1967. Circadian rhythms, space research, and manned space flight. *Life Science Space Research* 5:122–134.

Pollard JK. 1991. *Issues in Locomotive Crew Management and Scheduling.* USDOT Report #DOT/FRA/RRP-91-06. Washington, DC: U.S. DOT.

Poulton EC. 1972. *The Effects of Fatigue upon Sonar Detection, MRC.* NPRC Report N. OES 20-72. London: Royal Naval Personnel Research Committee.

Poulton EC, Hunt GM, Carpenter A, Edwards RS. 1978. The performance of junior hospital doctors following reduced sleep and long hours of work. *Ergonomics* 21(4):279–295.

Printup MB. 2000. The effects of fatigue on performance and safety. [Online]. Available: http://www.avweb.com/articles_fatigue [accessed October 18, 2002].

Public Citizen. 2002. *OSHA Denies Petition to Reduce Work Hours for Doctors-in-Training.* [Online]. Available: http://www.citizen.org/pressroom/release.cfm?ID=1239 [accessed November 1, 2002].

Putcha L, Berens KL, Marshburn TH, Ortega HJ, Billica RD. 1999. Pharmaceutical use by U.S. astronauts on space shuttle missions. *Aviation, Space, and Environmental Medicine* 70(7):705–708.

Quigley B. 1999. 10 DFR Part 26, PRM-26-2. *Federal Register* 64(230):67202–67205.

Ranter H, Luian F. 2002. *Aviation Safety Network, Accident Description.* Aviation Safety Network. [Online]. Available: http://www.aviationsafety.net/database1993_9co818-0.html [accessed October 17, 2002].

Reznick RK, Folse JR. 1985. Effect of sleep deprivation on the performance of surgical residents. *American Journal of Surgery* 154(5):520–525.

Rhodes W, Heslegrave R, Ujimoto KV, et al. 1996. *Impact of Shiftwork, and Overtime on Air Traffic Controllers—Phase II: Analysis of Shift Schedule Effects on Sleep, Performance, Physiology, and Social Issues.* Final Report TP 12816E. Canada: Transportation Department Centre.

Rosa R. 1995. Extended workshifts and excessive fatigue. *Behavior Research Methods Instruments and Computers* 17(1985):6–15.

Rosa R. 2001. *Examining Work Schedules for Fatigue: It's Not Just Hours of Work.* Hancock P, Desmond P, eds. Mahwah, MJ: Lawrence Earlbaum Associates. Pp. 513–528.

Rosa R, Colligan, M. 1988. Long workdays vs restdays: Assessing fatigue and alertness with a portable performance battery. *Human Factors* 30(3):305–317.

Rosekind MR, Smith RM, Miller DL, Co EL, Gregory KB, Webbon LL, Gander PH, Lebacqz V. 1995. Alertness management: Strategic naps in operational settings. *Journal of Sleep Research* 4(Supplement 2):62–66.

Rosekind MR, Gander PH, Gregory KB, Smith RM, Miller DL, Oyung R, Webbon LL, Johnson JM. 1997. Managing fatigue in operational settings 2: An integrated approach. *Hospital Topics* 75(3):31–75.

Rosekind MR, Gander PH, Connell LJ, Co EL. 1999. *Crew Factors in Flight Operations X: Alertness Management in Flight Operations.* U.S. DOT.

Rosekind MR, Co EL, Gregory KB, Miller DL. 2000. *Crew Factors in Flight Operations XIII: A Survey of Fatigue Factors in Corporate/Executive Aviation Operations.* Technical Memorandum No. 108839. Moffitt Field, CA: NASA Ames Research Center.

Russell B, Ehrenkranz NJ, Hyams PJ, Gribble CA. 1983. An outbreak of *Staphylococcus aureus* surgical wound infection associated with excess overtime employment of operating room personnel. *Am J of Infection Control* 11(2):63–67.

Ryman DH, Naitoh P, Englund CE. 1987. *Perceived Exertion Under Conditions of Sustained Work and Sleep Loss.* NHRC Report No. 87-9. San Diego, CA: U.S. Department of the Navy, Medical Research and Development Command, Health Research Center.

Santy PA, Kapanka H, Davis JR, Stewart DF. 1988. Analysis of sleep on shuttle missions. *Aviation, Space, and Environmental Medicine* 59(11(Part I)):1094–1097.

Schrader ES. 2000. Publisher's note. *OR Manager* 16:3.

Schuster, M. 1985. The impact of overtime work on industrial accident rates. *Industrial Relations* 24(2):234–246.

Seccombe I, Smith G. 1996. *In the Balance: Registered Nurse Supply and Demand.* Report No. 315. Brighton, UK: Institute of Manpower Studies, University of Sussex.

Silberger AB, Thrau SL, Marder WD. 1988. The changing environment of resident physicians. *Health Affairs* 7(2 Supplement):121–133.

Smith L, Folkard S, Poole CJM. 1994. Increased injuries on the night shift. *Lancet* 344(8930):1137–1139.

Smith-Coggins R, Rosekind MR, Buccino KR, Dinges DF, Moser RP. 1997. Rotating shiftwork schedules: Can we enhance physician adaptation to night shifts? *Acad Emerg Med* 4(10):951–961.

Storer JS, Floyd HH, Gill WL, Giusti CW, Ginsberg H. 1989. Effects of sleep deprivation on cognitive ability and skills of pediatrics residents. *Acad Med* 64(1):29–32.

Suk M. 2001. *The Medical Resident's Perspective.* Presented at the Sleep, Fatigue and Medical Training Conference, Alexandria, VA. October 28-29, 2001.

Sussman D, Coplen M. 2002. *Fatigue and Alertness in the United States Railroad Industry Part 1: The Nature of the Problem.* [Online]. Available: http://www.volpe.dot.gov/opsad/sataprbm.htnl [accessed September 9, 2002]. Volpe National Transportation Systems Center. U.S. DOT Research and Special Programs Administration.

Taffinder NJ, McManus IC, Gul Y, Russell RC, Darzi A. 1998. Effect of sleep deprivation on surgeons' dexterity on laparoscopy simulator. *Lancet* 352(9135):1191.

Thorpe KE. 1990. House staff supervision and working hours: Implications of regulatory change in New York State. *Journal of the American Medical Association* 263(23):3177–3181.

TiredNukes.org. [Online]. Available: http://www.tirednukes.org [accessed September 2002].

Travers WD. 2001. *Rulemaking Issue: Fatigue of Workers at Nuclear Power Plants.* U.S. Nuclear Regulatory Commission. [Online]. Available: http: //www.nrc.gov/reading-rm/doc-collections/commission/SECYS/2001/SECY2001-01131/2001-0113scy.html [accessed September 19, 2001].

Tucker P, Barton J, Folkard S. 1996. Comparison of eight and 12 hour shifts: Impacts on health, wellbeing, and alertness during the shift. *Occup Environ Med* 53(11):767–772.

Ugrovics A, Wright J. 1990. 12-Hour shifts: Does fatigue undermine ICU nursing judgments? *Nursing Management* 21(1):64A–64G.

Union of Concerned Scientists. 2000. *Overtime and Staffing Problems in the Commercial Nuclear Power Industry.* [Online]. Available: http:// www.UCSUSA.org/energy/find. overtime.html [accessed September 19, 2002].

United Transportation Union. 2001 (November 30). *History of Safety Regulations, Bus Department.* [Online]. Available: http:// www.utu.org/DEPTS/BUSFILES/BUSNEWS/BUS-SFT.htm [accessed September 20, 2002].

U.S. Coast Guard Research and Development Center. 1996. *Fatigue and Alertness in Merchant Marine Personnel: A Field Guide of Work and Sleep Patterns.* Groton, CT: U.S. Coast Guard Research and Development Center.

U.S. Congress Office of Technology Assessment. 1978. *Historical Industry and Safety Overview.* Washington, DC: U.S. Government Printing Office. Pp. 40–50.

U.S. Congress Office of Technology Assessment. 1991a. *Biological Rhythms and Work Schedules.* Washington, DC: U.S. Government Printing Office. Pp. 85–120.

U.S. Congress Office of Technology Assessment. 1991b. *Case Study: Nuclear Power Plant Control Room Operators.* Washington, DC: U.S. Government Printing Office. Pp. 142–152.

U.S. Congress Office of Technology Assessment. 1991c. *Case Study: The Military.* Washington, DC: U.S. Government Printing Office. Pp. 183–195.

U.S. Congress Office of Technology Assessment. 1991d. *Legal and Regulatory Issues.* Washington, DC: U.S. Government Printing Office. Pp. 121–140.

U.S. DOT (United States Department of Transportation). 2002. *Bibliography: Human Fatigue Research in Railroad Operations.* Federal Railroad Administration, U.S. DOT. [Online]. Available: http://www.fra.dot/gov/rdv/volpe/pubs/bibliogs/rndlist.html [accessed September 11, 2002].

U.S. Nuclear Regulatory Commission. 1980. *Nuclear Plant Staff Working Hours.* Circular No. 80-02. Washington, DC: U.S Nuclear Regulatory Commission.

U.S. Nuclear Regulatory Commission. 1991. *Nuclear Plant Staff Working Hours.* Information Notice No. 91-36. Washington, DC: U.S. Nuclear Regulatory Commission.

U.S. Nuclear Regulatory Commission. 2000a. *Assessment of the NRC's "Policy on Factors Causing Fatigue of Operating Personnel at Nuclear Reactors."* Washington, DC: U.S. Nuclear Regulatory Commission.

U.S. Nuclear Regulatory Commission. 2000b. (June 22). *Rulemaking Plan Nuclear Power Plant Personnel Fatigue and Working Hours Regulation.* Washington, DC: U.S. Nuclear Regulatory Commission.

Van-Griever A, Meijman T. 1987. The impact of abnormal hours of work on various modes of information processing: A process model on human costs of performance. *Ergonomics* 30(9):1287–1299.

Vega A, Gilbert MJ. 1997. Longer days, shorter weeks: Compressed work weeks in policing. *Public Personnel Management* 26(3):391–402.

Vila B. 1996. Probable connections between fatigue and the performance, health, and safety of patrol officers. *American Journal of Police* 15(2):51–92.

Vila B. 2000. *Tired Cops: The Importance of Managing Police Fatigue.* Washington, DC: Police Executive Research Forum.

Vila B, Kenney DJ. 2002. Tired cops: The prevalence and potential consequences of police fatigue. *NIJ* 248:16–21.

Wallace M, Greenwood KM. 1995. Twelve-hour shifts [editorial]. *Work and Stress* 9:105–108.

Walsh JK, Tepas DI, Moss PD. 1981. *The EEG Sleep of Night and Rotating Shift Workers.* Johnson LC, Tepas DI, Colquhon WP, Colligan MJ, eds. New York, NY: Spectrum. Pp. 371–381.

Weigner MB, Ancoli-Israel S. 2002. Sleep deprivation and clinical performance. *Journal of the American Medical Association* 287(8):955–957.

Weigner MB, Vora S, Herndon CN. 1998. *Evaluation of the Effects of Fatigue and Sleepiness on Clinical Performance in On-Call Anesthesia Residents during Actual Nighttime Cases and in Simulated Cases.* Scheffler AL, Zipperer LA, eds. Chicago, IL: National Patient Safety Foundation. Pp. 306–310.

Wesnes K, Walker M. 1997. Cognitive performance and mood after a weekend on call in a surgical unit. *British Journal of Surgery* 84(4):493–495.

Williamson AM, Gower CGI, Clarke BC. 1994. Changing the hours of shiftwork: A comparison of 8- and 12-hour shift rosters in a group of computer operators. *Ergonomics* 37(2):287–298.

Wojtczak-Jaroszowa J, Banaszkiewicz A. 1974. Physical work capacity during the day and at night. *Ergonomics* 17(2):193–198.

Word LE. 1987. *Observations from Three Years at the National Training Center.* USARI Research Product 87-02. Alexandria, VA: U.S. Department of the Army, Medical Research and Development Command, Research Institute for the Behavioral and Social Sciences.

Wylie C, Schultz T, Miller J, Mitler M, Mackie R. 1996. *Commercial Motor Vehicle Driver Fatigue and Alertness Study.* FHWA Report number: FHWA-MC-97-001, TC Report Number TP12876E. Montreal, Canada: Transportation Development Center. Prepared for the Federal Highway Administration, U.S. Department of Transportation; Trucking Research Institute, American Trucking Associations Foundation; and the Transportation Development Centre, Safety and Security, Transport Canada.

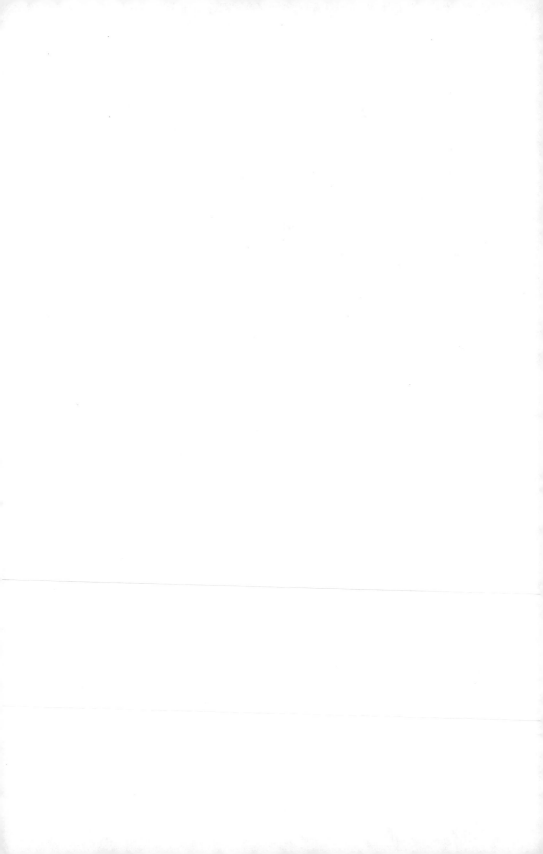

Index

E

Slips, 261n
Sloan-Kettering Institute, 37
Smart infusion pumps, 242
SNFs. *See* Skilled nursing facilities
Society for Critical Care Medicine, 269
Solutions
    need for internal and external, 245–248
    streamlining standards and standards
        compliance requirements, 247–248
    use of automation, 246–247
    work redesign, 245–246
SOPs. *See* Standard operating procedures
Staff turnover
    high, 42–43, 319–320
    minimizing, 193
Staffing, adequate, 16–17, 315
Staffing data needed, 198–201
    collecting valid and reliable, 11, 200–
        201
    from hospitals, 200–201
    from nursing homes, 198–200
Staffing levels, causal relationship with
    patient outcomes, 169–171
Staffing principles contributing to efficiency,
    188–196
    continually assessing staffing
        methodologies and their relationship
        to patient safety, 193
    incorporating admissions, discharges,
        and "less than 24-hour" patients into
        estimates of daily patient volume,
        189
    involving direct-care nursing staff in
        selecting, modifying, and evaluating
        staffing methods, 189–190
    minimizing staff turnover, 193
    providing for "on-time" staffing or
        demand elasticity to accommodate
        unpredicted variations in patient
        volume and/or acuity and resulting
        workload, 190–193
    using nursing staff from external
        agencies, 193
Standard operating procedures (SOPs), 365
Standardizing common work procedures
    and equipment, 258, 260–261
Standards and standards compliance
    requirements, streamlining, 247–248
Staphylococcus aureus, outbreaks of linked
    to overtime, 390–391

State boards of nursing, recommendations
    for, 13, 287
State regulatory bodies, recommendations
    for, 12–13
Step-down units
    acute care hospital staffing levels in, 172,
        178
    changes in workload in, 81
Streamlined physical plant layout, 258
Stress, impact of underestimated, 371
Successive days of sustained work hours,
    research needed on the effects of, 324
Suggestions, generating when standards of
    care are not being followed, 265
Summa Health System, 246
Surveillance of patients, 32, 34–36
    by direct-care nursing staff, 91–94
Sustained attention, in actively managing
    the process of change, 120–121
"Sustained operations," 229
Sustained work hours, research needed on
    the effects of successive days of, 324
Sustaining trust, 115–118, 137–139, 149,
    214, 292
Systematic experimentation, to generate new
    knowledge internally, 125
Systems approach, to understanding and
    reducing errors, 28

T

Task diversity in health care, 255
    implications for patient safety defenses,
        61
Team functioning, 341–383
    in areas of chronic illness and
        rehabilitation, 353
    creating effective teams and collaborative
        work relationships in the workplace,
        366–375
    early theories of, 342–344
    need for further research, 375–378
    teams and performance outcomes, 342–
        366
Team nursing, 80
Team-related factors, facilitating effective
    team development and performance,
    369
Technology, remaining alert to the
    limitations of and risks created by,
    266–267